3D Printing and Microfluidics in Dermatology

3D Printing and Microfluidics in Dermatology provides a thorough exploration and applications of three-dimensional (3D) printing and microfluidics within the field of dermatology. It investigates various methods utilized in these fields, such as 3D bio-printing, nano-transporters, microscopic fabrication, and device development.

The book not only examines practical applications but also delves into the design principles crucial for implementing these techniques using specific materials tailored to their intended purposes. Additionally, it addresses ethical concerns and regulatory considerations pertinent to these evolving technologies.

Key highlights include the following:

- A detailed insight into the utilization of 3D printing and microfluidic technologies for treating skin disorders.
- Exploration of design concepts necessary for effective implementation, considering the unique properties of materials involved.
- Coverage of diverse methodologies, ranging from 3D bioprinting to nano-transporters, microscopic fabrication, and device engineering.
- In-depth discussion on ethical considerations vital for the sustainable development of the industry.
- Investigation into advancements in material development, device design, fabrication techniques, and performance evaluation through preclinical and clinical studies.

This book targets graduate students and researchers in fields such as 3D printing, dermatology, drug delivery, bioengineering, and pharmaceutical sciences.

3D Printing and Microfluidics in Dermatology
Innovations in Drug Delivery

Edited by
Madhulika Pradhan
Krishna Yadav

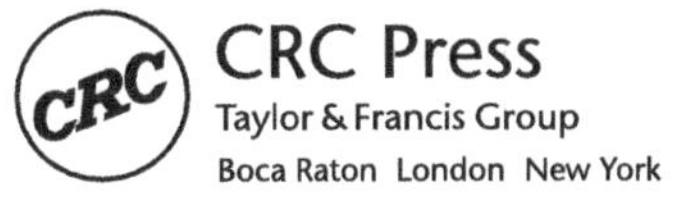

CRC Press
Taylor & Francis Group
Boca Raton London New York

CRC Press is an imprint of the
Taylor & Francis Group, an **informa** business

Designed cover image: Shutterstock

First edition published 2025
by CRC Press
2385 NW Executive Center Drive, Suite 320, Boca Raton FL 33431

and by CRC Press
4 Park Square, Milton Park, Abingdon, Oxon, OX14 4RN

CRC Press is an imprint of Taylor & Francis Group, LLC

© 2025 selection and editorial matter, Madhulika Pradhan and Krishna Yadav; individual chapters, the contributors

Reasonable efforts have been made to publish reliable data and information, but the author and publisher cannot assume responsibility for the validity of all materials or the consequences of their use. The authors and publishers have attempted to trace the copyright holders of all material reproduced in this publication and apologize to copyright holders if permission to publish in this form has not been obtained. If any copyright material has not been acknowledged please write and let us know so we may rectify in any future reprint.

Except as permitted under U.S. Copyright Law, no part of this book may be reprinted, reproduced, transmitted, or utilized in any form by any electronic, mechanical, or other means, now known or hereafter invented, including photocopying, microfilming, and recording, or in any information storage or retrieval system, without written permission from the publishers.

For permission to photocopy or use material electronically from this work, access www.copyright.com or contact the Copyright Clearance Center, Inc. (CCC), 222 Rosewood Drive, Danvers, MA 01923, 978-750-8400. For works that are not available on CCC please contact mpkbookspermissions@tandf.co.uk

Trademark notice: Product or corporate names may be trademarks or registered trademarks and are used only for identification and explanation without intent to infringe.

Library of Congress Cataloging-in-Publication Data
Names: Pradhan, Madhulika, editor. | Yadav, Krishna (Ph.D. in
Pharmaceutical Technology), editor.
Title: 3D printing and microfluidics in dermatology : innovations in drug
delivery / edited by Madhulika Pradhan and Krishna Yadav.
Other titles: Three-dimensional printing and microfluidics in dermatology
Description: First edition. | Boca Raton, FL : CRC Press, 2025. | Includes
bibliographical references and index.
Identifiers: LCCN 2024017761 (print) | LCCN 2024017762 (ebook) | ISBN
9781032634098 (hardback) | ISBN 9781032690957 (paperback) | ISBN
9781032690926 (ebook)
Subjects: MESH: Skin Diseases--therapy | Printing, Three-Dimensional |
Microfluidics | Bioprinting | Drug Delivery Systems | Tissue Engineering
Classification: LCC RL110 (print) | LCC RL110 (ebook) | NLM WR 650 | DDC
616.5/06--dc23/eng/20240703
LC record available at https://lccn.loc.gov/2024017761
LC ebook record available at https://lccn.loc.gov/2024017762

ISBN: 978-1-032-63409-8 (hbk)
ISBN: 978-1-032-69095-7 (pbk)
ISBN: 978-1-032-69092-6 (ebk)

DOI: 10.1201/9781032690926

Typeset in Times
by SPi Technologies India Pvt Ltd (Straive)

First, we thank **almighty God** for giving us this opportunity to serve the scientific fraternity through the book "**3D Printing and Microfluidics in Dermatology: Innovations in Drug Delivery**."

This book is dedicated to the guiding lights in our research and academic journey, **Dr. Manju Singh** and **Dr. Deependra Singh**. Your unwavering support, invaluable mentorship, and profound wisdom have been the driving forces behind the creation of this work. Your dedication to excellence, passion for knowledge, and commitment to nurturing young minds have inspired us every step of the way.

Our first book stands as a tribute to your mentorship, a token of gratitude for the knowledge you have imparted, and a testament to the profound impact you have had on our academic and professional lives. We are immensely grateful for the privilege of being mentored by two exceptional individuals whose passion for education and commitment to fostering the next generation of scholars continue to inspire us.

— Always your students

Contents

Preface

The convergence of 3D printing and microfluidics has ushered in a new era of possibilities in dermatology, marking a transformative juncture in the realm of drug delivery innovations. Our book, *3D Printing and Microfluidics in Dermatology: Innovations in Drug Delivery*, embarks on an exploration of this cutting-edge intersection, unraveling the revolutionary contributions these technologies offer to advance dermatological treatments.

In the evolving landscape of health care, the marriage of 3D printing and microfluidics has emerged as a pivotal force, presenting unprecedented opportunities for precision and customization in drug delivery for dermatological conditions. This book serves as a compass, guiding readers through the intricate details of these technologies and their applications, emphasizing their importance in revolutionizing therapeutic interventions for various skin-related ailments.

This comprehensive book is meticulously crafted to bridge the knowledge gap and provide a consolidated resource for researchers, clinicians, students, and industry professionals. It encapsulates the latest advancements, research findings, and practical applications of 3D printing and microfluidics in dermatology. By assembling contributions from leading experts in the field, our aim is to offer a cohesive and insightful journey into the innovations that hold the promise of reshaping dermatological drug delivery.

Our book is tailored for a diverse audience committed to advancing health care through technological innovation. It caters to researchers delving into the intricacies of 3D printing and microfluidics, clinicians seeking to integrate cutting-edge approaches into their practice, students eager to grasp the forefront of dermatological advancements, and industry professionals aiming to stay abreast of the latest trends. By fostering collaboration and understanding, we aspire to empower readers to harness the potential of 3D printing and microfluidics for improved patient outcomes and elevated standards of care in dermatology.

As you embark on this journey through the pages of *3D Printing and Microfluidics in Dermatology: Innovations in Drug Delivery*, we invite you to delve into the profound impact these technologies have on the future of dermatological treatments. May this book serve as a beacon of knowledge and inspiration, fostering innovation and driving positive change in the field of dermatology.

About the Editors

Dr. Madhulika Pradhan is a professor and principal at Gracious College of Pharmacy, Abhanpur, Chhattisgarh, India. She received her PhD degree in pharmaceutical technology from Pt. Ravishankar Shukla University, Raipur, India. She has more than 15 years of academic and research experience. She has published more than 40 papers and 6 book chapters in nationally and internationally recognized journals. She also holds an Australian patent and an Indian patent. In various conference sessions, she has won numerous accolades for excellence in research at the international, national, and state levels (Malaysia, India, etc.). In addition, she has garnered with International Travel Award for her research presentation in Malaysia, Singapore, Denmark, and the United States. She is a member of several professional bodies, including the Association of Pharmaceutical Teachers of India and the Indian Pharmacy Graduates Association. Her principal research interests involve developing novel drug delivery systems for dermal disorders such as psoriasis and other autoimmune skin disorders using modern statistical and computational tools. She is an active reviewer of various journals.

Dr. Krishna Yadav is an assistant professor and active researcher at Department of Pharmaceutics, Rungta College of Pharmaceutical Sciences and Research, Bhilai, Chhattisgarh, India, with 8 years of academic and research experience. He holds a PhD in Pharmaceutical Technology from Pt. Ravishankar Shukla University, Raipur, India. He has numerous published research articles, reviews, and book chapters in both national and international journals and books. Dr. Yadav holds an Australian patent and an Indian patent and has received various international-, national-, and state-level awards for research excellence. He is a member of several professional bodies. His primary research focuses on innovative formulation and drug delivery techniques, particularly targeting, such as psoriasis, breast cancer, bone disorders, and other conditions. Dr. Yadav is actively involved in the screening and evaluation of novel pharmacological agents and formulation development using advanced drug delivery systems like nanovesicles, solid lipid nanoparticles, nanostructured lipid carriers, exosomes, carbon quantum dots, and others. His expertise includes bioanalytical techniques, pharmacokinetics, advanced statistics, and proficiency in various biological platforms.

Contributors

Ajazuddin
Rungta College of Pharmaceutical
Sciences and Research
Bhilai, India

Hemant Badwaik
Shri Shankaracharya Institute of
Pharmaceutical Science and Research
Bhilai, India

Madhuri Baghel
Apollo College of Pharmacy
Durg, India

Monika Bhairam
Columbia Institute of Pharmacy
Tekari, Raipur, India

Harish Bhardwaj
University Institute of Pharmacy
Pt. Ravishankar Shukla University
Raipur, India

Pankaj Kumar Bhatt
Lloyd Institute of Management and
Technology
Greater Noida, India

Shashikant Chandrakar
Columbia Institute of Pharmacy
Raipur, India

Nagendra Singh Chauhan
Drugs Testing Laboratory Avam
Anusandhan Kendra (AYUSH)
Government Ayurvedic College
Raipur, India

Vineet Devangan
Chhattisgarh Swami Vivekanand
Technical University
Utai, India

Dhansay Dewangan
Swami Atmanand Government English
Medium Model College
Korba, India

Swati Dubey
Department Of Pharmacy
Indira Gandhi National Tribal University
Amarkantak, India

Bina Gidwani
Columbia Institute of Pharmacy
Tekari, Raipur, India

Tapan Kumar Giri
Department of Pharmaceutical
Technology
Jadavpur University
Kolkata, India

S Princely Ebenezer Gnanakani
Department of Pharmaceutical
Biotechnology
Parul Institute of Pharmacy, Parul
University
Gujarat, India

Sachin Gupta
Department of Pharmacy
Agra Public College of Higher
Education and Research Centre
Artauni, Agra, India

Parag Jain
The University of Texas Health Science
    Center at Houston
School of Dentistry
Houston, TX, USA

Ritesh Jain
Department of Pharmacology, School of
    Pharmacy
Chouksey Engineering College
Bilaspur, India

Rajendra Kumar Jangde
University Institute of Pharmacy
Pt. Ravishankar Shukla University
Raipur, India

Ramakant Joshi
Amity Institute of Pharmacy
Amity University Madhya Pradesh
Gwalior, India

Monika Kaurav
Department of Pharmaceutics
KIET School of Pharmacy
KIET Group of Institutions
Ghaziabad, India

J John Kirubakaran
Department of Pharmacy Practice
Parul Institute of Pharmacy, Parul
    University
Gujarat, India

Ganesh Kumar
SLT Institute of Pharmacy
Guru Ghasidas Vishwavidyalaya
Bilaspur, India

Leena Kumari
Department of Pharmaceutical
    Technology
NSHM Knowledge Campus
Kolkata, India
Sunita Minz

Department of Pharmacy
Indira Gandhi National Tribal
University
Amarkantak, India

Achal Mishra
Institute of Pharmacy
Guru Ghasidas Vishwavidyalaya (a
    central University)
Bilaspur, India

Kushagra Nagori
Rungta College of Pharmaceutical
    Sciences and Research
Bhilai, India

Kartik T. Nakhate
Shri Vile Parle Kelavani Mandal's
    Institute of Pharmacy (SVKM-IOP)
Dhule, India

Ashish Kumar Pandey
Shri Shankaracharya Technical
    Campus
Faculty of Pharmaceutical Science
Bhilai, India

Ravindra Kumar Pandey
Columbia Institute of Pharmacy
Raipur, India

Madhulika Pradhan
Gracious College of Pharmacy
Abhanpur, India

Wasim Raza
Central Laboratory Facility
Chhattisgarh Council of Science and
    Technology
Raipur, India

Kantrol Kumar Sahu
Institute of Pharmaceutical Research
GLA University
Mathura, India

Pravin Kumar Sahu
School of Pharmacy
Chouksey Engineering College
Bilaspur, India

Varsha Sahu
Department of Pharmaceutical
Sciences
Utkal University
Bhubaneswar, India

Kalyani Sakure
Rungta College of Pharmaceutical
    Sciences and Research
Kohka, India

Khomendra Kumar Sarwa
Department of Pharmacy
Government Girls Polytechnic
Raipur, India

Geetika Sharma
Department of Pharmacy
Indira Gandhi National Tribal University
Amarkantak, India

Kiran Sharma
School of Dentistry and Medical
    Sciences
Charles Sturt University
Orange, NSW, Australia

Mukesh Kumar Sharma
Rungta College of Pharmaceutical
    Sciences and Research
Bhilai, India

Rashnita Sharma
Rungta Institute of Pharmaceutical
    Education and Research
Bhilai, India

Barnali Maiti Sinha
School of Pharmacy
Techno India University
Kolkata, India

Deependra Singh
University Institute of Pharmacy
Pt. Ravishankar Shukla University
Raipur, India

Manju Rawat Singh
University Institute of Pharmacy
Pt. Ravishankar Shukla University
Raipur, India

Shalini Singh
Department Of Pharmacy
Indira Gandhi National Tribal University
Amarkantak, India

Shiv Shankar Shukla
Columbia Institute of Pharmacy
Tekari, Raipur, India

Alok Singh Thakur
Shri Shankaracharya Institute of
    Pharmaceutical Science and Research
Bhilai, India

Rakesh Tirkey
University Institute of Pharmacy
Pt. Ravishankar Shukla University
Raipur, India

Anshita Shukla
Rungta Institute of Pharmaceutical
    Education and Research
Bhilai, India

Astha Verma
Shri Rawatpura Sarkar Institute of
    Pharmacy
Kumhari, Durg, India

Dipti Verma
Chhattisgarh Swami Vivekanand
    Technical University
Utai, India

Ravi Verma
Institute of Pharmaceutical Research,
    GLA University
Mathura, India

Shekhar Verma
Institute of Pharmacy
Guru Ghasidas Vishwavidyalaya (a
    central University)
Bilaspur, India

R Vijayalakshmi
Department of Pharmaceutical Analysis
GIET School of Pharmacy
Chaitanya Knowledge City,
Rajahmundry, India

Umesh Vishwakarma
School of Engineering
O P Jindal University
Raigarh, India

Amber Vyas
University Institute of Pharmacy
Pt. Ravishankar Shukla University
Raipur, India

Krishna Yadav
Department of Pharmaceutics
Rungta College of Pharmaceutical
    Sciences and Research
Bhilai, Chhattisgarh, India

1 The Basic Concept of 3D Printing and Its Application in Dermatological Conditions

Mukesh Kumar Sharma and Ajazuddin
Rungta College of Pharmaceutical Sciences and Research,
Bhilai, India

Umesh Vishwakarma
O P Jindal University, Raigarh, India

Vineet Devangan and Dipti Verma
Chhattisgarh Swami Vivekanand Technical University,
Utai, India

Parag Jain
The University of Texas Health Science Center at Houston,
Houston, United States

1.1 INTRODUCTION TO 3D PRINTING TECHNOLOGY

1.1.1 OVERVIEW AND PRINCIPLE OF 3D PRINTING TECHNOLOGY OR ADDITIVE MANUFACTURING

Additive manufacturing (AM), commonly known as three-dimensional (3D) printing, is a revolutionary technology that transforms digital design files into physical objects by adding material layer by layer (1, 2). Unlike traditional subtractive manufacturing processes that involve cutting away material from a solid block, AM builds objects layer by layer, enabling the creation of complex geometries and intricate

DOI: 10.1201/9781032690926-1

designs that were once impractical or impossible to produce (3). The fundamental principle of AM is to add material in a controlled manner to create a 3D object. This contrasts with subtractive manufacturing, where the material is removed to achieve the desired shape. AM processes vary, but they all generally involve the following steps (4):

- Digital Design: The process begins with a 3D digital model created using computer-aided design (CAD) software (4).
- Slicing: The digital model is sliced into thin horizontal cross sections using slicing software. Each slice represents a layer of the final object.
- Layer-by-Layer Printing: The 3D printer reads the sliced file and starts building the object layer by layer. This involves depositing or curing material (such as plastic, metal, or resin) according to the design specifications.
- Fusing and Solidification: Depending on the technology, the material is fused, cured, or solidified to create a cohesive layer. This layer adheres to the previous layer and gradually builds up the final object (5).

1.2 AM TECHNOLOGIES, APPLICATIONS, AND CHALLENGES

1.2.1 AM TECHNOLOGIES

1.2.1.1 Fused Deposition Modeling

Fused deposition modeling (FDM) is one of the most common 3D printing technologies. It involves extruding thermoplastic filament layer by layer to create objects. FDM is widely used for rapid prototyping and creating functional parts (6).

1.2.1.2 Stereolithography

In stereolithography (SLA), layers of liquid resin are solidified with the help of an ultraviolet (UV) laser. Its ability to create things with a high level of detail and a flawless surface finish has made it a favorite for uses where such characteristics are important (7).

1.2.1.3 Selective Laser Sintering

To build complicated shapes and useful items with good mechanical qualities, selective laser sintering (SLS) uses a laser to selectively fuse powdered materials, such as plastics or metals (8).

1.2.1.4 Direct Metal Laser Sintering

Direct metal laser sintering (DMLS) is a similar process to SLS that employs a laser to sinter metal powder, creating completely dense metal objects that can be used in aerospace, automotive, and medical settings (9).

1.2.1.5 Binder Jetting

With binder jetting, a binding agent is deposited onto powdered material layers. It can be used to create color prototypes, metal parts, and sand molds (10).

1.2.1.6 Electron Beam Melting

Electron beam melting (EBM) is a process in which metal powder is melted by an electron beam, yielding a product with high strength and durability. The aerospace and medical industries rely heavily on it.

1.2.1.7 Material Jetting

Similar to inkjet printing, material jetting uses UV light to harden tiny droplets of material. It is put to use in the fabrication of exact and comprehensive models (10).

1.2.1.8 Digital Light Processing

Digital light processing (DLP) is a hybrid between SLA and FDM in terms of speed and precision; it involves the use of a digital light projector to cure liquid photopolymer resin in successive layers (11).

1.2.2 APPLICATIONS OF AM

AM is used to produce lightweight, complex, and efficient aerospace components, such as engine parts and structural elements (12, 13). Customized implants, prosthetics, surgical tools, and patient-specific models are produced using AM, improving patient outcomes, and reducing surgery time.

Rapid prototyping, tooling, and manufacturing of lightweight and optimized parts are common in the automotive industry. AM also enables the creation of customized and unique consumer products, from fashion accessories to home décor. Large-scale 3D printers can create building components and prototypes, speeding up the construction process (14). AM is also used for producing dental crowns, bridges, and orthodontic appliances with high precision. Artists and designers create intricate sculptures, jewelry, and other artistic pieces using AM.

1.2.3 CHALLENGES OF AM

Available materials for AM are still limited compared to traditional manufacturing methods. Developing new materials with desired properties is a challenge. Many AM parts require post-processing, such as support removal, surface finishing, and heat treatment, which can add time and cost to the production process.

In addition, ensuring consistent quality and repeatability across multiple AM prints can be challenging due to variations in material properties and process parameters. While AM excels in customization and low-volume production, it can be slower and less cost-effective for mass production. Designing for AM requires a different approach due to certain geometric and structural limitations unique to the layer-by-layer manufacturing process. The initial investment in AM equipment, materials, and post-processing can be relatively high, impacting the cost-effectiveness of small-scale production.

Industries like aerospace and medical need to meet strict regulations and certifications, which can be challenging due to the relatively new nature of AM. The mechanical properties of AM materials might not always match those of traditionally manufactured materials, requiring validation and testing (15).

1.3 MATERIALS AND TECHNIQUES IN DERMATOLOGICAL 3D PRINTING

Dermatological 3D printing involves the use of AM techniques to create skin-related structures, models, and medical devices. This technology has applications in research, education, medical training, and even patient-specific treatment. Here are some of the materials and techniques used in dermatological 3D printing (15).

1.3.1 BIOCOMPATIBLE MATERIALS FOR DERMATOLOGY

- Photopolymers: These are light-sensitive liquid resins that solidify when exposed to UV light. They are often used in SLA and DLP printers to create highly detailed and accurate models (2).
- Thermoplastic Polymers: Materials like polylactic acid (PLA) and polyethylene terephthalate (PETG) are commonly used in FDM printers. These printers are widely accessible and can produce anatomical models and prosthetic devices.
- Hydrogels: Hydrogels are a type of biocompatible substance that, like human tissue, can retain water. They are used in the construction of pliable and malleable models meant to stand in for human skin in the pursuit of knowledge (16, 17).
- Bioprinting Materials: Tissue engineering and regenerative medicine are only two of the cutting-edge fields that use bioinks made of living cells and supporting biomaterials to print replacement tissues. For drug testing and transplanting, these materials can be used to produce living skin tissue models (18).

1.3.2 AN OVERVIEW OF 3D PRINTING TECHNIQUES IN DERMATOLOGY

The common 3D printing techniques in dermatology are as follows (3):

- SLA
- FDM
- DLP
- Bioprinting
- Multi-Material Printing
- Color Printing
- Post-Processing

1.4 3D PRINTING APPLICATIONS IN PROSTHETICS AND ORTHOTICS

Since 3D printing allows the production of unique and inexpensive devices, it has had a profound effect on the field of prosthetics and orthotics. Examples of how 3D printing is being used in orthotics and prosthetics are provided in the following subsections.

1.4.1 PROSTHETICS (19)

Three-dimensional printing has made it possible to create prosthetics that are uniquely shaped for each user, increasing their level of comfort and efficiency. Prosthetic prototypes can be developed more quickly because of rapid prototyping, which allows for inexpensive design iterations and modifications. Three-dimensional printing enables the production of personalized and aesthetic covers for prosthetic limbs, allowing users to express their style and preferences. Prosthetic sockets, connectors, and joints can also be 3D-printed with the appropriate materials to provide the necessary rigidity and pliability.

Traditional prosthetics can be costly, especially if modifications are required. In developing nations, 3D printing has made prostheses more affordable and accessible. Three-dimensional printing can create auxiliary devices, such as attachments for holding objects or tools, enhancing the prosthetic user's capabilities.

1.4.2 ORTHOTICS (20)

Using 3D scanning and printing, orthotic devices like braces and splints can be custom-made to fit the patient's unique anatomy and therapy goals. When compared to traditionally manufactured devices, 3D-printed orthotics can offer superior fit and comfort. Supportive and permeable lattice designs are just one example of the various geometries that may be printed with 3D printing.

Three-dimensional printing makes it possible to create orthotics that are both lightweight and durable. In addition, children who are still developing often benefit from a combination of orthotic devices. Modifications may be made quickly and cheaply as they develop thanks to 3D printing. Physical therapy and rehabilitation can benefit from the use of individualized 3D-printed equipment and supports, which can lead to better patient outcomes. The optimal design allows orthotics to be tailored to a patient's unique needs, such as providing arch support for those with flat feet.

1.5 3D-PRINTED DERMAL SUBSTITUTES FOR BURNS

Accidents that cause burns can cause irreparable damage to the skin and the tissues beneath it, necessitating intensive medical treatment to facilitate the patient's appropriate healing and recovery (21). Dermal substitutes that are created using 3D-printing technology have emerged as a cutting-edge alternative for resolving the one-of-a-kind problems caused by burn injuries. These replacements provide a personalized and regenerative approach to wound healing, with the goals of enhancing patients' quality of life, reducing the likelihood of scarring, and improving overall outcomes (22).

1.5.1 KEY COMPONENTS AND STEPS

In terms of size, severity, and location, every burn injury is different. Patient-specific dermal prostheses can now be printed with 3D-printing technology. To create a unique scaffold, it is necessary to take precise measurements or 3D scans of the burn area.

Scaffold structures are 3D-printed layer by layer using biocompatible materials like natural polymers or synthetic hydrogels. This scaffold provides a supportive structure for developing and repairing tissue (23). Integrating living cells like fibroblasts and keratinocytes into the scaffold increases the substitute's regeneration ability. Tissue repair, collagen production, and wound healing all rely on these cells to varying degrees.

The 3D-printed dermal replacement is put onto the burn wound with great care. By producing growth factors and encouraging cell migration, live cells aid in the healing process when included (3).

1.5.2 Benefits and Advantages

The use of 3D-printed dermal replacements offers personalized options for the treatment of burns, lowering the danger of infection, accelerating the healing process, and minimizing the possibility of problems at the donor site. Their capacity to promote tissue regeneration and lessen the formation of scar tissue contributes to improved cosmetic results. Even if the upfront costs could be substantial, there are long-term benefits that include cost-effectiveness and availability on demand (24). In addition, the technology of 3D printing opens up new doors for research into enhanced biomaterials and growth factors, which is another reason why it is a potential advance in the field of burn care (25).

1.5.3 Challenges and Ongoing Research

Ensuring biocompatibility, promoting vascularization, maintaining long-term stability, achieving scalability, and navigating regulatory hurdles are some of the challenges associated with 3D-printed dermal substitutes (26).

Ongoing research efforts are concentrated on the development of advanced biomaterials, the improvement of vascularization techniques, the conduct of clinical trials to evaluate the product's safety and efficacy, the automation and standardization of production processes, the exploration of immunomodulation strategies, and the establishment of methods for long-term performance monitoring. These efforts have the goal of resolving these issues and advancing the use of 3D-printed dermal replacements as efficient and easily accessible treatments for burn victims (27). The development of 3D-printed dermal substitutes for burns holds immense promise for revolutionizing burn treatment. By combining precision, regenerative potential, and reduced scarring, these substitutes offer hope for improved outcomes and enhanced quality of life for burn survivors.

1.6 3D-PRINTED DERMAL SUBSTITUTES FOR SKIN REPLACEMENT SURGERIES

Surgeries to replace damaged or diseased skin, as well as those performed for cosmetic purposes, frequently need exact solutions that are tailored to the individual requirements of the patient (16). It has recently come to light that 3D-printed dermal replacements are an innovative answer to these problems. These dermal substitutes offer personalized, regenerative, and functional alternatives for skin replacement surgery (28).

1.6.1 DESIGN AND FABRICATION PROCESS

Patient-Specific Design: Surgical procedures involving the replacement of skin must be individualized for each patient. To make sure the dermal substitute fits the patient's specific anatomy, 3D printing begins with the acquisition of precise 3D scans or measurements of the affected area.

Scaffold Generation: Layer-by-layer 3D printing of biocompatible materials like hydrogels, polymers, or biomaterials to create a scaffold. This scaffold serves as a support system for developing tissues (12).

Cell Incorporation Functional Integration (Optional): Integrating living cells like fibroblasts and keratinocytes into the scaffold increases its regeneration ability. These cells aid in the formation of collagen and the repair of damaged tissues. For better functional integration with the surrounding tissues, the 3D-printed alternative can sometimes be created with features like blood arteries or nerve paths (29).

1.6.2 ADVANTAGES AND BENEFITS

Three-dimensional-printed dermal substitutes offer a range of significant advantages and benefits for skin replacement surgeries:

- Customization
- Reduced Scarring
- Accelerated Healing
- Minimized Donor Site Morbidity
- Cosmetic Improvement
- Availability
- Research Potential

Three-dimensional-printed dermal substitutes are an exciting new development in skin replacement procedures due to their adaptability, reduced scarring, accelerated healing, less donor site morbidity, enhanced aesthetics, wider availability, and much room for future study (30, 31).

1.6.3 ONGOING RESEARCH AND CHALLENGES

Ongoing research and challenges in the field of 3D-printed dermal substitutes for skin replacement surgeries are crucial for advancing this technology:

- Biocompatibility and Integration
- Vascularization Long-Term Stability
- Scalability

- Regulatory Compliance
- Clinical Trials
- Immunomodulation
- Long-Term Monitoring

In summary, advancing 3D-printed dermal substitutes for skin replacement surgeries and realizing their full potential to improve patient outcomes requires addressing challenges related to biocompatibility, vascularization, stability, scalability, regulation, clinical validation, immunomodulation, and long-term monitoring (32).

1.7 CUSTOMIZED WOUND CARE SOLUTIONS

The use of 3D printing to create individualized wound care solutions holds great promise for accelerating the recovery from a wide range of wound types. Wound dressings, implants, and other individualized medical items can now be 3D-printed to meet each patient's personal needs. Here are some ways that 3D printing is being put to use in the growing field of individualized wound care.

1.7.1 PATIENT-SPECIFIC WOUND DRESSINGS (33)

Patients who suffer from chronic wounds, burns, or surgical incisions frequently require specialized dressings that offer ideal moisture balance and enhance the body's natural ability to recover.

Wound dressings of unique shapes and styles are now possible thanks to 3D printing. The wound site's shape can be used to create a custom dressing that provides optimal coverage and adherence (34). The integration of targeted therapeutic ingredients or drugs into the dressing is also made possible by 3D printing.

1.7.2 BIOACTIVE IMPLANTS FOR WOUND HEALING (22)

Implants may be necessary for patients with severe wounds, such as extensive burns or ulcers that do not heal, to facilitate tissue regeneration and wound closure (35).

Three-dimensional printing makes it possible to fabricate bioactive implants, such as scaffolds or matrices, that are an accurate representation of the natural environment of the tissue. These implants are capable of being customized to match the wound geometry of the patient and are also capable of being created to release growth factors or other therapeutic agents that promote the patient's body's natural ability to heal.

1.7.3 NEGATIVE PRESSURE WOUND THERAPY DEVICES

Negative pressure wound therapy (NPWT) is a method that makes use of suction to hasten the healing of wounds by eliminating excess fluid and promoting blood flow.

Three-dimensional printing makes it possible to create individualized non-invasive pressure wound therapy (NPWT) devices that are a perfect match for the wound site. These devices can be constructed with integrated channels that allow for uniform distribution of negative pressure, which significantly increases the efficacy of the therapy.

1.7.4 Compression Garments for Lymphedema

Lymphedema is a disorder that is characterized by swelling owing to poor lymphatic outflow. This swelling can occur anywhere on the body. Compression clothing is frequently worn to alleviate the edema.

Three-dimensional scanning of the problematic area can result in the fabrication of personalized compression garments that exert the appropriate amount of pressure on specific places. This can help alleviate pain and discomfort caused by the condition.

1.7.5 Customized Surgical Guides for Wound Closure (36)

Accurate surgical methods are required to successfully close complex wounds, such as those that involve tissue flaps.

To assist in the accurate closure of wounds, surgeons can utilize surgical guides that have been 3D-printed to fit the anatomy of the patient. These guides have the potential to assist in the better alignment of tissue layers, the reduction of tension on the wound, and the improvement of overall healing outcomes.

1.7.6 Patient-Specific Bandages and Splints

Patients suffering from fractures, sprains, or any other type of injury might benefit from immobilization and support provided by bandages and splints.

Three-dimensional printing makes it possible to produce individualized bandages and splints that conform precisely to the patient's unique body shape. These gadgets offer improved support and comfort while also facilitating the health and recovery process.

The use of 3D printing to create individualized wound care solutions enables a more individualized approach to therapy, which, in turn, increases the efficacy of therapies and eventually speeds up the healing process. By adapting medical procedures and bandages to the specific needs of each patient, medical professionals can boost the likelihood of successful outcomes and increase the level of patient comfort throughout the healing process (37).

1.8 IMPORTANCE OF CUSTOMIZED WOUND DRESSINGS

In recent years, the application of 3D-printing technology to the creation of individualized wound dressings has become increasingly important in the field of wound treatment and healthcare more generally. These dressings offer a number of advantages over conventional dressings that are made to fit everyone, which makes them an important innovation in the field of patient care. The following are some of the most important reasons why customized wound dressings produced by 3D printing are important (33).

1.8.1 Tailored Fit

The size, shape, depth, and placement of each wound are different from one another. Using 3D printing, it is possible to create wound dressings that are specifically adapted to the wound of each particular patient. This enhances the overall effectiveness of the dressing by ensuring optimal coverage, contact, and adhesion to the wound site (38).

1.8.2 Conformity to Wound Contours

Conformity to wound contours custom dressings can be constructed to conform completely to the contours of a wound, even if the wound is of an irregular shape or has varied depths. This is possible because of the versatility of the dressings. Because of this conformance, the dressing will continue to maintain direct touch with the wound bed, which is an essential component of effective wound healing.

1.8.3 Enhanced Healing Environment

Using 3D printing, unique characteristics can be included in bandages for individual wounds. Included in this category are compounds including growth hormones, antibacterial agents, and structures that encourage cellular adhesion. It is possible to minimize the danger of infection and promote tissue regeneration with specially tailored dressings.

1.8.4 Personalized Treatment

Individual patient wounds might exhibit a wide range of characteristics. Using 3D-printed bandages, doctors may tailor care to each patient based on their wound's unique characteristics and severity. Better results and faster recovery periods may result from this level of customization.

1.8.5 Cost-Effectiveness and Rapid Prototyping

Custom sizes and shapes can reduce wastage when 3D-printing wound dressings, but setup and material costs are higher. Improved wound healing and fewer issues may lead to long-term savings. With 3D printing, wound covers may be prototyped quickly. This lets doctors quickly test novel dressings and adjust based on patient feedback and in-clinic observations. This kind of design flexibility can improve wound care (10).

1.8.6 Complex Wound Management

It may be necessary to use dressings with more advanced features on certain wounds, such as burns and chronic ulcers. A few examples of this would be variable degrees of porosity, the regulated release of medicinal chemicals, and even the incorporation of sensors to monitor the patient's progress as they heal (39). The use of 3D printing makes it possible to incorporate such intricate design details onto dressings.

1.8.7 PATIENT COMFORT AND REDUCED INFECTION RISK

It may be necessary to use dressings with more advanced features on certain wounds, such as burns and chronic ulcers. A few examples of this would be variable degrees of porosity, the regulated release of medicinal chemicals, and even the incorporation of sensors to monitor the patient's progress as they heal. The use of 3D printing makes it possible to incorporate such intricate design details onto dressings.

Wound dressings made using 3D printing technology are an exciting new breakthrough with the potential to completely alter the wound care industry. Better patient outcomes, faster healing, and higher quality of life for persons living with wounds are all possible results of the further development of this technology.

1.9 3D-PRINTING SKIN GRAFTS AND TISSUE ENGINEERING (18)

Tissue engineering, which includes the production of skin grafts and other complicated tissues, is an area where 3D printing has shown significant promise. Using a combination of cells, biomaterials, and bioactive substances, tissue engineers create functional replacements for dysfunctional tissues caused by injury or disease (40). Here is an example of the usage of 3D printing in the field of tissue engineering and skin grafting.

1.9.1 SKIN GRAFTS AND WOUND HEALING

Grafts are frequently necessary in the treatment of severe burns, chronic wounds, and other skin injuries to speed up the healing process and minimize the formation of scars.

Using 3D bioprinting technology, skin cells and biomaterials may be precisely placed to produce skin grafts that are indistinguishable from natural skin. The epidermis and dermis are just two of the layers that can be incorporated into these grafts to aid in wound healing and tissue regeneration.

1.9.2 BIOPRINTING LIVING SKIN TISSUE

Laboratory-grown skin tissue has the potential to replace donor organs in transplant procedures and be used in drug testing.

To produce 3D printing structures that are analogous to the architecture of natural skin, bioprinters deposit layers of bio-ink that comprise skin cells and supporting elements. Bioprinting allows for the creation of skin-like structures that have enhanced functioning. This is achieved by manipulating the positioning and organization of the cells.

1.9.3 ORGAN-ON-A-CHIP MODELS

Researchers employ small models that duplicate tissue functions to investigate skin-related disorders as well as the effects of various drugs.

Using 3D printing allows for the creation of microfluidic devices that have 3D cell architectures and can simulate the layers of skin. These "organ-on-a-chip" models give researchers the ability to investigate intricate cellular interactions in a setting that can be precisely regulated.

1.9.4 Composite Tissue Constructs

Composite tissue constructs can be designed to restore function in situations involving complex defects that include numerous types of tissues.

Printing in 3D enables the accurate stacking of various cell types and biomaterials, which is necessary for the creation of composite tissues. For face reconstruction, for instance, layers of bone, muscle, and skin can be printed together to rebuild a facial structure that is fully functional.

1.9.5 Patient-Specific Implants

Patients who have lost tissue as a result of surgery or trauma require implants that are customized to their anatomies.

When combined with scanned anatomical data, the 3D-printing technology enables the creation of implants that are particular to each patient. Because of this, a precise fit is achieved, as well as an improved integration with the tissues in the surrounding area.

1.9.6 Drug Testing and Personalized Medicine

Three-dimensional-printed tissue models can be used for drug screening to predict patient-specific responses.

By printing tissue constructs with disease-specific cells, researchers can test drug efficacy and toxicity more accurately, leading to personalized treatment strategies.

1.9.7 Vascularization Challenges

Creating complex tissues requires a functional vascular network to supply nutrients and remove waste.

Researchers are developing methods to 3D-print vasculature within engineered tissues, allowing for the creation of larger and more complex structures.

While 3D printing in tissue engineering has made significant progress, challenges remain, such as achieving full vascularization, ensuring long-term functionality, and regulatory approvals for clinical applications. Nevertheless, the field holds immense potential to revolutionize regenerative medicine by providing customized, functional, and patient-specific solutions for various tissue-related challenges.

1.10 ADVANCES IN WOUND HEALING USING 3D PRINTING (41)

Advances in wound healing using 3D printing have brought forth innovative solutions that enhance the treatment, management, and recovery of various types of wounds.

Here are some notable advances in wound healing achieved through 3D-printing technology.

1.10.1 Customized Wound Dressings

Three-dimensional printing allows for the creation of personalized wound dressings that match the contours of the wound site. Customized dressings ensure better coverage, fit, and adherence. They can also incorporate specific materials, medications, or growth factors to enhance healing and reduce infection risk.

1.10.2 Bioactive Bandages and Scaffolds

Three-dimensional printing enables the fabrication of wound healing materials that incorporate bioactive agents like growth factors, antimicrobial agents, or stem cells. These materials promote tissue regeneration, reduce inflammation, and expedite wound closure. They offer targeted therapeutic effects to accelerate healing.

1.10.3 Bioprinting Skin Constructs

Bioprinting allows the creation of skin-like constructs with intricate structures, including epidermis, dermis, and vascular networks.

These constructs closely mimic native skin, making them suitable for grafts, wound coverage, and research. Bioprinted skin can promote wound closure, reduce scarring, and potentially replace traditional skin grafts.

1.10.4 Smart Wound Monitoring Devices

Three-dimensional printing can integrate sensors and electronics into wound dressings to create smart devices for real-time monitoring.

These devices can track factors like pH, temperature, bacterial presence, and moisture levels. Timely feedback helps health care providers adjust treatment plans and prevent complications.

1.10.5 Patient-Specific Implants and Scaffolds

Three-dimensional printing enables the creation of patient-specific implants or scaffolds for challenging wounds.

Implants and scaffolds can assist in wound closure, provide support during healing, and promote tissue regeneration. Customization improves fit and reduces the risk of complications.

1.10.6 Vascularized Constructs

Researchers are working on 3D-printed constructs with functional vascular networks to improve nutrient and oxygen delivery.

Vascularized constructs enhance the viability of larger tissue replacements, such as skin grafts or complex wound treatments, by preventing necrosis and supporting tissue growth.

1.10.7 DRUG DELIVERY SYSTEMS

Three-dimensional printing allows for the creation of wound-healing materials with controlled drug-release capabilities.

Controlled drug delivery directly to the wound site improves the effectiveness of medications, reduces systemic side effects, and ensures prolonged therapeutic effects.

1.10.8 POINT-OF-CARE SOLUTIONS

Portable 3D-printing devices can be used in point-of-care settings to create customized wound care solutions.

Health care providers can quickly produce patient-specific wound dressings, implants, or other devices on-demand, enhancing treatment efficiency and patient outcomes.

1.10.9 COLLABORATION BETWEEN DISCIPLINES

Three-dimensional printing fosters collaboration between wound care specialists, 3D-printing experts, and material scientists.

By combining expertise from various fields, innovative wound care solutions are developed faster, leading to improved patient care and outcomes.

These recent breakthroughs in wound healing made possible by 3D printing emphasize the possibility for a complete overhaul of current wound care procedures. The technology provides personalized and focused methods for wound therapy, which promotes quicker healing, fewer problems, and an overall improvement in the patient's well-being.

1.11 DERMATOLOGICAL MODELS AND SURGICAL PLANNING

Improved diagnostic accuracy, preoperative visualization, and patient outcomes have resulted from the use of 3D-printed models in dermatology and surgical planning. These models let dermatologists see their patients' skin problems and better prepare for extensive operations. Here is how dermatology and surgical planning are utilizing 3D-printed models (42):

- Patient Education: 3D-printed models of skin lesions, tumors, and other abnormalities help patients understand their condition. Patients can see the exact position, size, and depth of the problem, allowing them to make more educated treatment decisions.
- Preoperative Planning and Complex Wound Management: Surgeons can inspect 3D-printed models to evaluate the complexity of dermatological operations before they are performed. This paves the way for them to

prepare the best strategy, pick the best incision spots, and prepare for any necessary excisions or grafts. For complex wound cases, 3D-printed models offer a hands-on, 3D-printing representation that assists in developing tailored wound care strategies.

- Mohs Surgery Planning: Mohs surgery, used to remove skin cancer, needs precise planning. Surgeons can better remove malignant tissue while sparing healthy tissue with the use of 3D-printed models.
- Flap and Graft Planning: When skin grafts or flap procedures are necessary, doctors can use 3D-printed models to determine incision lines, evaluate tissue viability, and foresee complications.
- Prosthetic Development: 3D-printed models help with the development of lifelike prosthetics for people who have lost face features because of surgery, trauma, or congenital conditions.
- Scar Management and Customized Instruments and Tools: Using 3D models to predict the results of surgical scar modifications can help both patients and surgeons pick the best course of action. They also have improved accuracy and efficiency in procedures thanks to patient-specific instruments and tools produced with 3D printing.

When it comes to bettering patient outcomes, increasing surgical precision, and expanding medical education and research in the field of dermatology, 3D-printed dermatological models have proven to be useful. These models help patients make better decisions and have better outcomes by providing realistic representations of skin diseases and surgery procedures.

1.12 ROLE OF 3D-PRINTED MODELS IN DERMATOLOGY (43)

Diagnostics, treatment planning, patient education, and research have all benefited greatly from the use of 3D-printed models in dermatology. Examining the uses of 3D-printed models in the field of dermatology.

Diagnostic Accuracy, Planning, and Customized Treatment Approaches: It is much easier for dermatologists to visualize and evaluate complex skin lesions, tumors, and other dermatological abnormalities using models that have been produced using 3D-printing technology since these models are both tangible and realistic representations of the skin disorders in question. To plan complex treatments such as skin grafts, flap surgeries, and Mohs surgery, dermatologists can employ models that have been 3D-printed. Surgeons can better foresee obstacles and design methods for good surgery with the assistance of models. Dermatologists are now able to design patient-specific treatment plans with the help of 3D-printed models since these models enable them to compare a variety of treatment modalities and customize their treatments to meet the requirements of each specific patient.

Training and Education and Complex Case Visualization: Before working on actual patients, medical students, residents, and dermatology experts can practice procedures and polish their abilities on models that have been produced using 3D-printing technology. This is a significant teaching tool.

1.13 RESEARCH AND DEVELOPMENT

Dermatologists can employ 3D-printed models to imitate a variety of skin disorders for the sake of research, test out new treatment methods, and evaluate the responses of tissue in controlled environments.

Prosthetic and Implant Design creation of prostheses and Implants: Patients who have skin defects or conditions that require prostheses or implants can benefit from the use of 3D-printed models, which assist in the creation of individualized solutions that are an aesthetic match for the patient's natural appearance.

- Lesion and Tumor Mapping: Mapping the dimensions and depths of skin lesions tumors and accurate treatment planning and monitoring of disease progression are made possible with the use of 3D-printed models.
- Minimally Invasive Procedures: Injectables, fillers, and Other Minimally Invasive Treatments: In the field of cosmetic dermatology, 3D-printed models assist in guiding the precise placement of injectables and other minimally invasive treatments.
- Visualizing Treatment Progress: Visualizing the progression of treatment dermatologists are able to monitor the development of wound healing, skin grafts, and other therapies over time by comparing the real outcomes to models that have been made using 3D technology.
- Improved Communication: The ability to communicate treatment plans and outcomes with other health care professionals involved in the patient's care can be improved with the usage of 3D-printed models by dermatologists.

In dermatology, 3D-printed models are useful tools that improve diagnostic precision, therapeutic efficacy, patient communication, and academic progress. Patients and doctors alike will reap the benefits of this developing technology as it finds more uses in dermatology.

1.14 SURGICAL PLANNING AND PREOPERATIVE SIMULATION (19)

Improved patient outcomes and safety have resulted from surgeons' ability to design and simulate difficult procedures in advance by utilizing 3D printing. Here is a comprehensive look at how doctors are using 3D printing in preoperative simulation and planning:

- Patient-Specific Anatomical Models: Medical imaging data from computed tomography or magnetic resonance imaging scans can be used with 3D-printing technology to create anatomical models that are unique to each patient. These models allow surgeons to physically interact with the patient's anatomy and the interactions between parts, leading to a more thorough grasp of both.
- Complex Procedure Visualization: Surgeons can better visualize complex procedures with the help of 3D-printed models due to the models' haptic and 3D-printing portrayal of the anatomy.

- Treatment Planning: Surgeons employ 3D-printed models for treatment planning, assessing the ideal approach, and determining incision locations.

1.15 PATIENT EDUCATION AND COMMUNICATION (19)

The utilization of 3D-printed models has brought about a revolution in the field of dermatology about patient education and communication. The improved patient comprehension that results from the use of these tangible replicas enables doctors to show skin problems visibly and practically. Patients can now see and feel their individual illnesses, which improves engagement, informed decision-making, and treatment compliance. Patients can also feel their condition. These models help to close the information gap that exists between patients and their health care professionals, which ultimately results in more productive consultations and improved dermatological care. Here is how 3D printing contributes to patient education and communication:

- Visual and Tactile Understanding
- Clear Explanation of Conditions
- Treatment Option Visualization
- Surgical Procedure Understanding
- Anatomical Variation Awareness
- Personalized Treatment Discussions
- Reduced Anxiety and Fear
- Improved Communication
- Family and Caregiver Involvement
- Post-Procedure Expectations
- Pediatric and Geriatric Engagement
- Interactive Learning
- Compliance and Adherence

1.16 PERSONALIZED DRUG DELIVERY SYSTEMS

The ability to personalize medication administration to the specific requirements of individual patients has the potential to usher in a new era of medical innovation enabled by personalized drug delivery systems made possible by 3D printing. These technologies make it possible to precisely dose medications, control their release, and achieve better therapeutic results. Personalized drug delivery systems that are made using 3D printing offer a new degree of precision in the administration of medication, which improves both treatment outcomes and the patient experience. It is possible that, as the technology continues to advance, it will bring about a revolution in the pharmaceutical sector, as well as in the way pharmaceuticals are prescribed and distributed. Heres how personalized drug delivery systems are developed using 3D printing (44):

- Patient-Specific Data
- Treatment Planning

- Formulation Design
- 3D Printing of Tablets
- Dose Individualization
- Controlled Release Profiles
- Complex Dosage Forms
- Combination Therapies
- Pediatric and Geriatric Dosage
- Implantable Devices
- Tailored Release Kinetics
- Targeted Therapies
- Quick Prototyping
- Compliance Improvement

1.16.1 MICRONEEDLES FOR DERMATOLOGICAL DRUG DELIVERY

One potentially useful application of 3D-printing technology is the creation of microneedles for the delivery of drugs in dermatology. Microneedles are minuscule, minimally invasive devices that can penetrate the top layer of the skin without causing any discomfort. This allows them to deliver medications or other substances for a variety of medical applications, including dermatology. Here is how 3D printing is utilized to create microneedles for dermatological drug delivery.

The personalization of the design 3D printing enables the precise modification of microneedle designs in a variety of dimensions, including length, density, form, and arrangement. These designs are adaptable to meet the precise requirements of drug delivery as well as the requirements of individual patients. Biocompatible and biodegradable materials suitable for microneedle fabrication are chosen for 3D printing. These materials ensure safe and effective drug delivery without causing harm to the skin.

Microneedle arrays are printed layer by layer using 3D-printing techniques, such as SLA or DLP, to create intricate structures with micron-scale precision. Drugs or active compounds are incorporated into the microneedles during the printing process. These substances can include medications, cosmetics, or therapeutic agents for various dermatological conditions (44).

Dissolving microneedles gradually release the drug into the skin and dissolve after drug delivery. Patch-type microneedles remain in place and can be removed after a specified duration of drug release. Microneedles can be designed to release drugs in a controlled and sustained manner, ensuring optimal therapeutic levels over a specific period. Three-dimensional-printed microneedles can be tailored to deliver drugs to specific depths within the skin, targeting various layers or structures as needed for dermatological treatments.

Administration using microneedles does not cause pain because microneedles are constructed to cause no pain or only a minimum amount of discomfort; they are an appealing choice for individuals who have a low threshold for needle pricks. Increased efficacy microneedles enable the effective transport of medications to the deeper layers of the skin, which increases the efficiency of topical therapies. Microneedles allow for transdermal drug administration without the need for injections or other intrusive procedures. Because of this, they are ideal for a wide variety of patients. Cosmetic applications for microneedles include delivering cosmetic substances like hyaluronic acid, peptides, or growth factors for rejuvenation and skin enhancement (45).

Microneedles can be used to administer drugs for conditions like acne, psoriasis, atopic dermatitis, and localized pain relief. Because 3D printing enables quick prototyping and modifications in microneedle designs, it is possible to maximize the effectiveness of medication delivery parameters. Because of its high level of precision and adaptability, 3D printing is ideally suited as a technique to produce microneedles specifically designed for dermatological drug delivery. This method has the potential to increase the efficacy of topical medicines, improve patient comfort, and provide creative solutions for a variety of skin-related disorders.

1.16.2 ADVANCEMENTS IN TARGETED THERAPY (38)

Innovative methods for delivering medications and therapies directly to specific areas of the body have been developed thanks to advancements in targeted therapy that make use of 3D printing. These methods have the potential to improve therapeutic efficacy while simultaneously reducing the risk of adverse effects. The following are some important developments in targeted medicine that have been made possible by 3D printing (Figure 1.1).

- Personalized Drug Delivery: 3D printing allows for the creation of patient-specific drug delivery systems that match an individual's unique anatomy, ensuring optimal treatment outcomes.
- Complex Drug Release Profiles: Three-dimensional printing enables the fabrication of drug delivery devices with intricate geometries that can release medications in complex patterns, such as pulsatile or controlled-release profiles.
- Implantable Drug Delivery Systems: Medication-eluting stents and localized cancer therapy implants are two examples of 3D-printed implants that provide a platform for prolonged and localized medication release.
- Organ-Specific Drug Delivery: Organ-Specific Drug Delivery: Thanks to 3D printing, drug delivery devices can be designed to closely mimic the shape of target organs or tissues.
- Combination Therapies: Three-dimensional printing makes it possible to combine various medications into one delivery system, opening the door to treatments that attack multiple symptoms of an illness at once.
- Cancer Therapy Advancements: Improved methods of delivering chemotherapy and radiation therapy to tumors while sparing surrounding healthy tissue have been made possible by 3D-printed implants, catheters, and microstructures.
- Controlled Drug Release: By controlling the rate at which drugs are released, 3D-printed drug delivery devices can maintain stable therapeutic dosages throughout time.

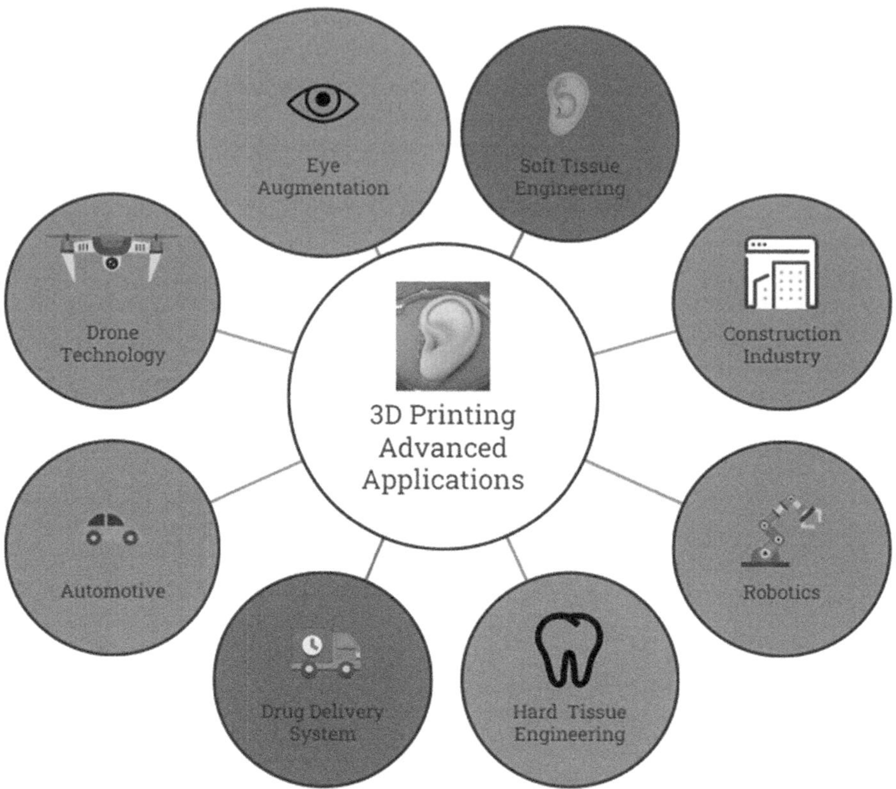

FIGURE 1.1 Advanced applications of 3D printing.

- Oral Drug Delivery Enhancement: Improved medication absorption and patient adherence thanks to 3D-printed oral drug delivery systems, such as tablets with controlled release profiles.
- Bone Regeneration and Repair: Growth factors, stem cells, or other therapeutic agents can be delivered to precise locations in need of bone regeneration and healing thanks to 3D-printed scaffolds.
- Wound Healing Applications: Bandages and dressings made with 3D printers can be infused with medication to treat specific wounds, ulcers, or burns.
- Neural Tissue Repair: Regeneration of Injured Neural Tissue: The use of 3D-printed nerve guides or scaffolds that are infused with neurotrophic factors has the potential to assist in the repair of injured neural tissue.
- Ocular Drug Delivery: Ocular Drug Delivery: Contact lenses or implants that have been created using 3D-printing technology have the potential to deliver pharmaceuticals directly to the eye, hence increasing the effectiveness of treatment for ocular disorders.
- Minimally Invasive Interventions: Three-dimensional-printed microdevices or catheters can be utilized for targeted drug distribution using minimally invasive procedures, hence minimizing the requirement for open surgeries.

- Patient-Specific Dosages: Patient-Specific Dosages: Three-dimensional printing makes it possible to create medication delivery systems with patient-specific dosages, which allows for treatment to be optimized depending on an individual's specific requirements. Exciting new possibilities exist for strengthening treatment outcomes, lowering the risk of adverse effects, and raising the level of patient comfort made possible by advances in targeted therapy made possible by 3D printing. The further development of this technology has the potential to bring about a sea change in the manner in which various medications and treatments are administered to treat a wide range of medical conditions.

1.16.3 Future Prospects and Challenges (38)

1.16.3.1 Future Prospects

The era of precision medicine, in which treatments are customized to an individual based on their genetic makeup, medical history, and unique requirements, is being ushered in by the advent of patient-specific drug delivery systems that can be printed using 3D-printing technology. Researchers are focused on building 3D-printed drug delivery devices with complicated release profiles, which will allow for more complex dosage regimens and greater therapeutic effects.

The capacity to combine numerous medications or therapeutic agents within a single 3D-printed device gives the promise for more effective combination therapies, addressing many elements of a disease simultaneously. This opens the door to the development of more effective combination therapies.

The development of organs-on-chips," or microdevices that duplicate the functions of organs, could be made easier with the help of 3D printing. These platforms would make it possible to assess the effectiveness and safety of drugs on patient-specific tissues, hence decreasing the necessity for testing on animals. In addition, the implants that are produced using 3D-printing technology could be used to treat cancer by delivering chemotherapeutic drugs directly to tumors while avoiding healthy tissue. This strategy may result in medicines that are more effective while causing less harm to patients (38).

The use of medications to direct the formation of new tissues or organs is an example of regenerative medicine. Combining 3D printing with personalized drug delivery could hasten the pace of technological advancements in this field.

Moreover, microdevices and implants that are created using 3D-printing technology have the potential to revolutionize minimally invasive therapies by enabling accurate drug delivery without the need for extensive surgical procedures. The potential for 3D-printed medical devices and implants will increase as research into materials that are biocompatible, functional, and biodegradable is continued. The approval procedure for medical devices that are manufactured using 3D printing can be streamlined with the help of clearer regulatory pathways, which will also assure patient safety.

The quality of printed medical equipment will improve because of developments in 3D-printing technology, which will lead to greater resolutions and smoother surface finishes. The use of more complex combination therapies is made possible by the fact that 3D printing makes it possible to incorporate a variety of substances, including medications and cells, into a single device. The use of 3D printing could eventually result in the local production of medical devices, which would cut down on lead times and provide clinical settings with more timely solutions (45).

The use of artificial intelligence (AI) algorithms can lead to more efficient and effective 3D printing in the medical industry by optimizing designs, materials, and production processes. The advent of realistic training models made possible by 3D printing could herald a new era in medical education. These models would enable students to perfect their skills before entering the clinical setting. Three-dimensional printing has the potential to bring medical solutions to remote and underserved areas where traditional medical infrastructure is lacking.

1.16.3.2 Challenges

Developing personalized medicine delivery systems entails navigating challenges such as complex manufacturing methods and stringent regulatory approval processes. Ensuring the safety and effectiveness of these systems is of utmost importance. Biocompatible materials are essential in 3D printing to prevent adverse reactions or immune responses when interacting with the human body. Quality control is a persistent challenge due to the intricate structures of 3D-printed drug delivery systems, demanding robust processes for reliability.

Scaling up production while maintaining accuracy and quality poses a significant challenge, as does ensuring the long-term stability of 3D-printed drug delivery systems, particularly for slow-release medications. Large-scale clinical trials are essential for validating the safety and efficacy of personalized drug delivery systems but come with the drawbacks of being time-consuming and costly.

Ethical concerns surrounding personalized medicine include questions about data privacy, ownership, and potential misuse of patient-specific information. Creating personalized drug delivery systems necessitates interdisciplinary collaboration, involving professionals from engineering, pharmacy, medicine, and materials science. The cost considerations of personalized 3D printing, which can be more expensive than conventional manufacturing processes, raise concerns about the affordability and availability of individualized medical care.

The enormous potential for 3D-printed, individually tailored medicine delivery systems, especially given current technological developments, necessitates overcoming obstacles related to regulation, quality control, and interdisciplinary collaboration. While the medical industry has made significant progress with 3D printing, challenges persist, and there are promising avenues for further exploration. The advancement of personalized medicine and health care through 3D printing holds the potential for revolutionizing these fields as technology continues to advance.

1.17 LIMITATIONS AND TECHNICAL CONSTRAINTS (46)

The use of 3D printing in several disciplines, including medicine and health care, is hindered by its inherent restrictions as well as by the technical constraints that come with it. Despite its many benefits, 3D printing is not without its drawbacks.

1.17.1 LIMITATIONS AND CONSTRAINTS ASSOCIATED WITH 3D PRINTING

- Material Limitations: However, there are still barriers to overcome in terms of biocompatibility, mechanical qualities, and material combinations despite the growing number of options for 3D printing. It can be difficult to identify the optimal material for a certain need.
- Resolution and Surface Finish: Some 3D-printing methods make it challenging to achieve high-resolution and flawless surface finishes. This restriction can be a concern in contexts where precision or smoothness is essential.
- Print Speed: Time is often an issue when 3D printing large or complicated objects. Limitations in print speed may make 3D printing impractical for bulk production or time-sensitive uses.
- Size Constraints: Larger things cannot be created on a 3D printer since the construction platform is too small. Printing large objects in pieces and then assembling them could introduce structural flaws.
- Post-Processing: Post-processing activities such as cleaning, support removal, and surface finishing are necessary for many 3D-printed goods. These procedures may increase production costs and lead times.
- Accuracy and Tolerance: Printer calibration, material qualities, and ambient conditions are only a few of the sources of potential error during 3D printing.
- Material Compatibility: There are a variety of different 3D-printing technologies, and not all materials are compatible with each one. It can be difficult to successfully match the appropriate material with the printing method that is needed.
- Regulatory Approval: Medical equipment that is manufactured using a 3D printer is subject to rigorous regulatory requirements regarding their safety and effectiveness. Providing evidence that an organization complies with these criteria can be a difficult and time-consuming process.
- Design Constraints: The capabilities of the 3D printer, which might include features such as overhang angles, support structures, and layer thickness, can place limitations on the design of an object that is to be manufactured via 3D printing.
- Cost: Even though 3D printing allows for customization, the process can often be more expensive than traditional manufacturing processes, particularly when it comes to producing items in big quantities.
- Intellectual Property and Counterfeiting: The simplicity of 3D printing can raise worries about the potential for intellectual property infringement as well as the possibility of fake products being sold.
- Limited Multi-Material Integration: It can be difficult to combine several materials or components, each of which has its unique qualities, into a single product that has been created using a 3D printer. This may necessitate post-processing or additional assembly stages.
- Limited Mass Production: In some cases, conventional manufacturing techniques, like as injection molding, may be preferable to 3D printing when it comes to volume production.

The transformational potential of 3D printing should not be overlooked, but neither should its limitations and restraints. Many of these restrictions are being removed as a result of constant technological improvement brought about by research, development, and new ideas.

1.18 SUMMARY OF 3D PRINTING IN DERMATOLOGY

In the realm of dermatology, 3D printing has emerged as a game-changing technology, giving creative solutions for a variety of patient care and treatment facets that were previously unaddressed. It makes it possible to create individualized medical equipment, surgical guides, prosthetics, and models, all of which improve diagnostic precision, surgical accuracy, and overall patient outcomes. The management of dermatological disorders is being revolutionized by 3D printing, which uses patient-specific data as its primary resource. The following are important applications (Figure 1.2):

- Customized Medical Devices and Wound Care Solutions: The use of 3D printing makes it possible to produce individualized medical devices such as prosthetics, orthotics, and wound care solutions that may completely conform to the patient's anatomy, hence increasing the patient's level of comfort and functioning. Wound dressings and skin grafts that are created using 3D-printing technology provide patients with a variety of wound geometries and healing requirements with the opportunity for personalized treatment options.
- Surgical Planning and Simulation: To improve accuracy and lower the risk of problems during surgery, dermatologists employ models that have been made using 3D-printing technology to design and simulate procedures.
- Patient Education: The use of visual aids produced through 3D printing enables dermatologists to convey treatment plans and processes more effectively to patients, hence increasing patients' levels of comprehension and participation.
- Cosmetic and Aesthetic Applications: Three-dimensional printing assists in surgical planning, implant design, and modeling for cosmetic procedures, leading to improved outcomes in dermatological aesthetics.
- Targeted Drug Delivery: Three-dimensional-printed drug delivery systems offer personalized treatment regimens, ensuring precise drug release profiles for dermatological conditions.
- Tissue Engineering and Bioprinting: The field of bioprinting holds promise for creating functional skin tissues and even organs, opening possibilities for regenerative medicine.
- Regulatory and Safety Considerations: Regulatory bodies play a crucial role in ensuring the safety and effectiveness of 3D-printed medical devices, driving the need for compliance with standards and guidelines.
- Challenges and Future Directions: Despite its potential, challenges like material selection, regulatory approval, and post-processing remain. The future holds promise in areas like bioprinting, AI integration, and sustainable practices. In essence, 3D printing is reshaping dermatology by offering

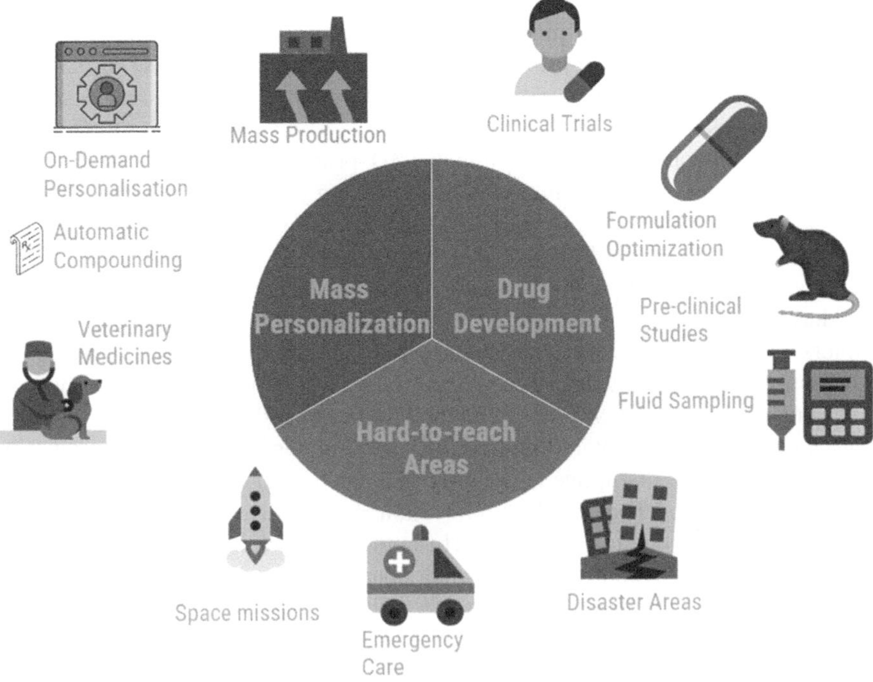

FIGURE 1.2 Different models of 3D-printing tissue and organs and applications of 3D printing in pharmaceutical and health care systems.

patient-centered, precise, and customized solutions for various medical and aesthetic needs. As research and technology continue to advance, the role of 3D printing in dermatology is set to expand, benefiting both patients and health care professionals.

1.19 CONCLUSION

In recent revelations, 3D printing has emerged as a transformative technology poised to reshape various business sectors, including medicine, industry, and aerospace. The ability to construct intricate, unique products with precision and speed opens up avenues for creativity and problem-solving. This technological advancement is fundamentally changing the landscape of design, production, and interaction across diverse fields, from personalized medical equipment to complex architectural structures. Notably, 3D printing is revolutionizing the medical and healthcare industries, ushering in a new era of patient care customization. The technology enables the personalization of implant devices, surgical guides, prosthetics, and drug delivery systems, providing medical professionals with precise tools for surgery planning, diagnostics, and research in areas like tissue engineering. Additionally, 3D printing fosters patient engagement and education through tangible visual aids. Looking ahead, the future of 3D printing presents both exciting possibilities and challenges.

Material advancements are anticipated to expand the technology's applications, with researchers discovering new materials boasting improved features like biocompatibility and sustainability. Bioprinting breakthroughs hold the promise of transforming transplantation and regenerative medicine by producing functional tissues and organs.

Mass customization, made feasible by 3D printing, ensures products can be tailored to specific requirements without sacrificing efficiency. Industry collaboration, particularly between healthcare and manufacturing, is expected to yield cross-disciplinary discoveries. Regulatory frameworks will evolve to address novel challenges posed by 3D-printed products, ensuring safety and quality standards.

Education and training are poised to witness the widespread integration of 3D printers across all levels, fostering experiential learning and creative thinking. The technology's potential extends to space exploration and sustainability, contributing to environmentally responsible industrial practices and aiding in the production of tools, equipment, and shelters for space missions. In conclusion, 3D printing stands as an innovative and disruptive force, altering industries and expanding the realm of what is conceivable. Its potential for innovation, personalization, and process optimization is only beginning to be realized. The continued pursuit of study, collaboration, and technological developments will undoubtedly ensure 3D printing's profound impact on the future in diverse ways.

ACKNOWLEDGMENT

The authors would like to acknowledge their affiliated institution.

CONFLICT OF INTEREST

None.

REFERENCES

1. Haleem A, Javaid M, Khan RH, Suman R. 3D printing applications in bone tissue engineering. *Journal of Clinical Orthopaedics and Trauma* 2020 Feb 1;11:S118–24.
2. Yadav K, Pradhan M, Singh D, Singh MR. Targeting autoimmune disorders through metal nanoformulation in overcoming the fences of conventional treatment approaches. In: Rezaei N, editor. *Translational Autoimmunity*. Academic Press; 2022. p. 361–93. (Translational Immunology; vol. 2). Available from: https://www.sciencedirect.com/science/article/pii/B9780128243909000177
3. Arif ZU, Khalid MY, Noroozi R, Hossain M, Shi HTH, Tariq A, et al. Additive manufacturing of sustainable biomaterials for biomedical applications. *Asian Journal of Pharmaceutical Sciences* 2023 May 1;18(3):100812.
4. Mohammed AA, Algahtani MS, Ahmad MZ, Ahmad J, Kotta S. 3D printing in medicine: Technology overview and drug delivery applications. *Annals of 3D Printed Medicine*. 2021 Dec 1;4:100037.
5. Bae S, Kim H, Lee Y, Xu X, Park JS, Zheng Y, et al. Roll-to-roll production of 30-inch graphene films for transparent electrodes. *Nature Nanotechnology* 2010;5(8):574–8.

6. Yu J, Xu Y, Li S, Seifert GV., Becker ML. Three-dimensional printing of nano hydroxyapatite/poly(ester urea) composite scaffolds with enhanced bioactivity. *Biomacromolecules* 2017 Dec 11;18(12):4171–83.

7. Lee SJ, Zhu W, Nowicki M, Lee G, Heo DN, Kim J, et al. 3D printing nano conductive multi-walled carbon nanotube scaffolds for nerve regeneration. *Journal of Neural Engineering* 2018 Feb 1;15(1):016018.

8. Hassan M, Dave K, Chandrawati R, Dehghani F, Gomes VG. 3D printing of biopolymer nanocomposites for tissue engineering: Nanomaterials, processing and structure-function relation. *European Polymer Journal* 2019 Dec 1;121:109340.

9. Băilă DI, Ghionea IG, Mocioiu OC, Ćuković S, Ulmeanu ME, Tarbă CI, et al. Design of handle elevators and ATR spectrum of material manufactured by stereolithography. *IFIP Advances in Information and Communication Technology* 2016;492:309–18.

10. Ligon SC, Liska R, Stampfl J, Gurr M, Mülhaupt R. Polymers for 3D printing and customized additive manufacturing. *Chemical Reviews* 2017 Aug 9;117(15):10212–90.

11. Heller C, Schwentenwein M, Russmueller G, Varga F, Stampfl J, Liska R. Vinyl esters: Low cytotoxicity monomers for the fabrication of biocompatible 3D scaffolds by lithography based additive manufacturing. *Journal of Polymer Science, Part A: Polymer Chemistry* 2009 Dec 15;47(24):6941–54.

12. Mauro N, Andrea Utzeri M, Sciortino A, Cannas M, Messina F, Cavallaro G, et al. Printable thermo- and photo-stable poly(D,L-lactide)/carbon nanodots nanocomposites via heterophase melt-extrusion transesterification. *Chemical Engineering Journal* 2022 Sep 1;443:136525.

13. Suryanarayana C. Mechanical alloying and milling. *Progress in Materials Science* 2001;46:1–184.

14. Williams JM, Adewunmi A, Schek RM, Flanagan CL, Krebsbach PH, Feinberg SE, et al. Bone tissue engineering using polycaprolactone scaffolds fabricated via selective laser sintering. *Biomaterials* 2005 Aug;26(23):4817–27.

15. Jamróz W, Szafraniec J, Kurek M, Jachowicz R. 3D printing in pharmaceutical and medical applications. *Pharmaceutical Research* 2018;35(9):1–22.

16. Singh D, Pradhan M, Nag M, Singh MR. Vesicular system: Versatile carrier for transdermal delivery of bioactives. *Artificial Cells, Nanomedicine, and Biotechnology* 2015;43(4):282–90.

17. Sahu K, Minz S, Pradhan M, Kaurav M, Yadav K. Antiviral nanomaterials as potential targets for malaria prevention and treatment. In: Thangadurai D, Islam S, Adetunji CO, editors. *Viral and Antiviral Nanomaterials.* 1st ed. CRC Press; 2022. p. 401–24.

18. Murphy SV, Atala A. 3D bioprinting of tissues and organs. *Nature Biotechnology* 2014;32(8):773–85.

19. Chae MP, Rozen WM, McMenamin PG, Findlay MW, Spychal RT, Hunter-Smith DJ. Emerging applications of bedside 3D printing in plastic surgery. *Frontiers in Surgery* 2015 Jun 16;2:25.

20. Scarpa M, Hesse S, Bradley SJ. M1 muscarinic acetylcholine receptors: A therapeutic strategy for symptomatic and disease-modifying effects in Alzheimer's disease? *Advances in Pharmacology* 2020;88:277–310.

21. Yadav H, Mahalvar A, Pradhan M, Yadav K, Kumar Sahu K, Yadav R. Exploring the potential of phytochemicals and nanomaterial: A boon to antimicrobial treatment. *Medicine in Drug Discovery.* 2023;17:100151. Available from: https://www.sciencedirect.com/science/article/pii/S2590098623000015

22. Kähäri VM, Saarialho-Kere U. Matrix metalloproteinases in skin. *Experimental Dermatology.* 1997;6(5):199–213.

23. Wong JY, Pfahnl AC. 3D printing of surgical instruments for long-duration space missions. *Aviation Space and Environmental Medicine* 2014;85(7):758–63.

24. Yadav R, Pradhan M, Yadav K, Mahalvar A, Yadav H. Present scenarios and future prospects of herbal nanomedicine for antifungal therapy. *Journal of Drug Delivery Science and Technology* 2022;74:103430.

25. Murphy SV, Skardal A, Atala A. Evaluation of hydrogels for bio-printing applications. *Journal of Biomedical Materials Research - Part A* 2013 Jan;101 A(1):272–84.

26. Jakus AE, Secor EB, Rutz AL, Jordan SW, Hersam MC, Shah RN. Three-dimensional printing of high-content graphene scaffolds for electronic and biomedical applications. *ACS Nano* 2015 Apr 28;9(4):4636–48.

27. Daly R, Harrington TS, Martin GD, Hutchings IM. Inkjet printing for pharmaceutics - A review of research and manufacturing. *International Journal of Pharmaceutics* 2015 Oct 30;494(2):554–67.

28. Park JH, Choi SO, Seo S, Choy Y Bin, Prausnitz MR. A microneedle roller for transdermal drug delivery. *European Journal of Pharmaceutics and Biopharmaceutics* 2010 Oct;76(2):282–9.

29. Sakes A, Hovland K, Smit G, Geraedts J, Breedveld P. Design of a novel three-dimensional-printed two degrees-of-freedom steerable electrosurgical grasper for minimally invasive surgery. *Journal of Medical Devices, Transactions of the ASME* 2018 Mar 1;12(1).

30. Li S, Kim Y, Lee JW, Prausnitz MR. Microneedle patch tattoos. *iScience*. 2022 Oct 21;25(10):1–14.

31. Kim YC, Park JH, Prausnitz MR. Microneedles for drug and vaccine delivery. *Advanced Drug Delivery Reviews* 2012 Nov;64(14):1547–68.

32. Moore LE, Vucen S, Moore AC. Trends in drug- and vaccine-based dissolvable microneedle materials and methods of fabrication. *European Journal of Pharmaceutics and Biopharmaceutics* 2022 Apr 1;173:54–72.

33. Leppiniemi J, Lahtinen P, Paajanen A, Mahlberg R, Metsä-Kortelainen S, Pinomaa T, et al. 3D-printable bioactivated nanocellulose-alginate hydrogels. *ACS Applied Materials and Interfaces* 2017 Jul 5;9(26):21959–70.

34. Yadav K, Singh D, Singh MR. Nanovesicles delivery approach for targeting steroid mediated mechanism of antipsoriatic therapeutics. *Journal of Drug Delivery Science and Technology* 2021;65:102688. Available from: https://www.sciencedirect.com/science/article/pii/S1773224721003683

35. Singh SK, Dwivedi SD, Yadav K, Shah K, Chauhan NS, Pradhan M, et al. Novel biotherapeutics targeting biomolecular and cellular approaches in diabetic wound healing. *Biomedicines* 2023;11(2). Available from: https://www.mdpi.com/2227-9059/11/2/613

36. Gupta P. Natural products as inhibitors of matrix metalloproteinases. *Natural Products Chemistry & Research* 2016;4(1):6836.

37. Kaleev AA, Kashapov LN, Kashapov NF, Kashapov RN. Application of reverse engineering in the medical industry. *IOP Conference Series: Materials Science and Engineering* 2017 Sep 28;240(1):012030.

38. Palo M, Holländer J, Suominen J, Yliruusi J, Sandler N. 3D printed drug delivery devices: Perspectives and technical challenges. *Expert Review of Medical Devices* 2017 Sep 2;14(9):685–96.

39. Sahu KK, Kaurav M, Bhatt P, Minz S, Pradhan M, Khan J, et al. 5 - Utility of nanomaterials in wound management. In: Solanki PR, Kumar A, Pratap Singh R, Singh J, Singh RB editors. *Nanotechnological Aspects for Next-Generation Wound Management.* Academic Press; 2024. p. 101–30. Available from: https://www.sciencedirect.com/science/article/pii/B978032399165000006X

40. Yadav K, Sahu KK, Gnanakani SPE, Sure P, Vijayalakshmi R, et al. Biomedical applications of nanomaterials in the advancement of nucleic acid therapy: Mechanistic challenges, delivery strategies, and therapeutic applications. *International Journal of Biological Macromolecules* 2023;241:124582. Available from: https://www.sciencedirect.com/science/article/pii/S0141813023014769

41. Sun H, Ma X. α5-nAChR modulates nicotine-induced cell migration and invasion in A549 lung cancer cells. *Experimental and Toxicologic Pathology* 2015;67(9):477–82.

42. Lee KE, Park JE, Jung E, Ryu J, Kim YJ, Youm JK, et al. A study of facial wrinkles improvement effect of veratric acid from cauliflower mushroom through photoprotective mechanisms against UVB irradiation. *Archives of Dermatological Research* 2016;308(3):183–92.

43. Sharma M, Sharma M. Influence of culture media on mycelial growth and sporulation of some soil dermatophytes compared to their clinical isolates. *Journal of Microbiology and Antimicrobials* 2011;3(8):196–200.

44. Hirobe S, Azukizawa H, Hanafusa T, Matsuo K, Quan YS, Kamiyama F, et al. Clinical study and stability assessment of a novel transcutaneous influenza vaccination using a dissolving microneedle patch. *Biomaterials* 2015 Jul 1;57:50–8.

45. Raphael AP, Crichton ML, Falconer RJ, Meliga S, Chen X, Fernando GJP, et al. Formulations for microprojection/microneedle vaccine delivery: Structure, strength and release profiles. *Journal of Controlled Release* 2016 Mar 10;225:40–52.

46. Sears NA, Seshadri DR, Dhavalikar PS, Cosgriff-Hernandez E. A review of three-dimensional printing in tissue engineering. *Tissue Engineering - Part B: Reviews* 2016 Aug 1;22(4):298–310.

2 Bioink as Integral Material for 3D Printing

Kushagra Nagori, Rashnita Sharma, and Anshita Shukla
Rungta Institute of Pharmaceutical Education and Research, Bhilai, India

Kartik T. Nakhate
Shri Vile Parle Kelavani Mandal's Institute of Pharmacy (SVKM-IOP), Dhule, India

Dhansay Dewangan
Swami Atmanand Government English Medium Model College, Korba, India

2.1 INTRODUCTION

Skin is the body's outermost covering and is extremely prone to trauma and damage. The normal physiologic reaction to damage, known as wound healing, is essential for patient survival. The market offers a wide range of wound healing treatments, the bulk of which consists of biosynthetic dressings for wounds (1). Regardless of the positive clinical results, treating various types of wounds can be difficult. For instance, burn wounds, a common type of wound, are extremely dehydrated and demand a moist environment. Additionally, the majority of wound dressings do not assist the scarless wound healing of skin appendages including hair follicles, sweat glands, and natural colors, which are crucial for the characteristic skin functionality and appearance (2–4). Among the effects are bone imperfections, provoking illnesses, wounds, and adversely affected tissues that cause harm to the human body's organs and joints' ability to perform and remain useful (5). Therefore, investigations into wound healing have concentrated on creating cutting-edge wound dressings that enable scarless recovery while also reducing patients' psychological and physical discomfort (6). It has been an unrealistic expectation for many to imagine that damaged tissues or organs can fully recover and regain their abilities, which are now plausible through approaches like tissue engineering and regenerative medicine. Tissue engineering builds constructions that can heal or replace injured or contaminated organs and tissues by mixing cells, scaffolds that act as structured patterns for cell aggregation, and growth agents (7). Figure 2.1 illustrates the procedure for producing

DOI: 10.1201/9781032690926-2

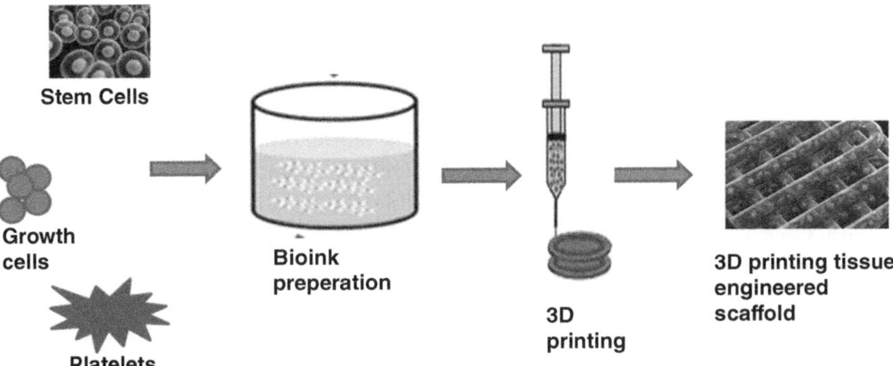

FIGURE 2.1 The diagram showcases the optimal steps for fabricating 3D-printed tissue scaffolds using bioinks. It illustrates the procedure for the design and bio-fabrication of tissue constructs from bioinks mimicking the native tissue parts.

bioink-based tissue engineering scaffolds. Tissue engineering has been advocated as a preferable substitute for impaired tissue by integrating scientific procedures with suitable standards of design with other regenerative medicine approaches, such as cell-based therapy and immunomodulation to enhance organ healing or in vivo tissue (8). Numerous researchers included fibroblast, mesenchymal stem cells, or keratinocytes in the bioink to address the regenerative medicine approach (9). One of the newest technologies, 3D bioprinting (tissue/organ printing), is widely utilized in regenerative medicine and tissue engineering to create complex tissue structures that closely match original tissues and organs. To produce organs or tissues that function, bioprinting involves layer-by-layer deposition of biomaterials containing cells in a specified structural framework. A specific configuration of microarchitecture is necessary for a successful macro tissue because it must offer the necessary mechanical support, a sufficient supply of supplemental nutrients for basic cell types, and, once embedded, the ability to rebuild efficiently (8). This method combines biomaterials, living cells, and controlled motor systems to construct complex structures, and has demonstrated higher precision control over the completed products compared to other currently available techniques. As an additive manufacturing (AM) technology, 3D bioprinting is solely based on biomaterials, enclosing cells on a micro to nanoscale to create constructs that are distinct from tissue. The main goal of using AM in tissue engineering is to create parts with arbitrary geometrical complexity at a low tooling cost and quick turnaround (9). The 3D-printed tissue engineering structures are often made using rapid prototyping capabilities, biodegradability, and biocompatibility as crucial key aspects (10). These 3D-printable structures have the ability to advance the pharmacology, toxicology, and medication development of skin-related conditions as well as skin restoration and wound healing (11). Primary human dermal fibroblasts were employed in a collagen hydrogel in the first skin bioprinting investigation, which was published in 2009 (12). The bioink used for printing is an important component of 3D bioprinting. For living cells to be accepted, this bioink should be extremely biocompatible and mechanically durable after printing and have a great printing resolution. Hydrogels are the most frequently utilized bioink materials in 3D bioprinting. This is primarily because they can store living cells, have chemical structures that can be changed, and have mechanical, adjustable, and biodegradable capabilities that can produce prints with good resolution. Three-dimensional bioprinting enables precise fabrication using cells, synthetic or natural hydrogels like collagen, alginate and cellulose, and biomolecules. The cost-effective mass manufacturing of biocompatible tissues that closely resemble their natural environment is made possible by 3D bioprinting (13). The main procedures in fabrication are imaging the desired tissue, making a model utilizing computer-aided design (CAD) software, sectioning biomaterial and formulating a bioink, optimizing bioprinting parameters for 3D tissue creation,and maturing printed products in vitro to create constructs with biomimetic histology (14). Complex 3D tissue architectures can be generated and developed using challenging geometrical data in CAD acquired from medical imaging techniques such as magnetic resonance imaging (MRI), X-ray imaging, and microcomputerized tomography (CT) scans. The use of 3D bioprinting in the biomedical industry has several benefits, including the construction of customized designs for individual patients, definite proclamation, cost feasibility, ease, flow controllability, and quick on-demand creation of complicated structures (15). For 3D printing of live cells, inkjet bioprinting and direct ink writing (DIW) are often preferred over other 3D-printing techniques like laser-induced forward transfer (LIFT) stereolithography (SLA), selective laser sintering (SLS), and fused deposition modeling (FDM) (16). The bioprinting of tissues and organs is now done using a variety of methods, including pneumatic bioprinting, microwave bioprinting, acoustic bioprinting, electro-hydrodynamic bioprinting, and others(17). Laser-based bioprinting, inkjet-based bioprinting, and extrusion-based bioprinting are the three basic technological solutions for bioprinting (14). Drops of cell suspension are deposited using drop-on-demand thermal, piezoelectric, and electromagnetic methods in inkjet-based bioprinting. A high-resolution structure can be produced using inkjet-based 3D bioprinting easily and inexpensively, with the ability to alter the concentration gradient. Instead of using droplets, extrusion-based bioprinting dispenses a constant stream of bioink using a mechanical or pneumatic mechanism. The basic principles of LIFT technology, which uses a pulsed laser beam focused on an energy-absorbing ribbon layer to create high-pressure bubbles that drive cell-containing materials onto the substrate, are the foundation of laser-based bioprinting (14).Three-dimensional bioprinting is a more clinically useful technology for the deposition of multiple kinds of matrix and cells into histologically healthy and functional skin. Bioprinting of skin can be approached one of two ways. The first method includes situ bioprinting, which involves printing precultured cells directly into the wound site in order to promote skin maturation there, and the second method is in vitro bioprinting, where the skin construct is printed, allowed to grow, and then applied to the area of the wound (14).

2.2 COMPOSITION

Regardless of the bioprinting technology, the composition, or cell type has a significant impact on the bioprinted skin substitute's biocompatibility, mechanical integrity, rheology, biodegradability, and antibacterial activity. The ability of hydrogels, which are three-dimensional networks of hydrophilic polymer chains, to provide a moist environment and a cell carrier, has led to encouraging wound healing effects. Synthetic polymers are the two primary types of hydrogels utilized for skin bioprinting. (e.g., PCL [polycaprolactone], PEG [polyethylene glycol], etc.) along with two types of natural polymers (e.g., collagen, alginate, gelatin) (18). Table 2.1 provides a brief overview of the various biomaterials used as bioinks in 3D printing. To preserve the appropriate shape in a repeatable manner, an optimal hydrogel for printing must remain liquid during printing and solidify after printing (19).

2.2.1 AGAROSE-BASED BIOINKS

The marine polysaccharide agarose is sourced from seaweed, which is a highly valued biopolymer in the biomedical area with exceptional gel-forming capabilities. It is utilized for a variety of purposes. Agarose is a polymer with a linear chain that contains repeated agarose units. The backbone chain of agarose is composed of the disaccharides D-galactose and 3,6-anhydro-L-galactopyranose. The researchers used human mesenchymal stem cells (hMSCs) in their study to evaluate it, and the constructs gave high cell survival up to 95% higher than the natural agarose gel. The degree of carboxylation can be adjusted to produce distinct gels with varying mechanical properties depending on the tissue or organ in question (41, 42). As a bioink, chemically modified agarose, such as carboxylated agarose, was employed to create mechanically adjustable 3D tissue constructions. According to Kreimendahl et al. (2017), agarose-based bioinks are made of distinct amounts of fibrinogen and collagen. They demonstrated that these agarose-based mixed biomaterials may form stable 3D structures and promote endothelial cell development and fibroblast (21). According to Daly et al., agarose gel was tested against three additional hydrogels that were used as bioinks in 3D printing for cartilage tissue engineering in order to assess their biocompatibility and printability toward the production of fibrocartilage cells or cartilage (43).

2.2.2 BIOINKS BASED ON ALGINATE

Alginate is commonly referred to as alginic acid or algin. It is a cheap, naturally occurring biopolymer obtained from brown algae. Alginates are negatively charged polysaccharides that, when injected into living organisms do not obscure or cause a significant inflammatory reaction. The repeated units of the alginate polymer are made up of the monomers -L-guluronic acid and (1–4)-D-mannuronic acid. While (L-4)-D-mannuronic acid and a mixture of (L-4)-L-guluronic acid and (L-4)-D-mannuronic acid assist in enhancing the material's flexibility, (1–4)-D-mannuronic acid aids in the formation of gel (44, 45). By employing capillary forces, the alginate biopolymers can retain other molecules and water while allowing them to diffuse from the inside out. This quality makes these bioinks ideal for 3D bioprinting (46, 47). Using an alginate-based hydrogel material, Gao et al. (2015) revealed a coaxial method that can 3D-print high-potency constructions with micro-channels for nutrient delivery (37). Similar to this, Jia et al. (2016) revealed a blended bioink system based on alginate that may be utilized to print 3D objects directly (48). To

TABLE 2.1

List of Biomaterials Employed as Bioink for 3D Printing

Biomaterial	Printing Technology	Bioink Concentration	Cells	Target Tissue	Crosslinking	Advantages	Disadvantages	References
Alginate	Pneumatic extrusion-based bioprinting	1-2%	Bone marrow stomal cells	Human lipoaspirate derived adipose	Ionic	Quick and simple gelation and high stability	Reduced cell–cell contact and biodegradation	(19, 20)
Agarose	Extrusion based bioprinting	2%	Human endothelial cells, Smooth muscle cells	Vascular TE	Thermal	Quick gelation, high cell viability, and good printability	Decreased stability and weak mechanical characteristics	(21, 22)
Collagen	Extrusion-based bioprinting	0.223%	NIH 3T3fibroblasts	Liver, Heart muscle	Thermal	Promotes the adherence of cells and proliferation	Limited solubility, Inadequate, mechanical qualities and slow gelation period	(23, 24)
Fibrin	Extrusion-based bioprinting	10mg/ml	L-929 cells	Bone	Enzymatic	Rapid angiogenesis and quick gelation	Inadequate mechanical stability and clogs quickly	(25, 26)
Gelatin	Extrusion-based bioprinting	10-20%	Keratinocytes, Fibroblasts, Progenitor cells	Brain, Cardiac tissue, skin	UV exposure	Reduced antigenicity and low expense	Least stable, weak mechanical strength and heat resistant	(27, 28)
Silk	Extrusion-based bioprinting	5-10%w/v	Fibroblasts		Physical	Low price, strong cell adhesion, less immunogenicity, high biocompatibility, and strong mechanical characteristics	To achieve the best rheology and printability, more polymers must be combined.	(29, 30)

Hyaluronic acid	Extrusion-based bioprinting	0.5% w/v	Keratinocytes, Fibroblasts	Human adipose stem cells	UV	High moisture retention and promotes proliferation	Rapid deterioration and weak mechanical stability	(31, 32)
Chitosan	Extrusion based bioprinting		Keratinocytes, Fibroblasts		Polyethylene glycol (PEG)	Moderate gelation issues and antimicrobial	• Weak solubility • Poor mechanical strength	(33, 34)
Decellularized extracellular matrix (dECM)	Extrusion-based bioprinting	3%	Human adipose stem cells		Thermal	Similar to ECM and strong cell adhesion	Tissues are an accessible, lengthy process	(35, 36)
Polyethylene glycol	Extrusion-based bioprinting	10%	hMSCs	Nose, Ear	UV	Reproducibility simple chemical alterations	Reduced cell contact and weak mechanical strength	(37, 38)
Polycaprolactone	Extrusion-based bioprinting		Human bone marrow–derived MSCs	Cartilage bone		Biodegradable and bioresorable		(39)
PVP	Extrusion-based bioprinting		MSCs	Cartilage-like tissue		Nontoxic, water-soluble		(40)

create diverse 3D-printed structures for tissue engineering, various polymers, such as PCL (43, 49, 50), poloxamer, hydroxyapatite, gelatin, and others were combined with alginate. Alginates have been utilized to create 3D constructions of brain tissue. Using a range of biomaterials, including alginate, carboxymethyl-chitosan, and agarose, a 3D construct with stem cells and its insitu growth of stem cells was printed. In another study, alginate was coupled with a 4-arm poly(ethylene glycol)-tetra-acrylate (PEGTA) and gelatin methacryloyl (GelMA) to develop biomimetic 3D-bioprinted materials for vascular tissue engineering. The bioink was first ionically crosslinked with calcium ions (alginate) and then subjected to light (GelMA and PEGTA) to generate stable structures. Including PEGTA assisted the bioink in being tuned or rectified in order to get the requisite mechanical or rheological properties for the bioprinting of intricate multilayer hollow 3D structures. The combination of bioinks created an ideal environment for the formation of highly organized, stable, and perfusable vascular structures by endothelial and stem cells. They stated that using this technique would make it easier for researchers to create more vascularized tissue constructions for use in tissue engineering (48).

2.2.3 Cellulose

It is the main structural constituent of plant cell walls which is a complex carbohydrate made up of multiple glucose units. Nanocellulosic materials are considered extrudable precursors for three-dimensional printing due to their exceptional biocompatibility and stiffness, including the fact that they are readily available, compostable, renewable, and inexpensive (51). Torres-Rendon et al. 3D-bioprinted living structures using cellulose nanofibrils, and they showed that the hydrogels could be processed into complicated designs that may be used as a model for freestanding cell constructions. (52). Kirk et al. demonstrated cellulose nanocrystal-based inks for bioprinting and created 3D-printed textured cellular architectures (53). To enhance the printability and shape fidelity of a bioink formulation, cellulose derivatives can be used as rheology modifiers.

2.2.4 Collagen

One essential component of extracellular matrix (ECM) composed of natural biomaterials is collagen (51, 54). Because of its exceptional biocompatibility, it has been employed as a bioink material in 3D bioprinting, either alone or in combination (51, 55). Temperature changes, pH shifts, or even the use of the vitamin riboflavin can crosslink this biopolymer (56, 57). In comparison to collagen that has not been crosslinked, they have greater tensile strength and viscoelastic characteristics (54, 58). By comparison, collagen must crosslink or gel for at least 30 minutes at 37 °C. Collagen is difficult to use in 3D printing when used alone, but mixing collagen with other gelation materials may help to solve this problem. Furthermore, for use in 3D bioprinting, the mechanical properties of collagen materials can be enhanced by altering the amounts of other polymers added (58, 59). Yang et al. (2017) created 3D structures containing chondrocytes using collagen and sodium alginate as a bioink. Moreover, they showed how the combination effectively prevented the chondrocytes from dedifferentiating into other cell phenotypes and promoted increased cell attachment and proliferation. The printed construct's mechanical qualities were improved, according to the results. Overall, they claimed that for applications involving cartilage tissue creation, a combination of alginate and collagen can be favored (60).

2.2.5 CHITOSAN

A polymer called chitosan is extracted from the tough outer shell of shellfish like prawns, crabs, and lobster. Chitosan is composed of randomly distributed (1–4)-linked D-glucosamine (deacetylated unit) and N-acetyl-D-glucosamine (acetylated unit). Chitin can be converted into chitosan, which can be employed as a gel-forming substance. Additionally, it is said to have antimicrobial and wound-healing qualities (61, 62). For tissue engineering investigations, chitosan has gained widespread use as a biodegradable substance (55). It is eventually explored as a thermoresponsive hydrogel and used as a bioink in 3D printing (61, 63). Intini et al. reported on the biofabrication of skin tissue constructions utilizing chitosan as a bioink, where the authors looked into the toxicity and biocompatibility of human fibroblasts and keratinocytes (33). Furthermore, when the aforementioned 3D-printed constructs were implanted at a wound site made in streptozotocin-induced diabetic rats, it was discovered that both spontaneous healing and improved wound healing compared to a commercial patch were displayed by the constructs. Miguel et al. studied the feasibility of combining electrospinning and 3D printing to build an asymmetric 3D skin construct in an intriguing work (55).

2.2.6 GELATIN

The most common natural polymer is generated by acidic or basic hydrolysis of animal bones or skin. Gelatin is biocompatible, biodegradable, and affordable, and at lower temperatures, it forms a hydrogel. Shi et al. created gelatin-based constructs for skin tissue engineering using the extrusion-free-forming approach (64, 65). The scientists here showed that the physicochemical characteristics of the structures that look a lot like human skin tissue may be fine-tuned using a three-stage crosslinking technique. For skin bioprinting, polyelectrolyte chitosan gelatin hydrogels were created in one study (66). Here, the authors demonstrated strong build gel states, good printability, and effective in vitro cellular responses. Another intriguing study described the utilization of a fibrin-gelatin hybrid hydrogel biopaper in skin bioprinting by Hakam et al. (2016). According to the findings, a composition that contains fibrin gelatin in an identical ratio offers a printable formulation.

2.2.7 SILK FIBROIN

Silk fibroin is a fibrous protein derived from cocoons of the silkworm *Bombyx mori* and a variety of spider species. Humans have always appreciated silk fibroin fibers for their glossy appeal as a fabric. Silk has grown into an advanced fiber and gained importance as a biomedical material as its exceptional mechanical, physical, chemical, and biological properties have been discovered. Sutures, surgical meshes, and other therapeutic applications of silk, as well as a variety of exciting biological applications, have all been thoroughly investigated (67). This exceptional biopolymer is a preferred material due to its affordability and abundance of demonstrated biocompatibility, tunable mechanical properties, and capacity to be processed into films, foams, and fibrous mats, among other things. Recent advancements in biomaterials research and technology have allowed silk fibroin to be used as a bioink in 3D bioprinting. According to studies conducted thus far, using silk as a bioink will improve soft tissue reconstruction's biocompatibility, tissue integration, and cell permeability. Xiong et al. described the utilization of 3D-printed gelatin sulfonated silk composite structures loaded with basic fibroblast growth factor 2 for wound healing applications in the context of skin fabrication (68). A full-thickness skin defect model was used throughout the in vitro and in vivo studies, which indicated that the 3D-printed constructions triggered epidermal development and dermal neovascularization. Admane et al. recently reported employing silk bioinks to directly 3D-bioprint full-thickness skin structures (69).

2.2.8　HYALURONIC ACID

Hyaluronic acid (HA), which is also known as hyaluronan, is a naturally occurring nonsulfated glycosaminoglycan, anionic in epithelial, neural, and connective tissues. Glycosaminoglycans are composed of polysaccharides, which are commonly referred to as unbranched, lengthy sugars or carbohydrates. HA is distinguished from other glycosaminoglycans by the fact that it is nonsulfated and originates in the plasma membrane rather than the Golgi apparatus. Because HA is a component of the ECM found in a variety of cartilage, tissues, and other connective tissues. HA-based biomaterials would be highly sought after (70). Ouyang et al. (71) introduced HA-based bioinks for 3D printing, which displayed good adhesive and mechanical properties. In another study, Poldervaart et al. reported the 3D printing of HA-based hydrogels that displayed high stability after printing with hMSCs (72). It is vital to investigate the various advantages of HA as a bioink.

2.2.9　FIBRIN

Blood contains a protein called fibrin, which aids in blood clotting. By treating thrombin with an enzyme, fibrinogen can be converted into fibrin hydrogel. Although this hydrogel has strong mechanical qualities, it has great biocompatibility and biodegradation properties (73). Fibrin is a tough, nonglobular fibrous protein that plays a role in blood coagulation. Because of its outstanding biocompatibility and biodegradability, fibrin is an appealing material for 3D-bioprinting applications (74). In the first significant instance of 3D fibrin bioprinting, fibrinogen was utilized to stabilize gelatin-based bioinks in 2007 (71, 75). Hinton et al. used a similar extrusion-based 3D printer and operating concept to print a Ca21-mediated alginate/fibrinogen hydrogel into a gelatin slurry bath containing thrombin (72, 76). By altering the amount of fibrinogen in the composite bioinks, it is straightforward to tune fibrinogen's printing characteristics for 3D organ bioprinting (77, 78). The polymerization of fibrinogen-containing composite bioinks and chemical crosslinking improves the stiffness and stability of printed stratified cell-laden 3D structures (79, 80).

2.2.10 ECM Based on Bioinks

The ECM is the composite structure in which cells are present. It is made up of various components, including glycosaminoglycans, elastin, collagen, chondroitin sulfate, and others. Decellularized ECM (dECM) resources are derived from the required tissues, where the ECM is left intact after the cells are sequentially removed (81). To make bioink for 3D printing, the collected ingredients are ground into a powder-like condition, dissolved in a buffer solution, and then used. Other polymeric hydrogels may also be added to the solution to increase the printability of the dECM-based bioinks. Pati et al. improved the printability of dECM bioink created from several tissue types using PCL. They then used it to print cell-based tissue structures in 3D. To avoid cell damage, dissolve the bioink formulation in an acidic buffer and regulate the pH of the solution. Following printing, the investigation demonstrated high construct functionality and cell survival (35). The same team has created a different technique for photo- and covalently crosslinking dECM biomaterials utilizing ultraviolet (UV) light and vitamin B2 as a covalent crosslinker. Cardio-myogenic differentiation and high cell viability were demonstrated by the 3D-printed constructs (82). For the construction of a cardiac patch, Jang et al. (2017) demonstrated 3D printing of dECM containing dual stem cells. The constructs had the potential to quickly vascularize while maintaining cell viability for a prolonged period (83). dECM offers good cell survival and functionality but compared to alternative hydrogel bioink formulations for 3D bioprinting, it is more expensive to isolate and quantify DNA and ECM components from the target tissue.

2.2.11 Cell Aggregates as Bioinks

They are composed of spherical cell aggregates, or spheroids, that were utilized to create 3D-printed things that contain tens of thousands of cells. Spheroids were distributed one at a time into biocompatible scaffolds and allowed to self-assemble before fusing. They also employed computer simulation studies to investigate the construction of structures (84). Without the usage of scaffolds, Yu et al. developed a new tissue spheroid bioink for 3D-bioprinting structures. Tissue fibers measuring up to 8 centimeters were created using fast cell fusion and virtually self-assembly without the need for any toxic chemicals as crosslinkers or support materials. These techniques generated constructions that resembled biological tissue and showed promise for use in the tissue engineering of articular cartilage (85). Another research investigation used a thermosensitive polymer gel as a substrate to form cell sheets or aggregates. The cells used the poly(N-isopropyl acrylamide) as a temporary substrate. Following successful cell growth on the substrate, the cell sheets were gently heated to separate them without altering the cell's matrix configuration. In 3D-bioprinting constructs, the sheets of split cells were utilized as bioinks. Because the ECM was retained, these bioinks performed better than regular cell aggregates. Comparing these findings to the cell viability and other tests conducted in this study, these findings are more encouraging (86).

2.2.12 GELLAN GUM

Water-soluble food component gellan gum (GG) is frequently used as a binding agent, to stabilize, or texturize processed foods. Similar to other gelling agents including xanthan gum, agar-agar, carrageenan, and guar gum, GG is an anionic microbial polysaccharide. Recently, GG has been investigated for application in bioprinting because of its distinct rheological behavior, biodegradability, and bio-compatibility (20). Gellan gum outperforms other hydrogels as a bioink due to its high gelling efficiency, shear thinning behavior, and inexpensive production costs (22, 23). For cartilage bioprinting, Mouser et al. recently created a bioink containing gelatin-methacryloyl and GG (87). To create 3D brain-like structures, Lozano et al. mixed primary neural cells with Arg-Gly-Asp (RGD)-peptide-modified GG (88). These results provide credence to the use of hydrogels based on GG for printing complex and useful 3D cell structures.

In addition, a list of biomaterials employed as bioink for 3D printing has been presented in Table 2.1.

2.3 REQUIREMENTS OF BIOINK FOR 3D PRINTING

When employing 3D bioprinting to create tissue or organ architectures, two different kinds of bioink materials are used. First, a cell-scaffold-based strategy, while the second is a cell-based approach without a scaffold (89). The first technique involves live cells and biomaterial that are mixed to form bioink, which is then printed to construct 3D tissue architectures. The scaffold biomaterial dissolves in this location, while the enclosed living cells proliferate and fill the space, forming predetermined tissue forms. Second, by comparison, directly printed living cells in a manner similar to how an embryo develops. A specific population of living cells forms the new tissues that are then arranged in a specified pattern to eventually produce fused, massively functioning tissue structures (90). Specific biological and biomaterial characteristics must be met by the optimum bioink formulation for a cell-scaffold-based approach. Biomaterials have printability, mechanical properties, biodegradability, surface-modifiable functional groups, and postprint maturation. The biomaterials as bioink used in 3D printing have been discussed in Table 2.1. The essential biological needs are biocompatibility, cytocompatibility cell bioactivity after printing, and economical production costs (56, 57). Considering the bioinks' printability, it is essential to understand the processing capabilities of the bioink formulation so that it should be able to keep the 3D-printed structure intact after being printed. The solution's viscosity, the bioink's surface tension, its ability to self-crosslink, and the surface properties of the printer nozzle are just a few of the aspects that influence the bioink's printing capability. Both live cell encapsulation and printing accuracy are significantly influenced by the viscosity and hydrophilicity of the bioink solution. The pressure needed for extrusion will be higher if the bioink formulation is extremely viscous, as well as the flow of polymer solution through the small nozzle aperture, as with the DIW approach, may be hampered. However, in comparison with formulations of lower viscosity solution, this increased viscosity feature may produce more stable 3D structures. With the use of pressure-aided microfabrication technique in DIW, Tirella et al. (28) investigated the effect of bioink viscosity in 3D printing. To show how viscosity and printing speed are related, they used pressure to produce incredibly stable printed objects. To make it simpler to use the same bioink in different commercially accessible printing equipment, the viscosity of the bioink formulation should also be adjustable. Droplet and inkjet printers require a solution viscosity of 10 mPas., but extrusion-based DIW requires a minimum of 30–6 107 mPas (16, 17, 44). However, a viscosity of 1–300 mPas is needed for laser-assisted printing (15, 17).

In order for extrusion and droplet-based printers to compensate for the high shear stress caused during printing, high-viscosity formulations, such as those used in bioink, must have a special shear thinning feature. The stiffness of the printed structure must sustain both the direct cellular behaviors and the 3D structure. As previously stated, the chosen biomaterial's biodegradation should coincide with that of the target tissue in order for the cells to eventually replace the decaying construct with their own newly formed ECMs as they grow and multiply. Furthermore, when implanted in vivo, the bioink formulation and breakdown end products should not instigate an immunological response in or against the host (91). Bioink materials should enable growth, better cell adhesion, and proliferation within the 3D construct, and it should also be simple to change the functional groups of biomaterials to contain and transport various biological signals or biomolecules (85). In addition to the various parameters discussed here, Gopinathan and Noh Biomaterials Research (2018) described the stiffness of the print substrate, which has a direct impact on cell viability, should also be emphasized (91). Scientists have recently become interested in the possibility of employing greater supramolecular activity polymeric biomaterials as bioinks for 3D-bioprinting applications. Combining these biomaterials may allow for faster printing, easier cell interaction management via surface properties, and more precise mechanical property modification via the use of multiple gradient biomaterials. Pekkanen et al. (2017) conducted a thorough investigation into the synthesis, characterization, and properties of such supramolecular polymeric biomaterials (86). High-resolution printing, viscoelastic properties, in situ gelation, affordability, availability, industrial scalability, mimicking internal tissue structures, mechanical integrity, immunological compatibility when implanted in vivo, a brief maturation period after printing, and the use of a variety of cell types are additional important desirable qualities for a bioink (27). The delivery of nourishment, metabolic wastes, and oxygen gas permeability are further important aspects. The selection of a successful bioink ingredient for 3D bioprinting depends on these essential factors. The critical parameters for selecting a bioink for 3D printing in biomaterial aspects as illustrated in Figure 2.2.

2.4 UTILIZING BIOINK FOR THE 3D PRINTING OF SKIN TISSUE EQUIVALENT

The skin of humans is jointly made up of various kinds of cells and contains an organized framework. It is the biggest organ in the body and is responsible for feeling pain, pressure, and temperature. Normally, the skin consists of three distinct parts:

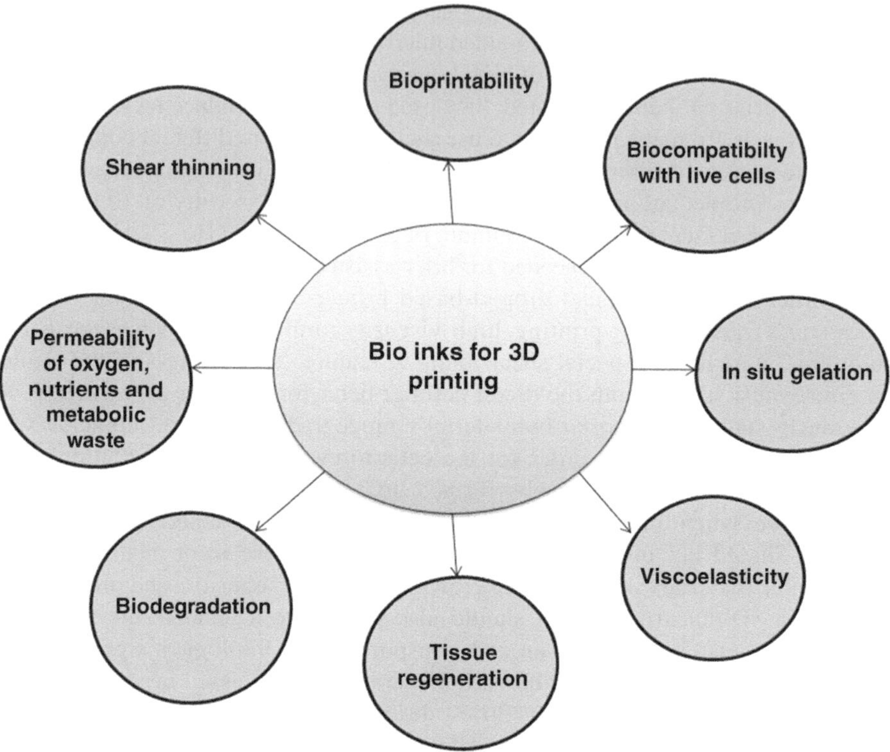

FIGURE 2.2   The schematic highlights essential criteria for bioink selection in biomaterial aspects for 3D printing. It covers factors like biocompatibility, rheological properties, cross-linking mechanisms, and cell interactions; crucial for successful tissue engineering applications, these key characteristics collectively ensure high-quality and accurate 3D prints.

- Epidermis: The outermost component of the skin acts as an impermeable layer and covers the appearance of the skin.
- Dermis: This layer of skin comprises hair follicles, connective tissue, and sweat glands.
- Hypodermis: It is a thicker subcutaneous tissue composed of connective tissue and fat.

In order to produce a skin-like part, 3D bioprinting necessitates the use of numerous kinds of cells in conjunction with particular biomaterials. This technology has the potential to cause pigmentation in the patient (92, 93).

In order to enable cell interaction, bioink offers crucial physical and chemical cues. These characteristics are good for cell growth and assist in carrying out the necessary tasks for a 3D-bioprinted skin. Bioink needs to sustain cells, should be biocompatible, and help functioning cells penetrate the skin. In order to make hydrogels, it needs natural substances like fibrin, collagen, and alginate. To produce a structure resembling skin, bioink uses living human cells that are printed (47, 94).

Biomaterials and cells used to create tissues are present in bioink, which ensures the survivability and usefulness of cells in 3D-printed designs. The bioink must print properly and have the necessary stiffness to maintain the 3D structure; additionally, the selected biomaterial must be biologically compatible. The bioink must have a shear thinning property since printing will cause high shear stress to form. The bio-degradation characteristic of bioink is crucial to take into account since, when cells develop and proliferate, they might add ECM of themselves to supplement the biological degradation component. Normally, biodegradation ought to match the tissue of interest. The host should not experience any immunological reactions as a result of the bioink. Additionally, a variety of biochemical signals or chemicals must be transmitted by the bioink to enhance the adhesion of cells and proliferation within the 3D tissue pattern (85).

In order to create bioink formulations for skin biofabrication, various types of biomaterials, mostly polymer-based are employed. These consist of mixtures with polymers derived from both synthetic and natural sources. Bioderived materials, often known as natural polymers, are materials made from biological sources. All naturally occurring polymers originate from plants, animals, and microbes. Among the natural polymers are starch, cellulose, fibrin, silk fibroin, natural rubber, collagen, chitosan, and others. Synthetic polymers are ones that have been produced artificially or in a laboratory. There are numerous uses for synthetic polymers in daily life. Polyvinyl chloride, polylactide, nylon, polycaprolactone, polyethylene, and so forth are some common examples of synthetic polymers. Compared to natural polymers, synthetic polymer structures may offer ideal conditions enabling the cells to develop, circulate, expand, and divide (51).

2.4.1 Skin Bioprinting Stages

The three stages of skin bioprinting are as follows:

(1) Skin preprinting
(2) Bioprinting
(3) Skin maturation

Skin preprinting stage entails the process of separating cells from a sample of skin, followed by cell division, differentiation, and the creation of bioink, which is composed of living cells and biological material supporting elements. When skin is healthy, primary cells can be separated, multiplied, and employed,but, when skin is wounded, it might be necessary for stem cells to divide into mesenchymal and epidermal cells. There are several ways to generate stem cells:mesenchymal, adipose, and stimulated pluripotent stem cells are among the sources.

In *bioprinting stage,*printed files containing precise information on surfaces for complex 3D models are transformed into stereolithography (STL)-type files, which have print head path parameters (95, 96). Those files can be constructed from clinical pictures utilizing information from CT and MRI scans, or they may be developed with computer-aided drug-design (CCAD) graphical layouts, which provide the accurate surface data required to recreate the intricate 3D model (97, 98). The STL design is divided into layers, and bioprinter tool routes are created by tracing the exterior and internal features of every layer to create the print head paths. The printer's resolution is based on each of these layers' thickness, which normally varies from 100 m to 500 m. The resolution depends on the type of printer being used; lower resolution yields greater quality but requires more time to print. In order to create a 3D tissue from a sequence of 2D layers, the bioprinter sequentially inserts the bioink after processing STL files. To produce high-fidelity bioprints, high-quality picture acquisition is required. Imaging software might be utilized to provide correct anatomical skin geometry, and clinical photos can display the dispersion of cells in vivo.

The *skin maturation* stage is the last step in the bioprinting process. This is important in the context of invitro bioprinting because the skin structures are delicate right after printing and should grow in a laboratory over a couple of days prior to being utilized for implantation. The damaged area of the body grows when the skin is bioprinted in situ (93).

2.5 APPLICATION

The use of 3D printing is expanding quickly across all industrial manufacturing sectors because of its benefits for improving production efficiency and lowering the cost and quantity of faults by preventing human mistakes (99, 100). Patients with a variety of specific conditions can benefit from 3D-bioprinted skin tissues as illustrated in Table 2.2. During surgery, it quickly restores the skin defect. It enables regenerative medicine in a standardized and automated manner. It stabilizes the wound quickly to encourage healing. Humans must have good health in order to function well. Reconstructive surgery and the treatment of burns can both benefit from 3D bioprinting. This affordable, transplantable human skin is made from viable human tissue. It is relevant for the creation of blood vessels and healthy cell activity (119, 120).

The need for skin biofabrication is still increasing due to the growing popularity of cosmetic/aesthetic surgeries, as well as the increased prevalence of obesity, diabetes, and aging populations. Skin bioprints are proposed as an alternate strategy for the following:

- Clinical applications of regenerative medicine include reconstructive surgery after extensive oncological resections, ulcerations, burn injuries, and chronic wounds.
- Modeling physiological and pathological circumstances, including aging, wound recovery, UV response, accessibility of the skin's obstacle, medical reaction, skin cancer, photoirradiation, genodermatoses, and inflammatory illnesses.
- The pharmaceutical and cosmetics industries (effectiveness and safety of active ingredients, drug absorption, metabolization of drugs, and customized treatments).

Additionally, bioprinted skin models could be used as a base for the creation of novel formulations. The use of animal testing in pharmaceutical and cosmetic industries to determine the safety and effectiveness of new formulae forces researchers in the

TABLE 2.2

Applications of 3D Bioprinting for Generating Skin

S.No.	Application Area	Findings	References
1	Functional Skin	• Impressive advancements in 3D bioprinting for human tissue. • It creates human tissue that functions as a biologically multilayered structure and is suitable during transplantation. • Bioprinting offers a cost-effective method for producing a functional layer of skin. • Produce human-like tissue instantly that is reliable after implantation.	(101–103)
2	Skin grafts	• The unpleasant skin transplant procedure can be replaced with this technique. • Capable of manufacturing blood vessels for skin transplants that resemble real living skin. • Minimizes the need for a donor and offers better care for skin grafting. • Utilized to create biological scaffolds that are sized and shaped to precisely suit the demands of the patient.	(104–106)
3	Curing burn wounds	• In actual practice, tissue engineering skin is created to treat burn injuries as a skin substitute. • It improves quality of life by promoting wound healing. • A more effective method of treating severe tissue burns. • A novel technique for efficient wound treatment with full-thickness skin wounds is 3D bioprinting.	(107, 108)
4	3D cell-laden	• Cell-laden hydrogels are developed through bioprinting, opening up new opportunities for cell treatment. • Using the tissue development platform, a range of issues is dealt with using cutting-edge technologies. • Skin made from cell-laden bioink has excellent anti-infection properties.	(109–111)
5	Reconstruction of complex Structure	• Using this technology's creative application, a complex skin graft structure is refabricated for clinical usage. • The design was created from a mixture of hydrogels, cells & collagen to perform the required functions. • Simple complex scaffolds are beneficial for producing complex functional tissues.	(112–114)
6	Reconstruction of nose wing	• With the use of this technology, the 3D complicated structure needed for a particular surgical skill can be restored. • It provides an innovative approach for reconstructing a skin-covered nose wing that can accommodate a full-thickness tissue donor for every individual. • Additionally employed for creating tissue analogs in a regulated manner.	(115, 116)

(Continued)

TABLE 2.2
(Continued)

S.No.	Application Area	Findings	References
7	Better functional responses	• 3D bioprinting is utilized to produce multilayer tissue in burn situations, improving the clinical result. • This is capable of creating tissue for a particular person utilizing information from injured individuals who were scanned with a variety of technologies. • Printed skin customized for each patient is capable of performing vital functions. • It facilitates the growth of tissue and organs by depositing living cells composed of bioink.	(114, 117, 118)

fields of cosmetology, pharmacy, and medicine to look for new solutions (121). In addition, Table 2.2. presents applications of 3D bioprinting for generating skin.

2.6 CURRENT CHALLENGES

An innovative feature of cell tissue technology known as 3D bioprinting has made it possible to create biomimicry on a scale never before possible. This biomimicry may eventually displace autografts, which are currently the gold standard. The study of pathology, drug screening, and regenerative medicine all benefit greatly from the form and function of biomimicry. Applications in vitro provide a high-throughput methodology that has been used to assess implant incorporation as well as clinical and toxicological situations. Animal testing for drugs and materials could be replaced with biomimetic microfluidic chips.

The needs for the bioink vary depending on the bioprinting technique, which might have a variety of implications for the cells that are being encapsulated. Inkjet bioprinting offers precise cell placement and excellent resolution. The bioink must be present in the smallest possible concentration, even though this could result in weak structural strength and insufficient cell entrapment. Skin and brain cells have been produced using this technology with great efficacy.

Extrusion-based printing provides the best practicable technique for vertical layout even if it has the least recorded cell lifespans among the other techniques. The shear tension that develops while printing is what causes the low survival. Extrusion printing's impact on the hydrogel both during and after printing is a crucial component. The hydrogel may lose its structural integrity as a result of the strong shear forces created during printing. Due to this, self-healing hydrogels were created, which, when subjected to shear, restore their mechanical integrity.

2.7 CONCLUSION AND FUTURE PERSPECTIVE

The recent development of 3D bioprinting as a form of biological engineering method offers hope for the abolition of organ shortage around the world. This technique is being used more frequently in a number of uses, including the creation of supports for tissue growth, customized medication treatment, and implants meant specifically for each patient. The technique remains in its beginning stages, however, had a tremendous potential to revolutionize applications in tissue engineering with further developments, even though the fast growth of software for 3D modeling allows for accurate geometric design of constructions and the creation of sophisticated bioprinters.

The ability to alter the form and behavior of the stimulus is constrained in the case of bioprinting. In the future, it will be enhanced by 4D-bioprinting technology that will produce naturally healthy tissue. Although 4D printing is still a relatively young sector, much effort is being put into it. However, it is quite difficult to accurately regulate the product transformation. In the future, mathematical modeling may be used to more accurately forecast how printed objects would behave in order to get around these restrictions. Future advancements in bioprinting technology will benefit people by enabling them to use them in healthcare settings.

ACKNOWLEDGMENTS

The authors express their sincere gratitude to the host institutions for generously providing all the necessary facilities throughout this study.

FUNDING

None.

CONFLICT OF INTEREST

None.

REFERENCES

1. Kordestani SS. *Atlas of Wound Healing: A Tissue Regeneration Approach.* Elsevier.2019;1–180.
2. Rowan MP, Cancio LC, Elster EA, Burmeister DM, Rose LF, Natesan S, et al.Burn wound healing and treatment: review and advancements. *Crit Care*. 2015 Jun 12 [cited 2023 Sep 14];19(1). Available from: https://pubmed.ncbi.nlm.nih.gov/26067660/
3. Auger FA, Lacroix D, Germain L. Skin substitutes and wound healing. *Skin Pharmacol Physiol*. 2009;22(2):94–102.
4. Shpichka A, Butnaru D, Bezrukov EA, Sukhanov RB, Atala A, Burdukovskii V, et al. Skin tissue regeneration for burn injury. *Stem Cell Res Ther*. 2019 Mar 15 [cited 2023 Sep 14];10(1):1–16. Available from: https://stemcellres.biomedcentral.com/articles/10.1186/s13287-019-1203-3
5. O'Brien FJ. Biomaterials & scaffolds for tissue engineering. *Mater Today*. 2011 [cited 2023 Sep 14];14(3):88–95. Available from: https://www.researchgate.net/publication/257555026_Biomaterials_scaffolds_for_tissue_engineering
6. Karppinen SM, Heljasvaara R, Gullberg D, Tasanen K, Pihlajaniemi T. Toward understanding scarless skin wound healing and pathological scarring [version 1; peer review: 2 approved]. *F1000Research*. 2019 [cited 2023 Sep 14];8. Available from: https://pubmed.ncbi.nlm.nih.gov/31231509/

7. Nerem RM, Sambanis A. Tissue engineering: from biology to biological substitutes. *Tissue Eng.*1995 Mar 1 [cited 2023 Sep 14];1(1):3–13. Available from: https://pubmed.ncbi.nlm.nih.gov/19877911/

8. Rivron NC, Rouwkema J, Truckenmüller R, Karperien M, De Boer J, Van Blitterswijk CA. Tissue assembly and organization: Developmental mechanisms in microfabricated tissues. *Biomaterials.* 2009 Oct 1;30(28):4851–8.

9. Elbert DL. Bottom-up tissue engineering. *Curr Opin Biotechnol.* 2011 Oct [cited 2023 Sep 14];22(5):674–80. Available from: https://pubmed.ncbi.nlm.nih.gov/21524904/

10. Mironov V, Kasyanov V, Markwald RR. Organ printing: From bioprinter to organ biofabrication line. *Curr Opin Biotechnol.* 2011 Oct 1;22(5):667–73.

11. Whyte DJ, Rajkhowa R, Allardyce B, Kouzani AZ. A review on the challenges of 3D printing of organic powders. *Bioprinting.*2019 Dec 1 [cited 2023 Sep 14];16. Available from: https://www.researchgate.net/publication/334413131_A_review_on_the_challenges_of_3D_printing_of_organic_powders

12. Koch L, Kuhn S, Sorg H, Gruene M, Schlie S, Gaebel R, et al. Laser printing of skin cells and human stem cells. *Tissue Eng Part C Methods.* 2010 Oct 1 [cited 2023 Sep 14];16(5):847–54. Available from: https://pubmed.ncbi.nlm.nih.gov/19883209/

13. Fayyazbakhsh F, Leu MC. sciencedirect sciencedirect sciencedirect a brief review on 3D bioprinted skin substitutes a brief review on 3D bioprinted skin substitutes. *Procedia Manuf.* 2020;48:790–6. Available from: https://doi.org/10.1016/j.promfg.2020.05.115

14. Gauthaman A, Krishnan A, Anju MS, Thomas LV, Kasoju N, Bhatt A. Chapter 8. Three-dimensional bioprinting of skin tissue equivalents using natural polymers as bioinks for potential applications in wound repair. *Natural Polymers in Wound Healing and Repair.* INC; 2022. 187–206 p. Available from: http://doi.org/10.1016/B978-0-323-90514-5.00013-4

15. Guillotin B, Souquet A, Catros S, Duocastella M, Pippenger B, Bellance S, et al. Laser assisted bioprinting of engineered tissue with high cell density and microscale organization. *Biomaterials.* 2010 Oct [cited 2023 Sep 15];31(28):7250–6. Available from: https://pubmed.ncbi.nlm.nih.gov/20580082/

16. Ozbolat IT, Peng W, Ozbolat V. Application areas of 3D bioprinting. *Drug Discov Today.* 2016 Aug 1 [cited 2023 Sep 15];21(8):1257–71. Available from: https://pubmed.ncbi.nlm.nih.gov/27086009/

17. Hölzl K, Lin S, Tytgat L, Van Vlierberghe S, Gu L, Ovsianikov A. Bioink properties before, during and after 3D bioprinting. *Biofabrication.* 2016 Sep 23 [cited 2023 Sep 15];8(3). Available from: https://pubmed.ncbi.nlm.nih.gov/27658612/

18. Yan WC, Davoodi P, Vijayavenkataraman S, Tian Y, Ng WC, Fuh JYH, et al. 3D bioprinting of skin tissue: From pre-processing to final product evaluation. *Adv Drug Deliv Rev.* 2018 Jul 1 [cited 2023 Sep 15];132:270–95. Available from: https://pubmed.ncbi.nlm.nih.gov/30055210/

19. Liu P, Shen H, Zhi Y, Si J, Shi J, Guo L, et al. 3D bioprinting and in vitro study of bilayered membranous construct with human cells-laden alginate/gelatin composite hydrogels. *Colloids Surf B Biointerfaces.* 2019 Sep 1 [cited 2023 Sep 15];181:1026–34. Available from: https://pubmed.ncbi.nlm.nih.gov/31382330/

20. Säljö K, Orrhult LS, Apelgren P, Markstedt K, Kölby L, Gatenholm P. Successful engraftment, vascularization, and In vivo survival of 3D-bioprinted human lipoaspirate-derived adipose tissue. *Bioprinting.* 2020 Mar 1;17:e00065.

21. Kreimendahl F, Köpf M, Thiebes AL, Duarte Campos DF, Blaeser A, Schmitz-Rode T, et al. Three-Dimensional Printing and Angiogenesis: Tailored Agarose-Type I Collagen Blends Comprise Three-Dimensional Printability and Angiogenesis Potential for Tissue-Engineered Substitutes. *Tissue Eng Part C Methods.* 2017 Oct 1 [cited 2023 Sep 15];23(10):604–15. Available from: https://pubmed.ncbi.nlm.nih.gov/28826357/

22. López-Marcial GR, Zeng AY, Osuna C, Dennis J, García JM, O'Connell GD. Agarose-Based Hydrogels as Suitable Bioprinting Materials for Tissue Engineering. *ACS Biomater Sci Eng*. 2018 Oct 8 [cited 2023 Sep 25];4(10):3610–6. Available from: https://pubs.acs.org/doi/abs/10.1021/acsbiomaterials.8b00903

23. Kim JE, Kim SH, Jung Y. Current status of three-dimensional printing inks for soft tissue regeneration. *Tissue Eng Regen Med*. 2016 Dec 1 [cited 2023 Sep 25];13(6):636–46. Available from: https://link.springer.com/article/10.1007/s13770-016-0125-8

24. Zhou D, Chen J, Liu B, Zhang X, Li X, Xu T. Bioinks for jet-based bioprinting. *Bioprinting*. 2019 Dec 1;16:e00060.

25. Xu T, Gregory CA, Molnar P, Cui X, Jalota S, Bhaduri SB, et al. Viability and electrophysiology of neural cell structures generated by the inkjet printing method. *Biomaterials*. 2006 Jul 1;27(19):3580–8.

26. de Melo BAG, Jodat YA, Cruz EM, Benincasa JC, Shin SR, Porcionatto MA. Strategies to use fibrinogen as bioink for 3D bioprinting fibrin-based soft and hard tissues. *Acta Biomater*. 2020 Nov 1;117:60–76.

27. Duan B, Hockaday LA, Kang KH, Butcher JT. 3D Bioprinting of heterogeneous aortic valve conduits with alginate/gelatin hydrogels. *J Biomed Mater Res Part A*. 2013 May 1 [cited 2023 Sep 25];101A(5):1255–64. Available from: https://onlinelibrary.wiley.com/doi/full/10.1002/jbm.a.34420

28. Liu P, Shen H, Zhi Y, Si J, Shi J, Guo L, et al. 3D bioprinting and in vitro study of bilayered membranous construct with human cells-laden alginate/gelatin composite hydrogels. *Colloids Surfaces B Biointerfaces*. 2019 Sep 1;181:1026–34.

29. Zheng Z, Wu J, Liu M, Wang H, Li C, Rodriguez MJ, et al. 3D Bioprinting of Self-Standing Silk-Based Bioink. *Adv Healthc Mater*. 2018 Mar 1 [cited 2023 Sep 25];7(6):1701026. Available from: https://onlinelibrary.wiley.com/doi/full/10.1002/adhm.201701026

30. Miguel SP, Cabral CSD, Moreira AF, Correia IJ. Production and characterization of a novel asymmetric 3D printed construct aimed for skin tissue regeneration. *Colloids Surfaces B Biointerfaces*. 2019 Sep 1;181:994–1003.

31. Law N, Doney B, Glover H, Qin Y, Aman ZM, Sercombe TB, et al. Characterisation of hyaluronic acid methylcellulose hydrogels for 3D bioprinting. *J Mech Behav Biomed Mater*. 2018 Jan 1;77:389–99.

32. Seol YJ, Lee H, Copus JS, Kang HW, Cho DW, Atala A, et al. 3D bioprinted biomask for facial skin reconstruction. *Bioprinting*. 2018 Jun 1;10:e00028.

33. Intini C, Elviri L, Cabral J, Mros S, Bergonzi C, Bianchera A, et al. 3D-printed chitosan-based scaffolds: An in vitro study of human skin cell growth and an in-vivo wound healing evaluation in experimental diabetes in rats. *Carbohydr Polym*. 2018 Nov 1 [cited 2023 Sep 15];199:593–602. Available from: https://pubmed.ncbi.nlm.nih.gov/30143167/

34. Hafezi F, Scoutaris N, Douroumis D, Boateng J. 3D printed chitosan dressing crosslinked with genipin for potential healing of chronic wounds. *Int J Pharm*. 2019 Apr 5;560:406–15.

35. Pati F, Jang J, Ha DH, Won Kim S, Rhie JW, Shim JH, et al. Printing three-dimensional tissue analogues with decellularized extracellular matrix bioink. *Nat Commun*. 2014 Jun 2 [cited 2023 Sep 17];5. Available from: https://pubmed.ncbi.nlm.nih.gov/24887553/

36. Jang J, Park HJ, Kim SW, Kim H, Park JY, Na SJ, et al. 3D printed complex tissue construct using stem cell-laden decellularized extracellular matrix bioinks for cardiac repair. *Biomaterials*. 2017 Jan 1 [cited 2023 Sep 17];112:264–74. Available from: https://pubmed.ncbi.nlm.nih.gov/27770630/

37. Gao Q, He Y, Fu JZ, Liu A, Ma L. Coaxial nozzle-assisted 3D bioprinting with built-in microchannels for nutrients delivery. *Biomaterials*. 2015 Aug 1;61:203–15.

38. Xin S, Chimene D, Garza JE, Gaharwar AK, Alge DL. Clickable PEG hydrogel microspheres as building blocks for 3D bioprinting. *Biomater Sci.* 2019 Feb 26 [cited 2023 Sep 25];7(3):1179–87. Available from: https://pubs.rsc.org/en/content/articlehtml/2019/bm/c8bm01286e

39. Nowicki M, Zhu W, Sarkar K, Rao R, Zhang LG. 3D printing multiphasic osteochondral tissue constructs with nano to micro features via PCL based bioink. *Bioprinting.* 2020 Mar 1;17:e00066.

40. Izgordu MS, Uzgur EI, Ulag S, Sahin A, Karademir Yilmaz B, Kilic B, et al. Investigation of 3D-Printed Polycaprolactone-/Polyvinylpyrrolidone-Based Constructs. *Cartilage.* 2021 Dec 1 [cited 2023 Sep 25];13(2_suppl):626S–635S. Available from: https://journals.sagepub.com/doi/full/10.1177/1947603519897302

41. Xiong JY, Narayanan J, Liu XY, Chong TK, Chen SB, Chung TS. Topology evolution and gelation mechanism of agarose gel. *J Phys Chem B.* 2005 Mar 31 [cited 2023 Sep 15];109(12):5638–43. Available from: https://pubmed.ncbi.nlm.nih.gov/16851608/

42. Fedorovich NE, De Wijn JR, Verbout AJ, Alblas J, Dhert WJA. Three-dimensional fiber deposition of cell-laden, viable, patterned constructs for bone tissue printing. *Tissue Eng Part A.* 2008 Jan 1 [cited 2023 Sep 15];14(1):127–33. Available from: https://pubmed.ncbi.nlm.nih.gov/18333811/

43. Daly AC, Critchley SE, Rencsok EM, Kelly DJ. A comparison of different bioinks for 3D bioprinting of fibrocartilage and hyaline cartilage. *Biofabrication.* 2016 Oct 7 [cited 2023 Sep 15];8(4). Available from: https://pubmed.ncbi.nlm.nih.gov/27716628/

44. Gudapati H, Dey M, Ozbolat I. A comprehensive review on droplet-based bioprinting: Past, present and future. *Biomaterials.* 2016 Sep 1 [cited 2023 Sep 15];102:20–42. Available from: https://pubmed.ncbi.nlm.nih.gov/27318933/

45. Moradali MF, Ghods S, Rehm BHA. Alginate biosynthesis and biotechnological production. *Springer Ser Biomater Sci Eng.* 2018 [cited 2023 Sep 15];11:1–25. Available from: https://link.springer.com/chapter/10.1007/978-981-10-6910-9_1

46. Axpe E, Oyen ML. Applications of Alginate-Based Bioinks in 3D Bioprinting. *Int J Mol Sci.* 2016 Dec 1 [cited 2023 Sep 15];17(12). Available from: https://pubmed.ncbi.nlm.nih.gov/27898010/

47. Noh I, Kim N, Tran HN, Lee J, Lee C. 3D printable hyaluronic acid-based hydrogel for its potential application as a bioink in tissue engineering. *Biomater Res.* 2019 Feb 6;23(1).

48. Jia W, Gungor-Ozkerim PS, Zhang YS, Yue K, Zhu K, Liu W, et al. Direct 3D bioprinting of perfusable vascular constructs using a blend bioink. *Biomaterials.* 2016 Nov 1 [cited 2023 Sep 15];106:58–68. Available from: https://pubmed.ncbi.nlm.nih.gov/27552316/

49. Shim JH, Lee JS, Kim JY, Cho DW. Bioprinting of a mechanically enhanced three-dimensional dual cell-laden construct for osteochondral tissue engineering using a multi-head tissue/organ building system. *JMiMi.* 2012 Aug [cited 2023 Sep 15];22(8):085014. Available from: https://ui.adsabs.harvard.edu/abs/2012JMiMi.22h5014S/abstract

50. Jang CH, Ahn SH, Yang GH, Kim GH. A MSCs-laden polycaprolactone/collagen scaffold for bone tissue regeneration. *RSC Adv.* 2016;6(8):6259–65.

51. Rodriguez-Pascual F, Slatter DA. Collagen cross-linking: insights on the evolution of metazoan extracellular matrix. *Sci Reports* 2016 61. 2016 Nov 23 [cited 2023 Sep 15];6(1):1–7. Available from: https://www.nature.com/articles/srep37374

52. Torres-Rendon JG, Köpf M, Gehlen D, Blaeser A, Fischer H, De Laporte L, et al. Cellulose nanofibril hydrogel tubes as sacrificial templates for freestanding tubular cell constructs. *Biomacromolecules.* 2016 Mar 14 [cited 2023 Sep 15];17(3):905–13. Available from: https://pubmed.ncbi.nlm.nih.gov/26812393/

53. Kirk KA, Othman A, Andreescu S. Nanomaterial-functionalized cellulose: Design, characterization and analytical applications. *Anal Sci.* 2018 [cited 2023 Sep 16];34(1):19–31. Available from: https://pubmed.ncbi.nlm.nih.gov/29321453/

54. Ferreira AM, Gentile P, Chiono V, Ciardelli G. Collagen for bone tissue regeneration. *Acta Biomater.* 2012 [cited 2023 Sep 15];8(9):3191–200. Available from: https://pubmed.ncbi.nlm.nih.gov/22705634/

55. van Uden S, Silva-Correia J, Oliveira JM, Reis RL. Current strategies for treatment of intervertebral disc degeneration: substitution and regeneration possibilities. *Biomater Res.* 2017 Oct 23 [cited 2023 Sep 15];21(1). Available from: https://pubmed.ncbi.nlm.nih.gov/29085662/

56. Wollensak G. Crosslinking treatment of progressive keratoconus: New hope. *Curr Opin Ophthalmol.* 2006 Aug [cited 2023 Sep 15];17(4):356–60. Available from: https://pubmed.ncbi.nlm.nih.gov/16900027/

57. Mrochen M. Current status of accelerated corneal cross-linking. *Indian J Ophthalmol.* 2013 Aug [cited 2023 Sep 15];61(8):428. Available from: https://journals.lww.com/ijo/pages/default.aspx/article.asp?issn=0301-4738;year=2013;volume=61;issue=8;spage=428;epage=429;aulast=Mrochen

58. Mori H, Shimizu K, Hara M. Dynamic viscoelastic properties of collagen gels with high mechanical strength. *Mater Sci Eng C Mater Biol Appl.* 2013 Aug 1 [cited 2023 Sep 15];33(6):3230–6. Available from: https://pubmed.ncbi.nlm.nih.gov/23706205/

59. Smith CM, Stone AL, Parkhill RL, Stewart RL, Simpkins MW, Kachurin AM, et al. Three-dimensional bioassembly tool for generating viable tissue-engineered constructs. *Tissue Eng.* 2004 Sep [cited 2023 Sep 15];10(9–10):1566–76. Available from: https://pubmed.ncbi.nlm.nih.gov/15588416/

60. Yang X, Lu Z, Wu H, Li W, Zheng L, Zhao J. Collagen-alginate as bioink for three-dimensional (3D) cell printing based cartilage tissue engineering. *Mater Sci Eng C Mater Biol Appl.* 2018 Feb 1 [cited 2023 Sep 15];83:195–201. Available from: https://pubmed.ncbi.nlm.nih.gov/29208279/

61. Roehm KD, Madihally SV. Bioprinted chitosan-gelatin thermosensitive hydrogels using an inexpensive 3D printer. *Biofabrication.* 2017 Jan 1 [cited 2023 Sep 15];10(1). Available from: https://pubmed.ncbi.nlm.nih.gov/29083312/

62. Dai T, Tanaka M, Huang YY, Hamblin MR. Chitosan preparations for wounds and burns: antimicrobial and wound-healing effects. *Expert Rev Anti Infect Ther.* 2011 Jul [cited 2023 Sep 15];9(7):857. Available from: /pmc/articles/PMC3188448/

63. Li S, Tian X, Fan J, Tong H, Ao Q, Wang X. Chitosans for tissue repair and organ three-dimensional (3D) bioprinting. *Micromachines.* 2019 Nov 1 [cited 2023 Sep 15];10(11). Available from: /pmc/articles/PMC6915415/

64. Shi L, Xiong L, Hu Y, Li W, Chen ZC, Liu K, et al. Three-dimensional printing alginate/gelatin scaffolds as dermal substitutes for skin tissue engineering. *Polym Eng Sci.* 2018 Oct 1;58(10):1782–90.

65. Shi Y, Xing TL, Zhang HB, Yin RX, Yang SM, Wei J, et al. Tyrosinase-doped bioink for 3D bioprinting of living skin constructs. *Biomed Mater.* 2018 Mar 6 [cited 2023 Sep 17];13(3). Available from: https://pubmed.ncbi.nlm.nih.gov/29307874/

66. Ng WL, Yeong WY, Naing MW. Development of Polyelectrolyte Chitosan-gelatin Hydrogels for Skin Bioprinting. *Procedia CIRP.* 2016 Jan 1;49:105–12.

67. Floren M, Bonani W, Dharmarajan A, Motta A, Migliaresi C, Tan W. Human mesenchymal stem cells cultured on silk hydrogels with variable stiffness and growth factor differentiate into mature smooth muscle cell phenotype. *Acta Biomater.* 2016 Feb 1 [cited 2023 Sep 15];31:156–66. Available from: https://pubmed.ncbi.nlm.nih.gov/26621695/

68. Xiong S, Zhang X, Lu P, Wu Y, Wang Q, Sun H, et al. A Gelatin-sulfonated Silk Composite Scaffold based on 3D Printing Technology Enhances Skin Regeneration by Stimulating Epidermal Growth and Dermal Neovascularization. *Sci Rep.* 2017 Dec 1 [cited 2023 Sep 15];7(1). Available from: https://pubmed.ncbi.nlm.nih.gov/28655891/

69. Admane P, Gupta AC, Jois P, Roy S, Lakshmanan C, Kalsi G, et al. Direct 3D bioprinted full-thickness skin constructs recapitulate regulatory signaling pathways and physiology of human skin. *Bioprinting.* 2019 [cited 2023 Sep 15];15:e00051. Available from: https://doi.org/10.1016/j.bprint.2019.e00051

70. Yoo HS, Lee EA, Yoon JJ, Park TG. Hyaluronic acid modified biodegradable scaffolds for cartilage tissue engineering. *Biomaterials.* 2005 May 1;26(14):1925–33.

71. Xu W, Wang X, Yan Y, Zheng W, Xiong Z, Lin F, et al.Rapid prototyping three-dimensional cell/gelatin/fibrinogen constructs for medical regeneration. *J Bioact Compat Polym.* 2007 Jul [cited 2023 Sep 15];22(4):363–77. Available from: https://www.researchgate.net/publication/239262799_Rapid_Prototyping_Three-Dimensional_CellGelatinFibrinogen_Constructs_for_Medical_Regeneration

72. Grigoryan B, Paulsen SJ, Corbett DC, Sazer DW, Fortin CL, Zaita AJ, et al. Multivascular networks and functional intravascular topologies within biocompatible hydrogels. *Science* (80-). 2019 May 3 [cited 2023 Sep 15];364(6439):458–64. Available from: https://www.science.org/doi/10.1126/science.aav9750

73. Cui X, Boland T. Human microvasculature fabrication using thermal inkjet printing technology. *Biomaterials.* 2009 Oct;30(31):6221–7.

74. Mosesson MW. Fibrinogen and fibrin structure and functions. *J Thromb Haemost.* 2005 Aug 1;3(8):1894–904.

75. Liu F, Liu C, Chen Q, Ao Q, Tian X, Fan J, et al.Progress in organ 3D bioprinting. *Int J Bioprinting.* 2018 [cited 2023 Sep 15];4(1). Available from: /pmc/articles/PMC7582006/

76. Noor N, Shapira A, Edri R, Gal I, Wertheim L, Dvir T. 3D printing of personalized thick and perfusable cardiac patches and hearts. *Adv Sci.* 2019 Jun 1 [cited 2023 Sep 15];6(11):1900344. Available from: https://onlinelibrary.wiley.com/doi/full/10.1002/advs.201900344

77. Wang X. Advanced polymers for three-dimensional (3D) organ bioprinting. *Micromachines.* 2019 Dec 1 [cited 2023 Sep 15];10(12). Available from: https://pubmed.ncbi.nlm.nih.gov/31775349/

78. Wang X. Intelligent Freeform manufacturing of complex organs. *Artif Organs.* 2012 Nov 1 [cited 2023 Sep 15];36(11):951–61. Available from: https://onlinelibrary.wiley.com/doi/full/10.1111/j.1525-1594.2012.01499.x

79. Yao R, Zhang R, Yan Y, Wang X. In vitro angiogenesis of 3D tissue engineered adipose tissue. 2009 Jan 1 [cited 2023 Sep 15];24(1):5–24. http://doi.org/101177/0883911508099367. Available from: https://journals.sagepub.com/doi/abs/10.1177/0883911508099367

80. Xu M, Wang X, Yan Y, Yao R, Ge Y. An cell-assembly derived physiological 3D model of the metabolic syndrome, based on adipose-derived stromal cells and a gelatin/alginate/fibrinogen matrix. *Biomaterials.* 2010 May [cited 2023 Sep 15];31(14):3868–77. Available from: https://pubmed.ncbi.nlm.nih.gov/20153520/

81. Jung JP, Bhuiyan DB, Ogle BM. Solid organ fabrication: comparison of decellularization to 3D bioprinting. *Biomater Res* 2016 201. 2016 Aug 31 [cited 2023 Sep 17];20(1):1–11. Available from: https://biomaterialsres.biomedcentral.com/articles/10.1186/s40824-016-0074-2

82. Ahn G, Min KH, Kim C, Lee JS, Kang D, Won JY, et al. Precise stacking of decellularized extracellular matrix based 3D cell-laden constructs by a 3D cell printing system equipped with heating modules. *Sci Rep.* 2017 Dec 1 [cited 2023 Sep 17];7(1). Available from: https://pubmed.ncbi.nlm.nih.gov/28819137/

83. Jang J, Kim TG, Kim BS, Kim SW, Kwon SM, Cho DW. Tailoring mechanical properties of decellularized extracellular matrix bioink by vitamin B2-induced photo-crosslinking. *Acta Biomater.* 2016 Mar 15 [cited 2023 Sep 17];33:88–95. Available from: https://pubmed.ncbi.nlm.nih.gov/26774760/

84. Zhou Y. The application of ultrasound in 3D bio-printing. *Molecules.* 2016 May 1;21(5).

85. Chen C, Bang S, Cho Y, Lee S, Lee I, Zhang SM, et al. Research trends in biomimetic medical materials for tissue engineering: 3D bioprinting, surface modification, nano/micro-technology and clinical aspects in tissue engineering of cartilage and bone. *Biomater Res.* 2016 May 4 [cited 2023 Sep 17];20(1):1–7. Available from: https://biomaterialsres.biomedcentral.com/articles/10.1186/s40824-016-0057-3

86. Pekkanen AM, Mondschein RJ, Williams CB, Long TE. 3D Printing Polymers with Supramolecular Functionality for Biological Applications. *Biomacromolecules.* 2017 Sep 11 [cited 2023 Sep 17];18(9):2669–87. Available from: https://pubmed.ncbi.nlm.nih.gov/28762718/

87. Mouser VHM, Melchels FPW, Visser J, Dhert WJA, Gawlitta D, Malda J. Yield stress determines bioprintability of hydrogels based on gelatin-methacryloyl and gellan gum for cartilage bioprinting. *Biofabrication.* 2016 Jul 18 [cited 2023 Sep 15];8(3). Available from: https://pubmed.ncbi.nlm.nih.gov/27431733/

88. Lozano R, Stevens L, Thompson BC, Gilmore KJ, Gorkin R, Stewart EM, et al. 3D printing of layered brain-like structures using peptide modified gellan gum substrates. *Biomaterials.* 2015 Oct 1 [cited 2023 Sep 15];67:264–73. Available from: https://pubmed.ncbi.nlm.nih.gov/26231917/

89. Kaushik SN, Kim B, Cruz Walma AM, Choi SC, Wu H, Mao JJ, et al. Biomimetic microenvironments for regenerative endodontics. *Biomater Res.* 2016 [cited 2023 Sep 17];20(1). Available from: /pmc/articles/PMC4890532/

90. Hospodiuk M, Dey M, Sosnoski D, Ozbolat IT. The bioink: A comprehensive review on bioprintable materials. *Biotechnol Adv.* 2017 Mar 1;35(2):217–39.

91. Tirella A, Orsini A, Vozzi G, Ahluwalia A. A phase diagram for microfabrication of geometrically controlled hydrogel scaffolds. *Biofabrication.* 2009 [cited 2023 Sep 17];1(4). Available from: https://pubmed.ncbi.nlm.nih.gov/20811111/

92. Skardal A, Mack D, Kapetanovic E, Atala A, Jackson JD, Yoo J, et al. Bioprinted Amniotic Fluid-Derived Stem Cells Accelerate Healing of Large Skin Wounds. *Stem Cells Transl Med.* 2012 Nov 1 [cited 2023 Sep 25];1(11):792–802. Available from: https://doi.org/10.5966/sctm.2012-0088

93. Varkey M, Visscher DO, Van Zuijlen PPM, Atala A, Yoo JJ. Skin bioprinting: the future of burn wound reconstruction? *Burn Trauma.* 2019 [cited 2023 Sep 25];7. Available from: https://pubmed.ncbi.nlm.nih.gov/30805375/

94. Athirasala A, Tahayeri A, Thrivikraman G, Franca CM, Monteiro N, Tran V, et al. A dentin-derived hydrogel bioink for 3D bioprinting of cell laden scaffolds for regenerative dentistry. *Biofabrication.* 2018 Jan 10 [cited 2023 Sep 25];10(2):024101. Available from: https://iopscience.iop.org/article/10.1088/1758-5090/aa9b4e

95. Mironov V, Visconti RP, Kasyanov V, Forgacs G, Drake CJ, Markwald RR. Organ printing: Tissue spheroids as building blocks. *Biomaterials.* 2009 Apr 1;30(12):2164–74.

96. Mondy WL, Cameron D, Timmermans JP, De Clerck N, Sasov A, Casteleyn C, et al. Computer-aided design of microvasculature systems for use in vascular scaffold production. *Biofabrication.* 2009 Sep 4 [cited 2023 Sep 26];1(3):035002. Available from: https://iopscience.iop.org/article/10.1088/1758-5082/1/3/035002

97. Arai K, Iwanaga S, Toda H, Genci C, Nishiyama Y, Nakamura M. Three-dimensional inkjet biofabrication based on designed images. *Biofabrication.* 2011 Sep 7 [cited 2023 Sep 26];3(3):034113. Available from: https://iopscience.iop.org/article/10.1088/1758-5082/3/3/034113

98. Keriquel V, Guillemot F, Arnault I, Guillotin B, Miraux S, Amédée J, et al. In vivo bio-printing for computer- and robotic-assisted medical intervention: preliminary study in mice. *Biofabrication*. 2010 Mar 10 [cited 2023 Sep 26];2(1):014101. Available from: https://iopscience.iop.org/article/10.1088/1758-5082/2/1/014101

99. Beg S, Almalki WH, Malik A, Farhan M, Aatif M, Rahman Z, et al. 3D printing for drug delivery and biomedical applications. *Drug Discov Today*. 2020 Sep 1;25(9):1668–81.

100. Palo M, Holländer J, Suominen J, Yliruusi J, Sandler N. 3D printed drug delivery devices: perspectives and technical challenges. *Expert Rev Med Devices*. 2017 Sep 2 [cited 2023 Sep 26];14(9):685–96. Available from: https://www.tandfonline.com/doi/abs/10.1080/17434440.2017.1363647

101. Cubo N, Garcia M, Del Cañizo JF, Velasco D, Jorcano JL. 3D bioprinting of functional human skin: production and in vivo analysis. *Biofabrication*. 2016 Dec 5 [cited 2023 Sep 26];9(1):015006. Available from: https://iopscience.iop.org/article/10.1088/175 8-5090/9/1/015006

102. Nordli HR, Chinga-Carrasco G, Rokstad AM, Pukstad B. Producing ultrapure wood cellulose nanofibrils and evaluating the cytotoxicity using human skin cells. *Carbohydr Polym*. 2016 Oct 5;150:65–73.

103. Kérourédan O, Ribot E, Fricain JC, Devillard R, Miraux S. Magnetic Resonance Imaging for tracking cellular patterns obtained by Laser-Assisted Bioprinting. *Sci Reports*. 2018 Oct 25 [cited 2023 Sep 26];8(1):1–10. Available from: https://www.nature.com/articles/s41598-018-34226-9

104. Biedermann T, Boettcher-Haberzeth S, Reichmann E. Tissue engineering of skin for wound coverage. *Eur J Pediatr Surg*. 2013 [cited 2023 Sep 26];23(5):375–82. Available from: http://www.thieme-connect.com/products/ejournals/html/10.1055/s-0033-1352529

105. Kucińska-Lipka J, Gubanska I, Janik H. Bacterial cellulose in the field of wound healing and regenerative medicine of skin: recent trends and future prospectives. *Polym Bull*. 2015 Sep 19 [cited 2023 Sep 26];72(9):2399–419. Available from: https://link.springer.com/article/10.1007/s00289-015-1407-3

106. Ghidini T. Regenerative medicine and 3D bioprinting for human space exploration and planet colonisation. *J Thorac Dis*. 2018 Jul 1 [cited 2023 Sep 26];10(Suppl 20):S2363. Available from: /pmc/articles/PMC6081368/

107. Cui H, Nowicki M, Fisher JP, Zhang LG. 3D Bioprinting for Organ Regeneration. *Adv Healthc Mater*. 2017 Jan 1 [cited 2023 Sep 26];6(1):1601118. Available from: https://onlinelibrary.wiley.com/doi/full/10.1002/adhm.201601118

108. Ma X, Yu C, Wang P, Xu W, Wan X, Lai CSE, et al. Rapid 3D bioprinting of decellular-ized extracellular matrix with regionally varied mechanical properties and biomimetic microarchitecture. *Biomaterials*. 2018 Dec 1;185:310–21.

109. Wu Z, Su X, Xu Y, Kong B, Sun W, Mi S. Bioprinting three-dimensional cell-laden tissue constructs with controllable degradation. *Sci Reports* 2016 61. 2016 Apr 19 [cited 2023 Sep 26];6(1):1–10. Available from: https://www.nature.com/articles/srep24474

110. Zhang HB, Xing TL, Yin RX, Shi Y, Yang SM, Zhang WJ. Three-dimensional bioprinting is not only about cell-laden structures. *Chinese J Traumatol - English Ed*. 2016 Aug 1;19(4):187–92.

111. Ong CS, Fukunishi T, Zhang H, Huang CY, Nashed A, Blazeski A, et al. Biomaterial-free three-dimensional bioprinting of cardiac tissue using human induced pluripotent stem cell derived cardiomyocytes. *Sci Reports* 2017 71. 2017 Jul 4 [cited 2023 Sep 26];7(1):1–11. Available from: https://www.nature.com/articles/s41598-017-05018-4

112. Hakkarainen T, Koivuniemi R, Kosonen M, Escobedo-Lucea C, Sanz-Garcia A, Vuola J, et al. Nanofibrillar cellulose wound dressing in skin graft donor site treatment. *J Control Release*. 2016 Dec 28;244:292–301.

113. Leberfinger AN, Ravnic DJ, Dhawan A, Ozbolat IT. Concise Review: Bioprinting of Stem Cells for Transplantable Tissue Fabrication. *Stem Cells Transl Med.* 2017 Oct 1 [cited 2023 Sep 26];6(10):1940–8. Available from: https://doi.org/10.1002/sctm.17-0148

114. Satpathy A, Datta P, Wu Y, Ayan B, Bayram E, Ozbolat IT. Developments with 3D bioprinting for novel drug discovery. *Expert Opin Drug Discov.* 2018 Dec 2 [cited 2023 Sep 26];13(12):1115–29. Available from: https://www.tandfonline.com/doi/abs/10.1080/17460441.2018.1542427

115. Kačarević ŽP, Rider PM, Alkildani S, Retnasingh S, Smeets R, Jung O, et al. An introduction to 3D bioprinting: Possibilities, challenges and future aspects. *Materials* 2018 Nov 6 [cited 2023 Sep 26];11(11):2199. Available from: https://www.mdpi.com/1996-1944/11/11/2199/htm

116. Sasmal P, Datta P, Wu Y, Ozbolat IT. 3D bioprinting for modelling vasculature. *Microphysiological Syst.* 2018 [cited 2023 Sep 26];2:1. Available from: /pmc/articles/PMC6436836/

117. Hsieh FY, Hsu SH. 3D bioprinting: A new insight into the therapeutic strategy of neural tissue regeneration. *Organogenesis* 2015 Jan 1 [cited 2023 Sep 26];11(4):153–8. Available from: https://www.tandfonline.com/doi/abs/10.1080/15476278.2015.1123360

118. Laternser S, Keller H, Leupin O, Rausch M, Graf-Hausner U, Rimann M. A novel microplate 3D bioprinting platform for the engineering of muscle and tendon tissues. *SLAS Technol.* 2018 Dec 1 [cited 2023 Sep 26];23(6):599–613. Available from: https://journals.sagepub.com/doi/full/10.1177/2472630318776594

119. Lee V, Singh G, Trasatti JP, Bjornsson C, Xu X, Tran TN, et al. Design and Fabrication of Human Skin by Three-Dimensional Bioprinting. https://home.liebertpub.com/tec. 2013 Dec 31 [cited 2023 Sep 26];20(6):473–84. Available from: https://www.liebertpub.com/doi/10.1089/ten.tec.2013.0335

120. Liu F, Chen Q, Liu C, Ao Q, Tian X, Fan J, et al. Natural Polymers for Organ 3D Bioprinting. *Polym.* 2018 Nov 16 [cited 2023 Sep 26];10(11):1278. Available from: https://www.mdpi.com/2073-4360/10/11/1278/htm

121. Smandri A, Nordin A, Hwei NM, Chin KY, Abd Aziz I, Fauzi MB. Natural 3D-Printed Bioinks for Skin Regeneration and Wound Healing: A Systematic Review. *Polym.* 2020 Aug 10 [cited 2023 Sep 26];12(8):1782. Available from: https://www.mdpi.com/2073-4360/12/8/1782/htm

3 Biomedical Application of 3D Printing

Harish Bhardwaj and Rajendra Kumar Jangde
Pt. Ravishankar Shukla University, Raipur, India

3.1 INTRODUCTION

There is a growing popularity of three-dimensional (3D) printing nowadays throughout the world. The application of 3D printing in the healthcare and pharmaceutical industries is growing in the biomedical sector (1). Additive manufacturing (AM) is another term for 3D printing, the first 3D-printing technique was introduced in the 1980s by Charles Hull. *AM* refers to a group of innovative technologies in 3D-printing physical objects that can be created using this technique. The use of 3D bioprinting, a modern technology that combines 3D printing with biology and computer-aided design (CAD) data can be used directly. A series of cross-sectional AM biomaterials are used to build it layer-by-layer on the substrate (2). It is compatible with biomaterials when inserted into the stomach; as a result, for the dispensing of tissues, automated dispensing systems are used. As 3D-bioprinting technology develops, the focus will be on the finished product, and the choice of biomaterials test dental applications need to use certain drugs for an extended period of high mechanical strength and biodegradability. A 3D-bioprinting method has the potential to solve a wide range of problems, including regenerative medicine, drug delivery, and biomedical applications of 3D printing, as illustrated in (Figure 3.1 and Table 3.1). Several studies have been conducted on the wide variety of 3D-bioprinting methods that are available, including inkjet bioprinting and 3D tissue printing (3). The most recent technology that produces revolutionary innovations and solves complex medical issues is additive manufacturing. Several promising results have been observed in regenerative medicine, implants, organ transplants, artificial tissue, and diagnosis (4). Due to advances in regenerative medicine and tissue engineering, it is now possible to regenerate damaged organs and tissues using 3D bioprinting. In 3D printing, bioink is the primary component and is essential for fabricating functional organs and tissues. In 3D printing, many essential characteristics must be taken into consideration when choosing bioinks (5).

A 3D printer is then used to construct the model layer by layer after it is cut horizontally into layers of photos; the thickness of a single layer of the construct depends on the method of 3D printing. Printed items must be superimposed layer by layer. Due to the technology's advantages in terms of economy and the environment, its capacity to produce intricate structures, and its suitability for large-scale industrial production, there is a lot of potential for 3D printing in biomedical fields (6). Biological macromolecular structures of the human body are replaced or

DOI: 10.1201/9781032690926-3

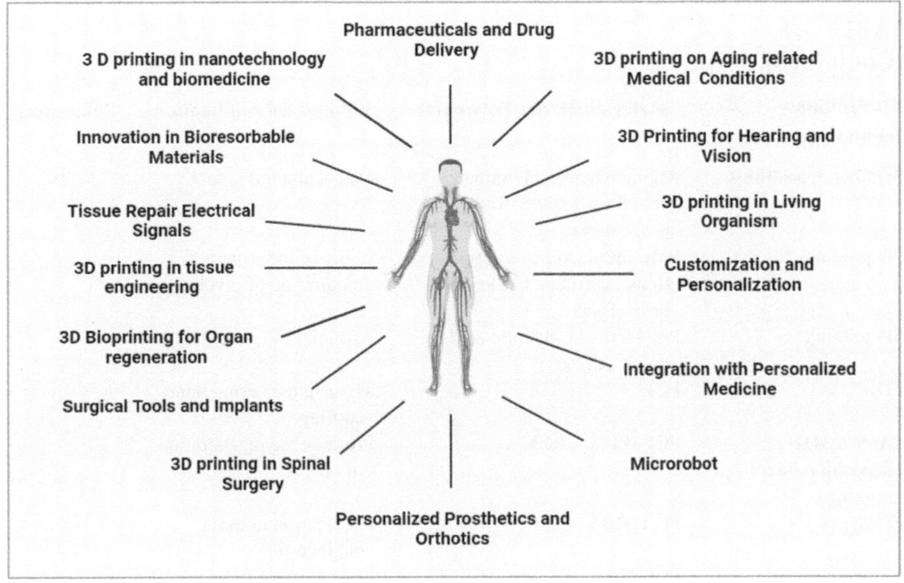

FIGURE 3.1 Biomedical application of 3D printing.

TABLE 3.1
Summary of Biomedical Application of 3D Printing

3D Printing Technology	Materials (Drug/Polymers)	Biomedical Application	References
Direct writing	Benzophenone/ polylactide/ Fe_3O_4	Cardiovascular Implants	(54)
Stereolithography laser sinter	PCL/HA Methacrylate polycaprolactone	Tracheal stent	
Fused deposition modeling (FDM)	Thermoplastic copolyester elastomer	Valve stent	
Photolithography	PLA-B-PEG-PLA/PIPAAm	Heart failure treatment	
Two-photon polymerization	Methacrylate, microrobot, gelatin	Drug delivery	
Microfluidic coaxial extrusion	Alginate glycerin hydrogel	Skin dressing	
Lasser matching screen printing	Sodium alginate, acrylamide, agarose	Patch	
FDM	Hyaluronic acid, polylactide	Orthopedic Implant	(37)
Plasma polymerization	Chitosan	Orthopedic Implant surface modification	
Stereolithography	Epoxide acrylate, soybean oil	Biomedical scaffolds	
Photolithography	PPF/Pnipam -AAc	Drug delivery	
Photopolymerization	PEG-diacrylate	Sensor	
Customized stereolithography (SLA)	Acrylate/graphene soyabean oil	Nerve Graft	

(*Continued*)

**TABLE 3.1
(Continued)**

3D Printing Technology	Materials (Drug/Polymers)	Biomedical Application	References
3D fiber depositions	Alginate hydrogel, human chondrocyte, and osteogenic progenitors	Osteochondral defect	(20)
3D printing	Polycaprolactone, adipose tissue, cartilage tissue, and heart tissue	Enhance the structural maturation of myoblast	
3D printing	Polylactic co-glycolic acid, polyurethane	Artificial blood vessels	
FDM	PCL	Tissue engineering bone cartilage	
Layer-by-layer deposition direct soaking	PCL, PDA, dECM	Promote the regeneration of nerve	
FDM	PLA, ABS	Application in tissue engineering	
Extrusion based	PCL/HA	Enhancement of bioactivity	
SLA	Diacrylate, riboflavin, ibuprofen, polyethylene,	Hydrogel	(17)
UV inkjet 3D-printed	Ropinirole, ethylene glycol diacrylate	Tablet	
FDM	Deflazacort, poly caprolactone	Nanocapsules	
3D-printed	Poly (lactide-co-glycolide), polycaprolactone 5-fluorouracil	Biodegradable patch	
SLA	Cold atmospheric plasma (CAD), PEGDA	Proliferation	(55)
FDM	TGF-β +PDA, SDF-1α, PCL	Improve biological performance	
3D bioploting	PLGA–copper-loaded ZIF-8 nanoparticles	Kill bacteria	
Binder jetting	Sand metal powder	Degradable metallic implant	(20)
Metal extrusion (FDM)	Hydrogel thermoplastic ceramics bioinks	Development of soft tissue, tissue, and organ culture	
Sheet laminations	Paper ceramics metal	Anatomical model	
Material jetting/inkjet	Photopolymers bioinks	Metallic implants, dental orthopedic and craniofacial, degradable rigid implants	
Binder jet printing	Mannitol polyvinyl pyrrolidone, colloidal silicon dioxide, paracetamol, and alizarin dye	Fast-dissolving drug delivery device	(18)
Pressure-assisted microsyringe (PAM)	Levetiracetam, polyvinyl pyrrolidone, vinyl acetate co-polymers	Controlled-release drug delivery	
SLA	Lidocaine hydrochloride, elastic resin	Site-specific drug delivery	
Direct powder extrusion	Tramadol, hydroxypropyl cellulose, polyethylene oxide	Modified release	

(*Continued*)

TABLE 3.1
(Continued)

3D Printing Technology	Materials (Drug/Polymers)	Biomedical Application	References
FDM	Blender filament polymers	Engineering customized products, medical aerospace	(56)
FDM	Carbohydrate particles, PLA	Bone regeneration	
FDM	Carbon fibers, polyether ether ketones	Orthopedic and dental applications	
Extrusion	Gliadin and PCL, mesoporus bioglass fibers	Tissue engineering	
Extrusion	Laponite, N -isopropyl acrylamide	Stimuli-responsive electrical device	
Digital light processing	Laponite XLG, 2-hydroxy ethyl methacrylate	Peripheral nerve repair	
Direct powder extrusion	Itraconazole, hydroxypropylecelulose	Modified release	(4)

regenerated using medical implants developed by humans. Implants made from a person's cells, which are produced from natural components extracted from other sections of the same body, were the first type of implants to be used for the treatment, but they are rather infrequently used because the field of spine prostheses is still in the development stages. The more popular method for treating spinal degeneration is arthroplasty, in which the intervertebral height must be preserved during these treatments. Biosynthesis and regeneration of bone tissue using cellular calcium hydroxyapatite (CHAp) and carbon nanotubes. As an application of biomaterial for medicinal purposes, column implants using CHAp have only begun to be used recently. The potential for biomedical uses, as well as biocompatibility, biologically derived cellular CHAp macromolecules, and their use biological cells of CHAp, has been shown for a number of implants, in contrast to synthetic CHAp. In the human body, sodium and potassium are naturally substituted by apatite because of their structure and biochemical macromolecules, and natural CHAps are comparable based on their chemical composition (7). A wide variety of tissues and organs can be reproduced using 3D bioprinting, including skin, blood vessels, hearts, and many more. As well as serving as an initial component for organ replacement, these tissues and organs can also serve as *in vitro* models for drug screening and pharmacokinetics, and various bioprinting techniques have been developed to address the complexity of organs (2).

Three-dimensional printing with biomedicine is a paradigm change in the health care system, which promises a patient-centered and individualized solution. By utilizing the capabilities of 3D printing, complexly designed structures and medical devices can be produced that are useful for human tissues. Scalability, biocompatibility, and regulatory structures are still problems, however. This book chapter discussed the present research and the potential for 3D printing to be applied to biomedical applications.

3.2   THE PRODUCTION OF NANOMATERIALS FOR USE IN VARIOUS BIOMEDICAL SECTORS

The use of nanomaterials in biomedical sectors has accelerated significantly over the past few decades; the incorporation of nanomaterials into 3D printing, such as polymer matrix 3D printing and composite biomaterial 3D printing, has been recognized as a beneficial strategy. Nanomaterials have been added to 3D-printed scaffolds for therapy and disease prevention; this combined strategy has various advantages. By combining 3D printing and nanomaterials, digital models can be directly created from digital data by using the science of gradually producing technology, which is the basis of 3D printing and is experiencing rapid growth and development in the pharmaceutical, health care, and medical research sectors. It was first mentioned in the early 2000s that dental implants and custom prosthetics may be made using 3D-printing technology. A large number of biomedical applications are now made possible because of 3D printing, and this technology has completely changed the medical industry. The manufacturing of surgical devices is heavily dependent on 3D printing. Furthermore, 3D printing may be utilized to create surgical models for prospective surgeons that offer a sharper picture of intricate anatomy, and this has substantial educational benefits for medical teaching and training. In addition to designing tailored prosthetics and developing pharmaceuticals, 3D printing is also employed in preclinical research for pacemaker implants and other medical devices. Three-dimensional printing is able to easily incorporate nanomaterials. A variety of nanomaterials are used in 3D printing, including metal nanoparticles, metal–oxide nanoparticles, metal–organic frameworks (MOFs), and upconversion nanoparticles.

3.2.1   Nanomaterial Based on Metal

Metal nanoparticles (MeNPs; such as gold, silver, copper), and metal–oxide nanoparticles (MONPs), metal–sulfide nanomaterials (MeSNs), liquid metal (LM) materials, MOFs, and composite nanoparticles (CNPs) have all been successfully incorporated into 3D-printing techniques to fabricate composite materials. The excellent conductivity, oxidation resistance, and chemical stability of gold and silver make them suitable nanoparticles for use in electronics and photonics. Nano-silver paste was used for electrode applications in a successful electric-field-driven microscale 3D-printing experiment. Due to the mechanical requirements of hard tissue, metals are expanding in the biomedical area, thus, there is a need for support, and prompt patient mobilization can be satisfied by the introduction of metal. Currently used clinical implants are made of metals, such as cobalt–chromium alloys, stainless steel, titanium alloys, or nitinol. MeNPs with distinct mechanical properties have been carefully explored in conjunction with 3D-printing methods in recent years. In order to create multifunctional hybrid materials for tumor therapy, antibacterial effect, tissue regeneration, and medical imaging, MeNPs, such as gold, silver, and copper nanoparticles are generally used in 3D printing techniques.

3.2.1.1 MONPs

In addition to pure metal nanoparticles, MONPs have also been noted as a significant improvement for 3D printing in the field of biomedicine. Particularly, the distinctive magnetic characteristics of iron-oxide nanoparticles (Fe_3O4 and g-Fe_2O_3) are of great interest in the diagnosis of diseases and the development of therapies.

3.2.1.2 MeSNs

MeSN nanoparticles have excellent photothermal conversion efficiency and near-infrared (NIR) absorption, which stimulates its application in cancer photothermal therapy and photoacoustic imaging.

3.2.1.3 LM

In distinction to hard-metal nanomaterials, LM materials derived from gallium (Ga) and its alloys, such as EGaIn (a eutectic alloy of Ga and indium) or Galinstan (a eutectic alloy of Ga, indium, and tin), have a fluidic nature.

3.2.1.4 MOFs

MOFs are an entirely novel type of networked mixture of nanomaterials made of functional organic linkers and metal ions/clusters. MOFs are interesting for drug delivery, bioimaging, biosensing, biocatalysis, and antibacterial applications due to their high porosity, stability, tunability, and advanced bio-related features.

3.2.1.5 CNPs

Scientists are extremely interested in CNPs, which are made up of two or more components. This is because they have more advanced characteristics and multifunctional properties than single-metal nanoparticles. These characteristics allow CNPs to have combined or noticeably distinct electrical, chemical, physical, and mechanical properties from materials that are a single component (8).

3.2.2 POLYMERS

The advantages of using polymers in 3D printing include their affordability, elasticity, lightweight, flexibility, and affordability. Among them are polycaprolactones and polylactones. There are many bioinert and biodegradable printing materials available that have been Food Drug Administration (FDA)–certified for biological applications, making them a popular choice for biomedical applications. The most common material used in extrusion-based printing is polylactic acid (PLA), which is low cost, biocompatible, and processable and has a slow degradation rate. A well-established biodegradable and compostable polyester, PLA, has rapidly developed into a commodity material over the past few decades due to its simple structure, cheap cost, and simplicity of 3D cell culture and activity evaluation. Understanding the PLA characteristics is essential to achieving appropriate chemical and biological qualities, which is necessary to give effective therapy for the biomedical application sector. Polymeric and nonpolymeric components can be mixed together to form copolymers. The degradation of PLA and its copolymers *in vivo* is usually more gradual without creating an infection or an inflammatory reaction. The characteristics of PLA include its thermal properties, solubility and miscibility, degradation, and crystallization behavior. Factors that can improve the properties of PLA and its copolymers, composites, and mixes in order to make them a better fit for use in various applications throughout the world (8).

3.2.3   BIOMEDICAL APPLICATIONS OF 3D-PRINTED SHAPE MEMORY POLYMERS

Biomedical applications for 3D-printed shape memory polymers (SMPs) with complicated architectures include occlusion devices, tracheal stents, cardiac stents, vascular stents, and bone scaffolds.

3.2.3.1   Cell Scaffolds

Currently, there are no effective treatments or clinically effective approaches for treating human body tissue loss, and tissue engineering has great promise for developing effective treatments. For scaffold-based bone engineering to succeed, a high-performing scaffold is crucial, and one of the main goals is to create scaffolds for bone tissue engineering that are desirable in shape and structural, physical, chemical, and biological ways for improved biological performance and bone tissue regeneration. Customized scaffolds are a highly desirable outcome of 3D printing for bone tissue development. The construction of organs or tissues often begins with cells. Significant advancements have been made in the study and creation of cell scaffolds in just a few decades utilizing basic materials like castor oil and soybean oil, several researchers have used 3D-printed cell scaffolds in clinical settings (9).

3.2.3.2   Vascular Stents

Coronary artery disease is characterized by narrowing or obstruction of coronary arteries. More than 7.2 million people worldwide die each year from this disease that affects the main blood vessels in the heart. The biomedical field has found many uses for 3D-printing technology, including the creation of medical devices, high-tech visualization, diagnosis planning, and surgical simulation. Three-dimensional printing is expected to transform the production of implantable bioresorbable drug-eluting scaffolds (stents). Bioresorbable scaffolds can be customized for individual needs in order to eliminate late thrombosis, enhance artery growth, and eliminate many other problems associated with stenting. Stents can be customized using 3D printing thanks to its rapid prototyping capabilities and efficiency. A stenotic or blocked blood vessel can be supported by an intravascular stent, usually composed of stainless-steel wire and Nitinol. Biodegradable and low-biotoxic SMP/biomaterials can be used in vascular stents. Stents for intravascular use can handle a variety of challenging issues. As a result, this technology is becoming more and more common in therapeutic settings (10).

3.2.3.3   Bone Scaffolds

An enormous number of patients require urgent care every year due to injuries sustained in car accidents, injuries sustained in traumas, burns, and congenital anomalies. The development of regenerative medicine was triggered in part by the shortage of donors, graft rejection, and other issues that prevented patients from having access to organs and tissues for replacement, repair, and regeneration. Although stem cell therapy cannot fill major tissue defects on its own, it is a vital component of regenerative medicine. Researchers combine stem cells with 3D-printed scaffolds to engineer bone tissue. The creation of biodegradable bone scaffolds has long been the main goal of tissue engineering. The biomaterials meet the performance requirements for implanted bone and offer mild healing conditions (9).

3.2.3.4 Tracheal Stents

A medical device called a tracheal stent is used to treat tracheal stenosis or tracheal damage. Non-degradable tracheal stents are used in a majority of clinical instances. Degradable tracheal stents have been researched as biodegradable materials, and their research and development have progressed. The tracheobronchial tree can be printed in three dimensions. The adult human trachea measures 10–13 cm, has 16–20 cm c-shaped cartilage anteriorly, and is membranous posteriorly; there are 1.5 and 4–4.5 cm of length between the right and left mainstem bronchi, respectively. Approximately 16–20 mm, 10–12 mm, and 8–12 mm are the internal diameters of the trachea and right and left mainstem bronchi, respectively, with a diameter of 9–18 mm, a length of 20–110 mm, and a thickness of 1–1.5 mm. Conventional mold injection techniques are used to create these stents. Customization is feasible, but because new molds must be made for every change in the design, producing these molds takes a lot of effort and money. There is a chance for using 3D printing to manufacture airway stents in this situation (11).

3.2.3.5 Cardiac Stents

A 3D-printed coronary artery model was used in cardiovascular computed tomography angiography research for the first time to demonstrate the potential of using 3D-printed coronary artery models for coronary stenting. To lessen the necessity for invasive angiography for surveillance, a variety of stent diameters should be implanted in future research. Cardiac stents have been increasingly popular in recent years as an effective treatment for arteriosclerosis. By combining fusion depositing modeling (FDM) with medical technology, Cabrera et al. created a stent that can be used during heart valve remodeling surgery, a minimally invasive procedure can be used to place the stent in the heart (12).

3.2.3.6 Occlusion Devices

Congenital heart disease is commonly associated with atrial septal defects (ASD), and treatment for structural heart disease with an implantable occluder is beneficial. The cardiac occluder, which seals the site of the heart defect, is a self-expanding double-umbrella structure. Lin et al. used composite PLA/Fe_3O_4 filaments to 4D-print the shape memory occludes with double-disc shapes (13).

3.2.4 Ceramics/Composites

Traditional methods to produce ceramics include injection molding, gel casting, and tape casting. To achieve densification, green pieces must be sintered at high temperatures. These traditional techniques have lengthy processing periods and expensive overheads. The need for molds in these processes to manufacture complicated geometries makes it challenging to create structures at the micro/nano level. The three types of feedstocks used for ceramic printing are slurry, powder, clay, and bulk solids. SiO_2, Al_2O_3, ZrO_2, and SiC are a few examples of ceramics utilized in additive manufacturing (AM). Zirconia (ZrO_2) is widely used in therapeutic applications, including bone and dental implants, because of its mechanical properties and resistance to fracture. Because of its poor cell affinity for bone regeneration and tissue binding and because of its shrinkage during heat treatment, ZrO_2 has limited clinical applications. Clinical applications require a balance between the mechanical qualities and cellular affinity to identify an acceptable ZrO_2–SiO_2 composite formula for ceramic 3D-printing techniques (14).

3.2.5 STIMULUS AND RESPONSIVE MATERIALS FOR BIOMEDICAL APPLICATIONS

There is a high demand for smart-responsive materials enabling the establishment of next-generation precision medicine in scientific fields, such as tissue regeneration, drug delivery, and diagnostics, that are responsive to outside stimuli, biological signals, or pathological abnormalities. The search for intelligent materials with novel features has also been fueled by global competition among multinational corporations. Cell-like structures for targeted medication delivery and tissue engineering two layers of lipid droplets (1,2-diphytanoyl sn-glycero-3-phosphocholine) with varying osmolarities spontaneously self-folded into a picoliter aqueous flower-shaped network and a hollow spherical are used (15).

3.3 APPLICATION OF 3D PRINTING IN THE MEDICAL FIELD

Researchers are developing permanent non-bioactive implants that are personalized, creating local bioactive scaffolds that are biodegradable, fabricating pathological organ models to aid in preoperative planning, printing tissues and organs with full-life functions directly and many other projects. These applications have made significant scientific progress, although they are still a long way from being widely adopted in medicine due to fundamental technical and scientific issues.

3.3.1 PREOPERATIVE PLANNING AND INTERVENTION ANALYSIS WITH ORGAN MODELS

Models of physical organs with high fidelity are essential in clinical therapy and medical education. Traditional manufacturing techniques, like casting or forging, waste a lot of time creating expensive tooling and never take into account patient individuality. Permanent implants, not the biological permanent medical implants that are frequently used in orthopedics and dentistry, need to be created from non-degradable biomaterial and provide strong biocompatibility following surgery. It is possible to fabricate complex implants in real time with great dimensional accuracy and rapid production cycles with 3D printing as opposed to creating implants using traditional machining techniques. Biodegradable and locally relevant scaffold tissues and organs can be produced in two ways if cells are directly influenced during development (16).

3.4   3D-PRINTING APPROACH IN DRUG DELIVERY SYSTEM

The term *drug delivery* concerns methods, applications, and tools, including formulations that securely deliver therapeutic compounds into the body as needed to provide their desired therapeutic effects. Targeted-release medication delivery methods have become increasingly popular over time, replacing immediate-release oral dose forms. To enhance product efficacy and safety, as well as to boost patient compliance, it quickly became clear that the release profile of the drug needed to be adjusted for its absorption, distribution, metabolization, and elimination. Pharmaceutical formulation development is dedicating increasing attention to 3D printing as a viable solution to several issues with traditional pharmaceutical unit operations. For example, the standard production process of milling, mixing, granulating, and compression can produce finished products with varying levels of drug loading, release, stability, and pharmaceutical dosage forms. In the pharmaceutical industry, 3D printing is becoming more popular as a means of creating patient-specific medication delivery systems that follow regulated dosages. Individual genetic variations in treatment responses drive the demand for personalized drug delivery systems. Thus, by customizing the drug or system, mass-produced pharmaceuticals can be reduced in adverse effects (17).

3.4.1   MULTIDRUG DELIVERY

Combinational drug delivery is possible by 3D printing, which makes it possible to multiply drugs into a single dosage form. Three-dimensional printing has the potential to change healthcare and enhance patient outcomes. Due to its potential benefits over customizing medications in individually regulated doses, 3D-printing technologies are already being used increasingly in drug delivery systems. With the help of 3D printing, drugs and excipients can be deposited precisely, potentially changing how drugs are designed, produced, and used. It can cover everything from the preclinical turn of events and clinical preliminary care to frontline medical treatment, including the medication improvement measure. Although 3D-printing technology offers therapeutic and economic benefits, its use in pharmaceutical goods is constrained by various technical and administrative issues (18).

3.4.2   PERSONALIZED DRUG DELIVERY

As a versatile 3D-printing technique, 3D printing has also gained popularity. It is a 3D-printing technique that is incredibly affordable and is employed by many different academic fields. Due to its flexible manufacturing capabilities, which allow for the manufacture of pharmaceutical items in virtually any shape, 3D printing has a significant potential to become the primary manufacturing method for pharmaceutical devices, in particular customized medicines and implants. When applied in pharmaceutics, offers the capacity to create dosage forms with complicated shapes, which might affect how a medicine releases its active ingredient. It works wonders at increasing the bioavailability and solubility of medications with low solubility and at muffling the harsh taste of active pharmaceutical ingredients (APIs). The use of 3D printing in the manufacturing of pharmaceuticals has several benefits, including design flexibility, cost-effectiveness, and excellent reproducibility (19).

3.4.3 TRANSDERMAL DELIVERY

Transdermal drug delivery uses the skin's circulation as a network of distribution for the gradual release of a variety of medications. Compared to medication delivery procedures that include ingesting, injecting, or inserting, this approach is noninvasive. Patches and microneedle arrays are the two most used transdermal medication delivery systems today. Patches act as a reservoir for medications that are passively released into deeper layer capillaries by continuously supplying a drug to the epidermis's upper layers. Microneedle arrays are made up of a patch with tiny, needle-like protrusions that pierce the epidermis. The danger of infection or other consequences associated with more intrusive equipment, such as a hypodermic needle, is decreased since the medicine can penetrate the skin more effectively without compromising its integrity. By enabling the creation of patches with complicated structures or patches carrying multiple medications at varied rates of release from the same patch, AM can be advantageous in the patch production process (20).

3.4.4 NASAL CAST IN NOSE-TO-BRAIN DELIVERY DEVELOPMENT

When medications are targeted at the central nervous system (CNS), instrument nose-to-brain administration has numerous advantages, including low latency, bypassing the blood–brain barrier, enhanced CNS bioavailability, noninvasiveness, less adverse effects, and avoidance of systemic toxicity. For severe brain pathologies, such as brain tumors, and neural degenerative disorders, such as Parkinson's disease (PD) and Alzheimer's disease (AD), it is an intriguing method of drug administration. The medicine must first enter the olfactory zone at the top of the nasal cavities, where it must then diffuse toward the brain through the nasal mucosa and olfactory neurons. This method of drug delivery calls for a considerable portion of the dose to be consistently deposited into the olfactory zone, which necessitates professional formulation expertise and a grasp of the intricate geometry of cavities. Nasal casts, often referred to as 3D-printed nasal cavities, are a useful technique for bridging and testing the formulation, nasal administration method, and the medication's travel to the nasal cavities to provide critical information regarding the effectiveness of a nasal drug product (21, 22).

3.4.5 THE STRUCTURE OF THE VASCULAR SYSTEM

To determine the resolution and biological characteristics of blood vessels, bioink, which consists of cells, nutrition, and growth factors, is used (23). The use of stents, surgical bypass transplantation, angioplasty, tissue-engineered vascular grafts, and nonbiodegradable conduits are now used as treatments for vascular regeneration.

Vascular regeneration can be achieved using endothelial cells, smooth muscle cells, stem cells, bioactive substances, biomaterials, and cell aggregates or spheroids as well as relevant cell aggregates. Building new vessels involves the use of vascular scaffolds, decellularizing vessels, and creating self-assembling vascular grafts, as well as using vessel reactors and introducing culture additives for vessel maturation. In recent years, vascular grafts have become increasingly popular a specific shape and function cannot be achieved through autologous implantation or allograft transplantation (24).

3.4.6 Vaccine Delivery

Three-dimensional-printing technology is rapidly becoming an effective strategy in vaccine development and delivery, including directly producing therapeutic drug and RNA vaccines. It can be predicted that there are great potential and commercial market prospects for 3D printing in vaccine delivery and exploration. In the area of cancer immunotherapy, there has been a lot of interest in the cancer vaccine platform. Here, immunoregulator-loaded 3D-printed scaffolds are created for improved cancer immunotherapy. The mass production of cancer vaccinations and customized designs are made possible by the accurate molding and rapid production processes enabled by 3D printing.

3.5 3D PRINTING APPLICATIONS IN AGING-RELATED MEDICAL CONDITIONS

3.5.1 The Nervous System

Neurodevelopmental disorder will replace cancer as the second-most lethal human disease by 2040, according to the World Health Organization. The development of therapeutically applicable treatments for various CNS illnesses has made little advancement. Comorbidities in older adults, the blood–brain barrier, and brain complexity are some of the difficulties that contribute to low success rates. Small and significant molecules are being delivered across the brain using a variety of invasive and noninvasive techniques. Because they provide benefits, including sustained and tailored delivery, patient compliance, and reduced side effects, biodegradable, implanted drug delivery devices have attracted a lot of attention. With the use of various materials and printing techniques, mechanically complex implants, forms, or release profiles can be created using the revolutionary additive manufacturing technique known as 3D printing.

3.5.2 AD

Globally, 75 million individuals are expected to have dementia by 2030, per the most recent data from the Alzheimer's Association International. AD is characterized by extracellular amyloid accumulation in the brain and intracellular protein hyperphosphorylation, which leads to intracellular fiber formation. AD is primarily characterized by cognitive dysfunction and memory impairment. As a result of inadequately controlled or aberrant protein aggregates, AD is usually caused by cytotoxic accumulation. Of all cases of neurodegenerative disease, 62% are caused by AD. In AD, the buildup of amyloid (A) plaques is a major cause of neurodegeneration that leads to necrosis and apoptosis of neurons. There is an increased expression and activity of beta- and gamma-secretase in AD patients, which regulates its generation another pathway linked to the pathophysiology of AD includes improper phosphorylation (25).

3.5.3 PD

The second most prevalent neurodegenerative condition after AD is PD. Resting tremors, motor bradykinesia, rigidity, and other symptoms of PD are caused by the inability to modulate motor movements. Among neurodegenerative disorders, Parkinson's disease is the most prevalent due to reduced dopamine levels in the basal ganglia. As a dopamine precursor, levodopa is capable of transporting medications. Levodopa-loaded scaffolds made of PLA and chitosan (CS) can be used to treat PD (26).

3.5.4 Amyotrophic Lateral Sclerosis

Amyotrophic lateral sclerosis (ALS), a rare neurological disease that affects both upper and lower motor neurons, is characterized by the progressive degradation of motor neurons in the brain and spinal cord ALS. The disease is a neurological condition that results in death within two to four years. Noninvasive ventilation (NIV) is a highly effective method for the treatment of ALS that can increase quality of life while also extending life by more than a year. Despite this effectiveness, patient adherence to NIV is subpar, which may be related to mask fit. By reducing mask leaks, lowering needed delivery pressures, and enhancing adherence to therapy, it was hypothesized that an improved mask fit made possible by facial scanning, and a 3D-printed interface might increase usage (27).

3.5.5 Osteoporosis

This degenerative bone disease affects middle-aged and elderly people frequently and is ranked among the top three geriatric diseases in the world. A patient has osteoporosis (OP) if their bone mineral density (BMD) T-score, which is used as a screening tool, is less than 2.5 standard deviations, and they have decreased BMD, bone strength, and bone durability. As a result of osteoporosis, bone tissue is reduced, bone shape is uneven, and bone fragility is increased, which increases the risk of secondary fractures. In most cases of geriatric OP, calcium absorption is impaired by tissue cellular hypofunction, which occurs after the age of 70. When it comes to idiopathic osteoporosis, which has no known etiology, adolescents are especially vulnerable. Most women who develop postmenopausal OP do so 5–10 years after menopause because of a drop in estrogen-induced calcitonin levels. This indirect inhibition of osteoclast function leads to bone resorption rather than bone production (28).

3.5.6   3D Printing Applications in Cardiovascular System

One of the leading causes of death for people over 65 years is cardiovascular disease, which is the most prevalent condition affecting older adults. The cardiovascular system is a complex network of blood vessels, the heart, and blood responsible for the circulation of nutrients and oxygens hormones and removing the vest products throughout the body.

3.5.6.1   Valvular Structural Heart Disease

Three-dimensional printing has been utilized to plan interventional and surgical procedures as well as diagnose valvular heart disease. In cases of aortic stenosis, 3D printed reproductions helped define the aortic architecture, with the size of the aortic valve, the shape of the root, the distribution of calcium, and the distance from the coronary arteries. To analyze hemodynamics across the aortic valve, there have also been functional models with flow across 3D-printed aortic valves developed. In patients with significant tortuosity or concurrent mitral valve prostheses, which can pose challenges during transcatheter valve deployment, these models have been used to assess their candidacy for transcatheter aortic valve replacement.

3.5.6.2   Non-valvular Structural Heart Disease

Patients with atrial fibrillation and significant bleeding risk now have a treatment alternative for reducing their risk of stroke known as percutaneous atrial appendage closure (LAA). However, because of the LAA's extreme variability in size and form, problems still exist. Aortic anatomy is properly portrayed in 3D models that may be 3D-printed and coupled to flow loops to improve physiologic replication. These models serve as a road map for endovascular methods and device selection, and they were especially useful in difficult scenarios like determining the best position to affix fenestrated stent grafts to prevent branch vessel occlusion.

3.5.6.3   Congenital Heart Disease

Congenital heart disease may be the area where 3D printing is used most extensively due to the significant anatomical variances and complexity. In comparison to conventional imaging, there is evidence that 3D-printed models assist in understanding the anatomy of congenital heart defects, such as complex ventricular septal defects and right ventricles with double outlets. For simple preoperative planning, 3D models of congenital heart abnormalities are available. The best baffle orientation was planned to use these models, which provided accurate results when compared to surgical findings (29).

3.5.7   3D Printing in the Treatment of Oral Cavity Diseases

Most tooth loss in older adults is caused by periodontal disease and dental caries as the gums recede and grow older and the exposed surface of the cervical root becomes more exposed, increasing the risk of caries (30). Since it is most practical and simple to administer medications via the oral route, it is frequently chosen by doctors and the majority of patients. Formulations for oral administration are generally less expensive than those made for other routes. Additionally, a lot of medications can be taken orally and supplied using a variety of dose forms, such as liquids, capsules, tablets, or chewable formulations. Traditional liquids such as solutions and suspensions and solids such as tablets and capsules dosing forms still have some limitations. Pediatric and geriatric patients have had swallowing issues with the solid form, which is one of its main drawbacks (31).

3.6 TISSUE ENGINEERING AND 3D BIOPRINTING

The potential for biomaterial production in tissue and organ bioengineering has made bioprinting technology. Since the skin is one of the most intricate, multilayered organs in the body, bioprinting is becoming increasingly important in rebuilding or regenerating burned skin. In addition to combining extrusion and inkjet modules, Kim et al. developed a new paradigm to produce 3D human skin. Combining two distinct bioprinting approaches proved to be a time-efficient way to complete this task. Albanna et al. have developed and validated a skin bioprinting method for quick on-site treatment of extensive wounds, regardless of the availability of several studies on skin creation. It has become more important to be able to regenerate tissues and organs to restore their functionality. As part of regenerative medicine, tissue engineering involves regenerating specific tissues *in vitro* or *in situ* to return them to their natural biological function. Scaffolds alone, cultured cells and other bioactive compounds alone, or both cells and scaffolds together. Traditional approaches to tissue engineering involve implanting scaffolds within or on scaffolds that mimic the body's natural extracellular matrix (ECM) the application of 3D printing in tissue engineering is shown in (Figure 3.2) (32).

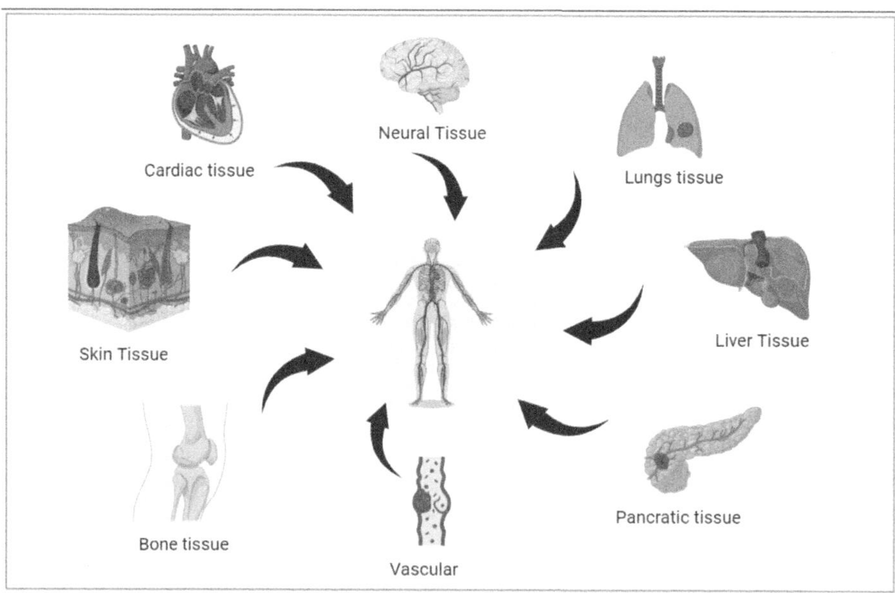

FIGURE 3.2   Application of 3D printing in tissue engineering.

3.7 INVESTIGATING THE EFFECTS OF 3D BIOPRINTING ON CANCER

The development of 3D bioprinting for use in cancer research has become a viable approach in several medical fields. One of the most important applications of 3D bioprinting is potential strategies that researchers have been exploring recently to get over the restrictions that currently exist in this sector. The biocompatibility of scaffold-free cellular spheroids makes them a startlingly important component of cancer research because they mimic the *in vivo* microenvironment of cancer cells (3).

3.8 TISSUE REPAIR ELECTRICAL SIGNAL

Biomaterials influence cell behaviors geometrically, electrically, thermally, and magnetically through their mechanical, electrical, thermal, and magnetic signals. To build biomimicking structures, fiber production techniques offer special benefits. Additionally, by incorporating conductivity into the fibers, it is possible to promote the transfer of internal and external electrical signals, which will improve tissue growth, differentiation, and cell adhesion. Numerous tissues and organs in the human body conduct metabolic and regenerative processes that are significantly influenced by neurovascular networks. Blood vessels are capable of carrying enough oxygen, nutrients, and biological components, while nerve fibers are responsible for sending excitation signals to specific cells. However, because the host neurovascular networks are so complex, conventional scaffolds are unable to quickly stimulate angiogenesis and innervation. A practical method for constructing biological scaffolds with biomimetic designs and multi-material compositions that are capable of controlling a variety of cell behaviors is 3D printing (32).

3.8.1 CARDIAC TISSUE ENGINEERING

The cause of more than 20 million deaths worldwide each year is cardiovascular disease. Heart valves, arteries, and myocardium, which are completely differentiated and load-bearing tissues, typically undergo replacement near the conclusion of the illness stage. Synchronous cardiac contraction is made possible by the anisotropic, interwoven fibrous network that makes up the myocardial ECM. This network allows for mechanical and electrical interaction between cardiac cardiomyocytes. The electrically active myocardium is replaced by inoperative scar tissue after a myocardial infarction, which makes it impossible for cells to communicate. In the meantime, a conductive patch attached to the heart can reconnect the interrupted current route, while mechanically supporting the thin ventricle wall. Cardiac tissue engineering is anticipated to restore the heart by producing functioning myocardial *in vitro*, even though the heart cannot repair and regenerate itself (33).

3.8.2 NERVE CONDUITS

In 3D printing, printing materials are carefully stacked one layer at a time, and the structures of arbitrary objects can be constructed quickly under computer control.

It is extensively used in the field of healthcare. One of the most clinical procedures in neurosurgery has always been the repair of peripheral nerve abnormalities. The main therapeutic option for peripheral nerve deficits at the moment is nerve autograft, even though this therapy is continually hampered by issues including limited donor availability, nerve distortion, dislocation, and mismatch of nerve diameter can result from loss of donor function. Besides creating synthetic nerve tissue *in vitro*, nerve conduits can be used to heal nerve injuries at short distances of 4 cm. In the conduit, proximal and distal nerve stumps are introduced into the two ends over time, allowing axon regeneration to begin at the proximal end and progress to the distal end with time. The most commonly used therapeutic technique for nerve repair is nerve autografts, even with limited tissue availability, mismatched tissue size, and donor site morbidity (34).

3.8.3 Bone Tissue Engineering

It was mostly extrusion-based procedures that were used to create the scaffolds. To create composites with a PLA matrix, hydroxyapatite was the bioceramic that was most frequently used. The studies used rats and six used rabbits, although it was challenging to compare them because of the wide range of experimental methods. According to the findings, composite scaffolds made of PLA and bioceramics have proven to be both mechanically and biologically robust. These scaffolds are capable of being used as bone grafts, which facilitate bone growth without causing harm to the bone, was clarified by preclinical research. It has been shown that PLA/bioceramics scaffolds are a hopeful alternative treatment for bone disease deformities (35). Because of their likeness to native ECM and ease of manufacture, bone tissue restoration has also been accomplished using fibrous scaffolds. Additionally, the expanding use of bone tissue containing conductive scaffolds creation is aided by the accelerated response of stem cells to electrical stimulation in osteogenic differentiation (36).

3.9 APPLICATIONS OF 3D BIOPRINTING FOR ORGAN REGENERATION

Three-dimensional bioprinting has emerged as an innovative technology with numerous applications, some of which are discussed in the following subsections.

3.9.1 Liver Tissues

In recent years, preoperative simulation-based training using 3D models has been used extensively in complex procedures; although there have been fewer documented instances, this is also true in liver surgery. The construction of realistic 3D-printed models is made possible by simulation-based training using 3D models, which offers reported advantages over, there are currently two methods for surgical simulation: *ex vivo* and animal models, as well as virtual reality. Three liver procedures were scheduled, and 3D simulators were constructed utilizing silicone molding and 3D-printing technologies (37). The 3D physical models replicated the real-world situation extremely well. They also demonstrated greater cost-effectiveness in comparison to other models. The only clinically approved treatment for people with usually necessary to undergo orthotopic liver transplantation for end-stage liver disease, despite the liver's remarkable capacity for self-regeneration. An additional method for creating liver tissue that can be used for drug testing and regeneration is 3D bioprinting for liver tissue engineering, naturally occurring polymers, such as silk, gelatin, alginate, and synthetic pluronic are greatly preferred (38).

3.9.2 SKIN TISSUES

Despite its self-healing mechanism for minor wounds, the skin is incapable of dealing with serious injuries, such as burns and deep wound infections, larger wounds can be filled in with bioprinted skin (39). Large-scale skin injuries frequently come with high morbidity and mortality or impeded wound healing that leads to the production of scars. Human adipose-derived stem cells (hADSCs) have been infused into a novel biomaterial to study the *in vivo* application of 3D-printed tissue-engineered skin substitute in wound healing. The extracellular matrix components of adipose tissue were decellularized, lyophilized, and solubilized to produce dermal extracellular matrix (dECM) pre-gel. It was found that wound healing in animals treated with 3D-printed skin substitutes that attenuated inflammatory responses, increased blood flow, stimulated re-epithelialization, collagen deposition, and angiogenesis, and stimulated collagen deposition and alignment, was accelerated (40).

3.10 3D PRINTING FOR BIOMEDICAL APPLICATIONS USING PHOTOCURING

The produced materials must have photosensitive properties in order for the 3D printing method to use photocuring. Photoinitiators, resin, and monomers are frequently found in printed materials. But for biomedical applications, a material's high biocompatibility is its most crucial quality. However, due to unreacted double bonds in photosensitive resins, most of them are cytotoxic, leftover photoinitiators, and other factors. Consequently, 3D printing using photocuring has gained wide applications as discussed in the following subsections.

3.10.1 APPLICATIONS IN INDIRECT OR TRANSIENT CONTACT WITH LIVING ORGANISMS

The biocompatibility capabilities of 3D-printing photocuring materials are still lacking as of right now. Therefore, the domains where the 3D-printing photocuring material can be used industrially on a big scale and without direct contact with living organisms are those. The highest usage of these is dental material created by 3D-printing photocuring. In part due to the low photosensitive resin biocompatibility, it has been challenging to employ photocurable 3D printing directly in humans up until now. Presently, inorganic materials make up the majority of 3D printing materials that can come into direct touch with human tissue through photocuring. Bone components with biological properties, such as biological glass and hydroxyapatite, must be combined with photosensitive resin because they are not photosensitive. The biological activity of items will therefore be significantly impacted after printing. The inorganic portion of the material is typically left after sintering to be used as a replacement material for bones, teeth, and others. After photocuring 3D printing, the resin is often removed to leave only the inorganic material (41).

3.10.2 3D PRINTING OF THE MEDICAL DEVICE

The present circumstance of the research field was thoroughly examined in this study. AM is categorized into commercially available devices in the medical field and surgical tools and guides play a crucial role. Hemostats and medical clamps are frequently used in surgical tools like retractors and are easily made utilizing AM technology (42). Recently, surgical instruments have become more popular in dentistry due to their excellent accuracy and customizability. Three-dimensional printing makes it possible to quickly produce patient-specific personalized anatomical models, surgical tools, rehabilitation supplies, and implants for example, for determining surgical access and practicing the surgery. These benefits increase the demand for 3D-printed medical products. The recent establishment of 3D printing facilities has reduced the distance between health care providers, medical facilities, and manufacturers of these devices, but it has also blurred the regulatory boundaries between them. Three-dimensional-printing proof-of-concept guidelines are being developed by the FDA in order to better prepare all stakeholders for the safe and efficient use of 3D printing in medical applications (43).

3.11   3D PRINTING IN SPINAL SURGERY

Anatomical knowledge is essential for surgeons working as specialists in spine surgery. 3D-printed replicas of the spine are helping in medical education. Three-dimensional-printed spine fracture models are useful for identifying complex spine fracture markers, practicing before surgery, and creating standardized training programs. The two types of models most frequently used to teach spinal anatomy are the bones of cadavers that have been specially treated and cast in plaster. Although cadaveric bones are sometimes difficult to obtain and are subject to ethical or legal concerns, a plaster mold is a single model that is not very precise (44, 45). Custom implants, anatomical models, molds for prosthetics production, and surgical guiding have all seen widespread applications since the advent of 3D printing and its advantages. Since there is now a wider range of production materials available and higher standards for precision and dependability, it is now possible to give patients customized medical equipment. Orthopedics and neurosurgery are two early and striking applications of the medical industry's use of 3D printing. By combining the possibilities of 3D printing with spinal surgery in 1999, D'Urso et al. made it possible to print correct patient-specific spinal morphology in physical form. Difficult local anatomical features and their relationship to one another inside the human body can be reproduced using the technology of 3D printing, simplifying difficult spinal surgery and improving functional repair. Currently, there are a number of ways in which 3D printing can be used in spine surgery, such as printing fracture models for preoperative planning and surgical simulation, manufacturing surgical instructions, bone-healing techniques, and patient education (46).

3.12 PERSONALIZED PROSTHETICS AND ORTHOTICS

Prostheses are devices that replace a lost body part's functionality, whereas orthoses are assistive devices that restore a body part's stability and movement in patients with neuromuscular and/or musculoskeletal problems. For users to be satisfied when treating patients, personalized orthotics and prosthetics (O and P) need to be fitted and comfortable devices, and a precise arrangement has been proven to be essential. Additionally, offering the patient suitable O-and-P equipment within four weeks of an amputation or other handicap greatly reduces user abandonment. Therefore, two essential elements that might considerably enhance patients' lives are a quick fabrication method and an easy fit of the O and P devices. The O and P devices are safe, dependable, and long-lasting for patients. The manufacture of high-performance O-and-P devices has recently been assessed by many researchers and experts in the field using AM technology, and a variety of customized foot orthoses have been produced (47).

3.13 3D PRINTING FOR HEARING AND VISION

The usage of 3D printing has revolutionized the field of assistive technology for those with hearing and vision impairments. There are many media accounts about amazing 3D printing; there are uses on Earth and in space, but it is a quiet and peacefully amazing innovation in producing hearing aids went almost completely not reported (48, 49). It is, in the words of *Forbes'* Rakesh Sharma, "The 3D Printing Revolution You Have Not Heard About." According to Phil Reeves, author of a study on 3D printing, more than 10,000,000 hearing aids were printed in 2013. By automating 3D printing and making it quick and patient-focused, a lot has changed in the manual, labor-intensive industry. Before 3D printing was introduced, the creation of hearing aids was an artisanal process that took about a week. (50). A concept for 3D-printing concrete is provided, taking into account technological, economic, and environmental factors. Although there are numerous examples of 3D-printed concrete constructions available around the globe, there are still significant technical and processing difficulties. Because they lack suitable rheological and stiffening qualities, high-performance cement-based materials currently on the market cannot be directly 3D-printed, they will benefit from new material palettes thanks to active stiffening control and active rheology control (51, 52).

3.14 3D PRINTING IN MICROROBOT

The development of novel functions for a growing number of biomedical applications is being developed cheers to research on microrobots, including drug delivery, surgery, tracking and imaging, and sensing. For these applications, it is becoming more common to use magnetic characteristics to regulate the mobility of microrobots. Microrobots can be built in many different designs, with a wide range of motions and capabilities. As an example, microswimmers, micro bowls (bowl-shaped microrobots), micro rockets (tubular micromachines propelled by bubbles), micro wheels (wheel-shaped rolling structures), microcarriers, and micro drillers are frequently used in microscale operations and drug delivery (53).

3.15 CONCLUSION

The potential for 3D printing in biomedicine enhances personalized treatments and improves patient outcomes. But for 3D printing to be widely used in biomedicine, it will be essential to address issues with scalability, material characteristics, and cost-effectiveness. The future of 3D printing in biomedicine will be designed by current research, which is essential in addressing these obstacles. It has several advantages, including increasing assembly speed and expense productivity. For the treatment of bone abnormalities, 3D-printed composite scaffolds offer a viable alternative. The tested implants appeared to be biocompatible and exhibited no adverse effects that could inhibit bone development. Future bioelectronics, implants, and medical equipment research and development using 3D printing. The use of reason would be most helpful for the development of hydrogel bioelectronics. Microrobots have gained interest because of their unique abilities to carry out responsibilities in parts of the human body that are difficult to access. In biomedical applications, they can deliver drugs, facilitate minimally invasive surgery, measure biosignatures, regenerate tissues, monitor particles, and detect diseases. The fundamental study of aging and elder care can now be conducted with the use of 3D printing, which has become a game-changing technology in the biomedical field.

ACKNOWLEDGMENTS

The authors express their sincere gratitude to the host institutions for generously providing all the necessary facilities throughout the course of this study.

FUNDING

None.

REFERENCES

1. Shahrubudin N, Lee TC, Ramlan R. An overview on 3D printing technology: Technological, materials, and applications. *Procedia Manufacturing*. Elsevier B.V.; 2019;35:1286–1296.
2. Gu Z, Fu J, Lin H, He Y. Development of 3D bioprinting: From printing methods to biomedical applications. *Asian Journal of Pharmaceutical Sciences*. Shenyang Pharmaceutical University; 2020;15:529–557.
3. Vanaei S, Parizi MS, Vanaei S, Salemizadehparizi F, Vanaei HR. An overview on materials and techniques in 3D bioprinting toward biomedical application. *Engineered Regeneration*. KeAi Communications Co.; 2021;2:1–18.
4. Ghilan A, Chiriac AP, Nita LE, Rusu AG, Neamtu I, Chiriac VM. Trends in 3D printing processes for biomedical field: Opportunities and challenges. *Journal of Polymers and the Environment*. Springer; 2020;28:1345–1367.

5. Gopinathan J, Noh I. Recent trends in bioinks for 3D printing. *Biomaterials Research.* BioMed Central Ltd.; 2018;22:11.

6. Yang W, Tu A, Ma Y, Li Z, Xu J, Lin M, Zhang K, Jing L, Fu C, Jiao Y, et al. Chitosan and whey protein bio-inks for 3d and 4d printing applications with particular focus on food industry. *Molecules.* MDPI; 2022;21:173.

7. Oladapo BI, Zahedi SA, Ismail SO, Omigbodun FT. 3D printing of PEEK and its composite to increase biointerfaces as a biomedical material - A review. *Colloids and Surfaces. B, Biointerfaces.* Elsevier B.V.; 2021;203:111726.

8. Ebrahimi F, Ramezani Dana H. Poly lactic acid (PLA) polymers: From properties to biomedical applications. *International Journal of Polymeric Materials and Polymeric Biomaterials.* Taylor and Francis Ltd.; 2022;71:1117–1130.

9. Su X, Wang T, Guo S. Applications of 3D printed bone tissue engineering scaffolds in the stem cell field. *Regenerative Therapy.* Japanese Society of Regenerative Medicine; 2021;16:63–72.

10. Hua W, Shi W, Mitchell K, Raymond L, Coulter R, Zhao D, Jin Y. 3D printing of biodegradable polymer vascular stents: A review. *Chinese Journal of Mechanical Engineering: Additive Manufacturing Frontiers* 2022;1:100020. doi: 10.1016/j.cjmeam.2022.100020

11. Cheng GZ, Folch E, Wilson A, Brik R, Garcia N, Estepar RSJ, Onieva JO, Gangadharan S, Majid A. 3D printing and personalized airway stents. *Pulmonary Therapy* 2017;3:59–66.

12. Sun Z, Jansen S. Personalized 3D printed coronary models in coronary stenting. *Quantitative Imaging in Medicine and Surgery* 2019;9:1356–1367. doi: 10.21037/qims.2019.06.21

13. Li YJ, Zhang FH, Liu YJ, Leng JS. 4D printed shape memory polymers and their structures for biomedical applications. *Sci China Technol Sci.* Springer Verlag; 2020;63:545–560.

14. Chang CH, Lin CY, Chang CH, Liu FH, Huang YT, Liao YS. Enhanced biomedical applicability of ZrO2–SiO2 ceramic composites in 3D printed bone scaffolds. *Scientific Reports* 2022;12:6845. doi: 10.1038/s41598-022-10731-w. Cited: in: PMID: 35477956.

15. Lui YS, Sow WT, Tan LP, Wu Y, Lai Y, Li H. 4D printing and stimuli-responsive materials in biomedical aspects. *Acta Biomaterialia.* Acta Materialia Inc; 2019;92:19–36.

16. Yan Q, Dong H, Su J, Han J, Song B, Wei Q, Shi Y. A review of 3D printing technology for medical applications. *Engineering.* Elsevier Ltd; 2018;4:729–742.

17. Horst DJ. 3D printing of pharmaceutical drug delivery systems. *Archives of Organic and Inorganic Chemical Sciences* 2018;1:1–5. doi: 10.32474/aoics.2018.01.000109

18. Mohapatra S, Kar RK, Biswal PK, Bindhani S. Approaches of 3D printing in current drug delivery. *Sensors International.* KeAi Communications Co.; 2022;3:100146.

19. Tan DK, Maniruzzaman M, Nokhodchi A. Advanced pharmaceutical applications of hot-melt extrusion coupled with fused deposition modelling (FDM) 3D printing for personalised drug delivery. *Pharmaceutics.* MDPI AG; 2018;10:203.

20. Ahangar P, Cooke ME, Weber MH, Rosenzweig DH. Current biomedical applications of 3D printing and additive manufacturing. *Applied Sciences (Switzerland).* MDPI AG; 2019;9:1713.

21. Cai MH, Chen XY, Fu LQ, Du WL, Yang X, Mou XZ, Hu PY. Design and development of hybrid hydrogels for biomedical applications: Recent trends in anticancer drug delivery and tissue engineering. *Frontiers in Bioengineering and Biotechnology.* Frontiers Media S.A.; 2021;9:630943.

22. Geraili A, Xing M, Mequanint K. Design and fabrication of drug-delivery systems toward adjustable release profiles for personalized treatment. *View.* John Wiley and Sons Inc; 2021;2:20200126.

23. Muldoon K, Song Y, Ahmad Z, Chen X, Chang MW. High precision 3D printing for micro to nano scale biomedical and electronic devices. *Micromachines (Basel)*. MDPI; 2022;13:642.

24. Wang P, Sun Y, Shi X, Shen H, Ning H, Liu H. 3D printing of tissue engineering scaffolds: A focus on vascular regeneration. *Bio-design and Manufacturing*. Springer; 2021;4:344–378.

25. Yefroyev DA, Jin S. Induced pluripotent stem cells for treatment of Alzheimer's and Parkinson's diseases. *Biomedicine*. MDPI; 2022;10:208.

26. Saylam E, Akkaya Y, Ilhan E, Cesur S, Guler E, Sahin A, Cam ME, Ekren N, Oktar FN, Gunduz O, et al. Levodopa-loaded 3D-printed poly (Lactic) acid/chitosan neural tissue scaffold as a promising drug delivery system for the treatment of Parkinson's disease. *Applied Sciences (Switzerland)*. 2021;11:10727. doi: 10.3390/app112210727

27. Goutman SA, Chen L, Plott JS, Vankoevering KK, Kurili A, Shih AJ, Green GE. A personalized approach to non-invasive ventilation masks in amyotrophic lateral sclerosis using facial scanning and 3D-printing. *Annals of 3D Printed Medicine* 2021;3:100027. doi: 10.1016/j.stlm.2021.100027

28. Wang B, Feng C, Pan J, Zhou S, Sun Z, Shao Y, Qu Y, Bao S, Li Y, Yang T. The effect of 3D printing metal materials on osteoporosis treatment. *BioMed Research International*. Hindawi Limited; 2021;2021:1–7.

29. El Sabbagh A, Eleid MF, Al-Hijji M, Anavekar NS, Holmes DR, Nkomo VT, Oderich GS, Cassivi SD, Said SM, Rihal CS, et al. The various applications of 3D printing in cardiovascular diseases. *Current Cardiology Reports*. Current Medicine Group LLC 1; 2018;20:1–9.

30. Ma M, Gu J, Wang DA, Bi S, Liu R, Zhang X, Yang J, Zhang Y. Applications of 3D printing in aging. *International Journal of Bioprinting* 2023;9. doi: 10.18063/ijb.732

31. Rodríguez-Pombo L, Awad A, Basit AW, Alvarez-Lorenzo C, Goyanes A. Innovations in chewable formulations: The novelty and applications of 3D printing in drug product design. *Pharmaceutics*. MDPI; 2022;14:1732.

32. Assad H, Assad A, Kumar A. Recent developments in 3D bio-printing and its biomedical applications. *Pharmaceutics*. MDPI; 2023;15:255.

33. Duan B. State-of-the-art review of 3D bioprinting for cardiovascular tissue engineering. *Annals of Biomedical Engineering*. Springer New York LLC; 2017;45:195–209.

34. Liu K, Yan L, Li R, Song Z, Ding J, Liu B, Chen X. 3D printed personalized nerve guide conduits for precision repair of peripheral nerve defects. *Advanced Science*. John Wiley and Sons Inc; 2022;9:2103875.

35. Alonso-Fernández I, Haugen HJ, López-Peña M, González-Cantalapiedra A, Muñoz F. Use of 3D-printed polylactic acid/bioceramic composite scaffolds for bone tissue engineering in preclinical in vivo studies: A systematic review. *Acta Biomaterialia*. Acta Materialia Inc; 2023;168:1–21.

36. Wei L, Wang S, Shan M, Li Y, Wang Y, Wang F, Wang L, Mao J. Conductive fibers for biomedical applications. *Bioactive Materials*. KeAi Communications Co.; 2023;22:343–364.

37. Vijayavenkataraman S, Yan WC, Lu WF, Wang CH, Fuh JYH. 3D bioprinting of tissues and organs for regenerative medicine. *Advanced Drug Delivery Reviews*. Elsevier B.V.; 2018;132:296–332.

38. Valls-Esteve A, Tejo-Otero A, Lustig-Gainza P, Buj-Corral I, Fenollosa-Artés F, Rubio-Palau J, Barber-Martinez de la Torre I, Munuera J, Fondevila C, Krauel L. Patient-specific 3D printed soft models for liver surgical planning and hands-on training. *Gels* 2023;9:339. doi: 10.3390/gels9040339

39. Agarwal K, Srinivasan V, Lather V, Pandita D, Vasanthan KS. Insights of 3D bioprinting and focusing the paradigm shift towards 4D printing for biomedical applications. *Journal of Materials Research* 2023;38:112–141. doi: 10.1557/s43578-022-00524-2

40. Fu H, Zhang D, Zeng J, Fu Q, Chen Z, Sun X, Yang Y, Li S, Chen M. Application of 3D-printed tissue-engineered skin substitute using innovative biomaterial loaded with human adipose-derived stem cells in wound healing. *International Journal of Bioprinting* 2022;9:394–406. doi: 10.18063/IJB.V9I2.674

41. Quan H, Zhang T, Xu H, Luo S, Nie J, Zhu X. Photo-curing 3D printing technique and its challenges. *Bioactive Materials*. KeAi Communications Co.; 2020;5:110–115.

42. Kumar R, Kumar M, Chohan JS. The role of additive manufacturing for biomedical applications: A critical review. *J Manuf Process* Elsevier Ltd; 2021;64:828–850.

43. Rojek I, Mikołajewski D, Dostatni E, Kopowski J. Specificity of 3D printing and AI-based optimization of medical devices using the example of a group of exoskeletons. *Applied Sciences (Switzerland)*. 2023;13:1060. doi: 10.3390/app13021060

44. Valls-Esteve A, Tejo-Otero A, Lustig-Gainza P, Buj-Corral I, Fenollosa-Artés F, Rubio-Palau J, Barber-Martinez de la Torre I, Munuera J, Fondevila C, Krauel L. Patient-specific 3D printed soft models for liver surgical planning and hands-on training. *Gels* 2023;9:339. doi: 10.3390/gels9040339

45. Goh GD, Sing SL, Lim YF, Thong JLJ, Peh ZK, Mogali SR, Yeong WY. Machine learning for 3D printed multi-materials tissue-mimicking anatomical models. *Materials and Design* 2021;211:110125. doi: 10.1016/j.matdes.2021.110125

46. Rojek I, Mikołajewski D, Dostatni E, Kopowski J. Specificity of 3D printing and AI-based optimization of medical devices using the example of a group of exoskeletons. *Applied Sciences (Switzerland)*. 2023;13:1060. doi: 10.3390/app13021060

47. Sakib-Uz-Zaman C, Khondoker MAH. Polymer-based additive manufacturing for orthotic and prosthetic devices: Industry outlook in Canada. *Polymers (Basel)*. MDPI; 2023;15:1506.

48. Haleem A, Javaid M. Polyether ether ketone (PEEK) and its manufacturing of customised 3D printed dentistry parts using additive manufacturing. *Clinical Epidemiology and Global Health* 2019;7:654–660. doi: 10.1016/j.cegh.2019.03.001

49. Rojek I, Mikołajewski D, Dostatni E, Kopowski J. Specificity of 3D printing and ai-based optimization of medical devices using the example of a group of exoskeletons. *Applied Sciences (Switzerland)*. 2023;13:1060. doi: 10.3390/app13021060

50. Dodziuk H. Applications of 3D printing in healthcare. *Kardiochirurgia i Torakochirurgia Polska*. Termedia Publishing House Ltd.; 2016;13:283–293.

51. Triacca A, Pitzanti G, Mathew E, Conti B, Dorati R, Lamprou DA. Stereolithography 3D printed implants: A preliminary investigation as potential local drug delivery systems to the ear. *International Journal of Pharmaceutics* 2022;616:121529. doi: 10.1016/j.ijpharm.2022.121529. Cited in: PMID: 35114311.

52. De Schutter G, Lesage K, Mechtcherine V, Nerella VN, Habert G, Agusti-Juan I. Vision of 3D printing with concrete—Technical, economic and environmental potentials. *Cement and Concrete Research*. Elsevier Ltd; 2018;63:25–36.

53. Sarabi MR, Karagoz AA, Yetisen AK, Tasoglu S. 3D-printed microrobots: Translational challenges. *Micromachines (Basel)*. 2023;14:1099. doi: 10.3390/mi14061099

54. Zhou W, Qiao Z, Nazarzadeh Zare E, Huang J, Zheng X, Sun X, Shao M, Wang H, Wang X, Chen D, et al. 4D-printed dynamic materials in biomedical applications: Chemistry, challenges, and their future perspectives in the clinical sector. *Journal of Medicinal Chemistry*. American Chemical Society; 2020;63:8003–8024.

55. Su X, Wang T, Guo S. Applications of 3D printed bone tissue engineering scaffolds in the stem cell field. *Regenerative Therapy*. Japanese Society of Regenerative Medicine; 2021;16:63–72.

56. Ding Z, Zhang Y, Guo P, Duan T, Cheng W, Guo Y, Zheng X, Lu G, Lu Q, Kaplan DL. Injectable desferrioxamine-laden silk nanofiber hydrogels for accelerating diabetic wound healing. *ACS Biomaterials Science & Engineering* 2021;7:1147–1158. doi: 10.1021/acsbiomaterials.0c01502. Cited: in: PMID: 33522800.

4 Recent Trends and Pharmaceutical Applications for 3D Printing in Dermal Drug Delivery

Ashish Kumar Pandey
Faculty of Pharmaceutical Sciences, Bhilai, India

Achal Mishra and Shekhar Verma
Guru Ghasidas Vishwavidyalaya (A Central University),
Bilaspur, India

4.1 INTRODUCTION

Addressing skin-related problems and diseases is of paramount importance given their widespread prevalence and impact on individuals' quality of life. Furthermore, the economic burden associated with skin disorders, particularly chronic wounds, highlights the need for innovative and effective treatment approaches.

Advancements in technology, such as three-dimensional (3D) printing, play a crucial role in developing novel solutions for skin-related issues. Additionally, ongoing research into areas like nanotechnology, biomaterials, and advanced imaging techniques is contributing to the development of more effective diagnostics and treatments for skin diseases.

Incorporating interdisciplinary approaches involving dermatologists, material scientists, engineers, and health care providers can lead to the creation of cutting-edge solutions that address the diverse range of skin conditions. Furthermore, the integration of telemedicine and digital health technologies can facilitate remote monitoring and consultation, ensuring timely and effective care for patients with skin disorders.

Skin-related problems and all types of skin diseases are very common problems for our world population as 70% of the world population is affected by these disorders (1).

Still, skin diseases stand as the fourth-most prevalent cause of human infirmity, posing a significant challenge to the Indian health care system. Additionally, the management of wounds, particularly chronic wounds, places a substantial burden on

DOI: 10.1201/9781032690926-4

health care, with global care costs fluctuating between US$20 and US$35 billion annually (2). Recognizing the substantial impact of these conditions, there is a strong push for the development and adoption of innovative technologies in the treatment of skin diseases and injuries (3). These advancements are seen as pivotal in addressing the prevalent health challenges and improving outcomes for individuals affected by dermatological conditions (4).

Today, dermal products are a lot more complex, varying from simple solutions and creams to multiphase, nanotechnology, and assisted technologies (5). In this scenario, 3D printing is a promising alternative for developing and producing biomedical and pharmaceutical products aimed at the treatment of skin disorders and skin injuries. This technology allows the design and control of specific desired properties, porosity, pore size, roughness, functional groups, size, shape, swelling, degradability profile, drug loading, and drug release profile (6, 7).

3D printing has emerged in the past years as an innovative and versatile platform for the development of new health care solutions. Three-dimensional printing enables the fabrication of complex geometries and structures, which can be especially valuable for creating specialized drug delivery systems, wound dressings, and other dermal products. This technology also facilitates rapid prototyping and iterative design, expediting the development process and allowing for quick adjustments based on feedback from preclinical or clinical trials. Three-dimensional printing is the construction of a 3D object from a computer-aided design (CAD) model (8). It can be done in a variety of processes in which material is deposited, joined, or solidified under computerized control, with all material being added together (such as bioplastics, drug solution, liquids, or powder grains being fused), typically layer by layer. In the field of dermal products, 3D printing holds immense potential for advancing the treatment of skin disorders and injuries. The benefits of 3D printing are reduced manufacturing costs, increased product customization, and improved product quality. Another benefit of 3D printing is the technology's ability to produce complex geometries with high precision and accuracy (9).

4.2 DERMAL DRUG DELIVERY ROUTES

Dermal administration is a crucial method for the local treatment of various diseases and injuries due to the barrier properties of the skin (Figure 4.1). This approach involves applying formulations directly onto the surface of the skin, and it offers several distinct advantages:

- Targeted Delivery to Specific Skin Sites: Dermal administration allows for precise targeting of various skin layers, including the stratum corneum, viable epidermis, dermis, pilosebaceous unit, hypodermis, and even deeper tissues. This precision is vital for addressing specific dermatological conditions effectively.
- Enhanced Drug Bioavailability: By bypassing the digestive system and first-pass metabolism, dermal administration can improve the bioavailability of drugs. This means that a higher proportion of the administered dose reaches the target site in a biologically active form (10).

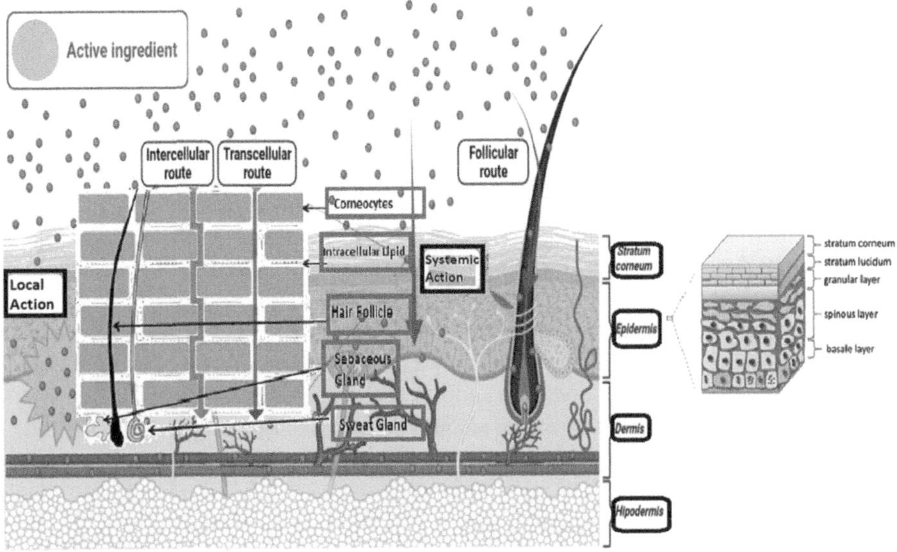

FIGURE 4.1 Structure of human skin and barrier (4).

- Patient Acceptance: Dermal delivery is generally well accepted by patients due to its noninvasive and painless nature. This can lead to higher compliance rates and better treatment outcomes.
- Localized Effects: The method allows for localized treatment, which means that the drug primarily affects the area where it is applied. This minimizes systemic exposure and reduces the potential for systemic toxicity or adverse effects.
- Improved Pharmacological and Physiological Response: Dermal administration can lead to a more predictable and sustained release of the drug, resulting in a better therapeutic response. This is particularly beneficial for medications with a narrow therapeutic window (11).
- Reduced Risk of Systemic Toxicity: Because the drug primarily acts locally, there is a lower risk of systemic toxicity compared to systemic administration methods. This is especially important for drugs with potential side effects.
- Minimized Exposure to Non-Desired Sites: Unlike systemic administration, which can lead to the distribution of the drug throughout the body, dermal administration limits drug exposure to non-desired sites, reducing the likelihood of unintended effects.

Overall, dermal administration is a valuable route for delivering medications to treat skin-related conditions. Its advantages in terms of patient acceptance, targeted delivery, enhanced bioavailability, and reduced systemic exposure make it a preferred option for many dermatological treatments (12). In this chapter, we focus on localized skin active ingredient delivery, which implies targeting specific skin layers while reducing systemic absorption (13).

The therapeutic effect of the dermally applied formulations relies on the following three steps (14):

- Release of the active ingredient from the formulation/dosage form: This is the initial step where the active pharmaceutical ingredient (API) is released from the dosage form (e.g., cream, gel, patch) into contact with the skin.
- Partition and distribution of the drug within the skin barrier, the SC, and permeation/diffusion through the SC: The API undergoes partitioning within the skin' outermost layer, the stratum corneum (SC), and then proceeds to permeate through it.
- Partitioning and diffusion from the SC to the viable epidermis and/or dermis: Once the API has passed through the SC, it may further partition and diffuse into the viable epidermis and/or the deeper dermal layers. It's at this stage that the active ingredient should reach its target site to produce the desired pharmacological effect.

The passage of drugs into the skin or through the skin involves three potential routes: This indicates that APIs can traverse the skin using various pathways:

- The transcellular route: This route involves the transport of drugs through the lipid matrix and corneocytes of the SC. It's essentially a path through the cells of the skin.
- The intercellular route: Here, the drug diffuses between the lipid matrix and the corneocytes, effectively moving between the cells of the SC.
- The transappendageal route: In this route, the drug is transported through the skin's appendages, such as hair follicles, sebaceous glands, or sweat glands. These are natural openings in the skin that can facilitate drug absorption.

Understanding these steps and routes is crucial for designing effective dermal formulations and delivery systems. It allows researchers and pharmaceutical developers to optimize formulations to enhance API absorption and therapeutic efficacy while minimizing the potential side effects or systemic exposure.

4.3 3D PRINTING TECHNOLOGY IN PHARMACEUTICAL FORMULATIONS

Three-dimensional printing is used extensively in organ and tissue engineering, disease, modeling, manufacturing of biomedical devices diagnostics, and the formulation and development of unique novel dosage forms (Figure 4.2). It has been utilized in the pharmaceutical industry's research and development and in process innovation technology to develop digitally controlled and personalized products by converting a concept into a prototype (additive manufacturing) using 3D CAD or magnetic resonance imaging. Three-dimensional structures can be printed on a functionalized surface characterized by a specific permeability, porosity, hydrophobicity, or hydrophilicity (15). This flexibility can offer many novel strategic approaches for the research and development of controlled-release drug delivery systems (16).

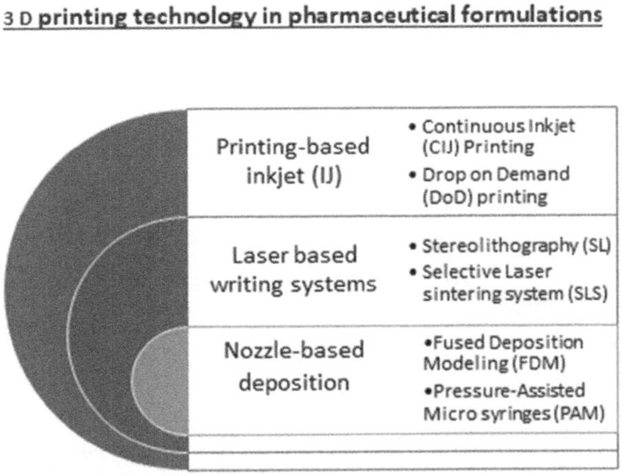

FIGURE 4.2   Types of 3D-printing technology in pharmaceuticals (8).

Based on the energy source, material source, and other mechanical characteristics, various 3D printing methods have been three designed (Figure 4.3) (20).

4.3.1 PRINTING-BASED INKJET

Two prominent approaches within inkjet technology are continuous inkjet (CIJ) printing and drop-on-demand (DoD) printing:

A. **CIJ Printing**: In CIJ printing, a continuous stream of ink is expelled through a nozzle, which creates a stream of droplets. A piezoelectric or thermal element is used to break this stream into individual droplets. An electrical charge is then applied to each droplet, selectively deflecting it onto the printing substrate or allowing it to continue its trajectory and be recycled. This process allows for a continuous stream of droplets to be generated and controlled (Figure 4.3A).

B. **DoD Printing**: In DoD printing, droplets are generated on demand, meaning that they are produced only when needed for printing. This is achieved by applying a force (such as a thermal pulse or piezoelectric pressure) to push a droplet from the nozzle. The droplet is then propelled toward the printing substrate. DoD technology offers precise control over droplet placement, making it particularly suitable for high-resolution printing.

CIJ and DoD (Figure 4.3B) are two distinct printing technologies with unique characteristics and applications (7). CIJ is well suited for high-speed printing tasks, thanks to its continuous stream of ink that enables rapid and consistent printing, making it commonly used in large-scale commercial operations such as packaging and labeling. By comparison, DoD printing provides precise control over droplet placement, making it ideal for high-resolution and intricate designs. It is often preferred for small-scale applications like electronics, textiles, and bioprinting, where

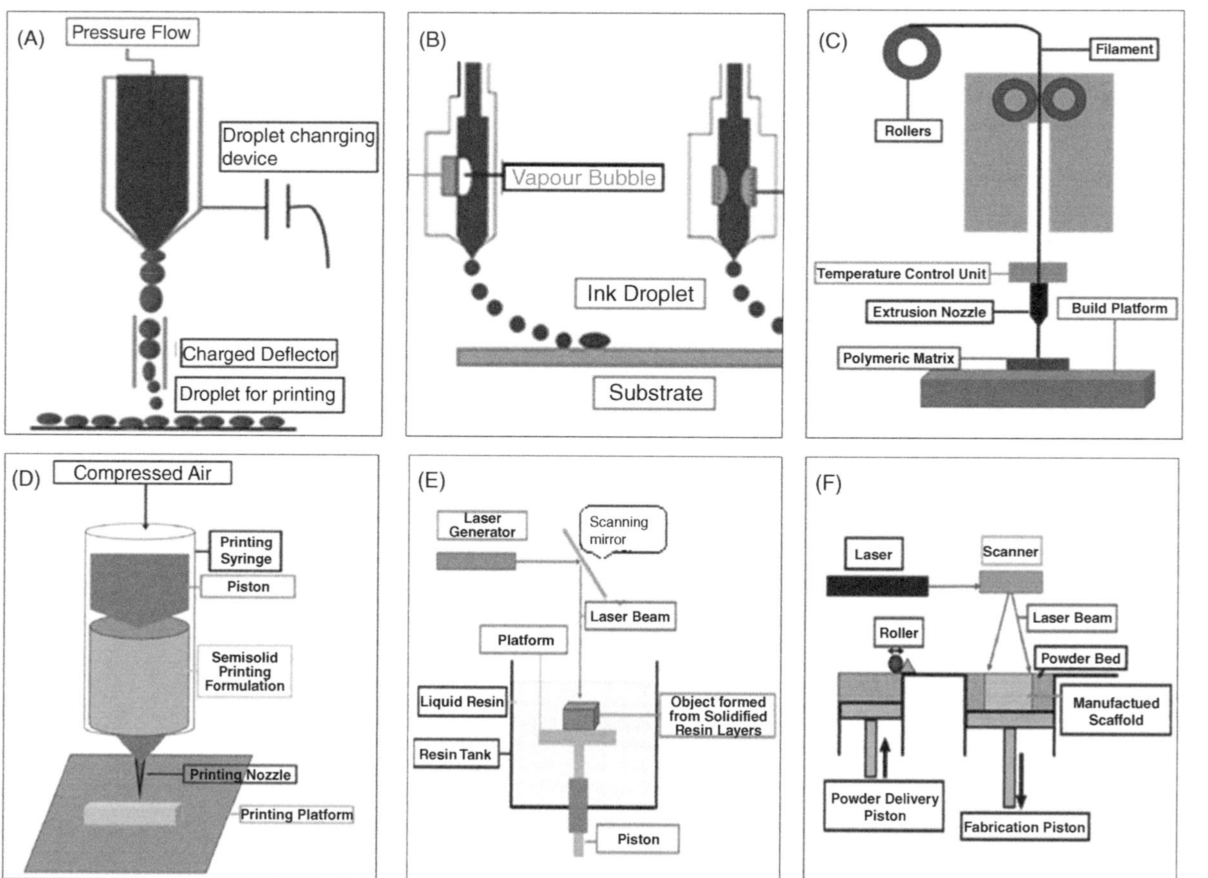

FIGURE 4.3   Pictorial representation of various 3D-printing methods. A. Continuous inkjet printing (10). B. Drop-on-demand printing (14). C. Fusion-based deposition modeling (17). D. Pressure-based assisted modeling (17). E. Stereolithography (18). F. Selective laser sintering system (19).

minimizing ink wastage is essential. Despite their differences, both CIJ and DoD printing technologies play critical roles in various industries, offering versatility and flexibility to achieve high-quality, digitally controlled printing results (21).

4.3.2 Nozzle-Based Deposition

A nozzle deposition system in 3D printing integrates the solid material with the binder before 3D printing and directly deposits the mixture through a small nozzle. This is divided into two subtypes based on the process including fused deposition modeling (FDM) and pressure-assisted microsyringes (PAM) (22).

- **FDM**: FDM is a widely used 3D printing technique whereby a thermoplastic material, often in the form of a filament, is heated until it becomes semi-liquid and is then extruded through a nozzle (Figure 4.3C). The material is then deposited layer by layer to build up the final 3D object. As the material cools, it solidifies, creating a stable structure (17, 22).
- **PAM**: This subtype of nozzle deposition system involves using microsyringes to precisely control the deposition of materials (Figure 4.3D). It is particularly valuable in bioprinting and other applications in which high precision and control over material deposition are crucial. The material may be in the form of a bioink, which can contain living cells or other biologically active components.

4.3.3 Laser-Based Writing Systems

4.3.3.1 Stereolithography

Rapid prototyping currently makes extensive use of stereolithography (SL), which was the first laser-based liquid resin polymerization technology developed. It is a technique that uses a computer-controlled laser beam to turn liquid polymer or resin into a solid, producing a 3D structure (Figure 4.3E) (17). The initial laser-based liquid resin polymerization method was called SL.

The process involves using a computer-controlled laser beam to solidify a liquid polymer or resin, creating a 3D structure layer by layer. This is achieved by selectively curing thin layers of liquid resin with an ultraviolet (UV) laser. The laser traces the cross-section of the object onto the liquid resin, solidifying it. The build platform then descends, and the process is repeated for the next layer. SLA is known for its high level of detail, making it suitable for producing intricate and complex parts. It's commonly used in industries such as aerospace, automotive, and health care for prototyping and creating master patterns for casting (18).

4.3.3.2 Selective Laser Sintering System

Selective laser sintering (SLS) technology has evolved (Figure 4.3F), leading to the development of variations like digital light processing (DLP) and continuous liquid interface production (CLIP), which use similar principles with slight variations in execution.

SLS provides several benefits over the earlier technology of 3D printing, the most significant of which is its remarkable resolution and avoidance of thermal procedures that can destroy specific drug molecules. The most common 3D-printing technologies for pharmaceutical applications are those listed earlier, which are further divided into subtypes based on materials and energy sources (23).

4.4 DERMAL DRUG DELIVERY SYSTEM AND CHALLENGES

Dermal administration describes the application of substances to the skin's surface for the localized treatment of diseases or wounds (18). The stratum corneum (SC), viable epidermis, dermis, pilosebaceous unit, hypodermis, and deeper tissues can all be targeted by site-specific drug delivery (19). The main advantages of this delivery route follow:

- Patient Acceptance: generally well received by patients due to its noninvasive and painless nature.
- Improved Drug Bioavailability: bypasses digestive processes, allowing a higher proportion of the drug to reach the target site in an active form.
- Enhanced Pharmacological and Physiological Response: provides a more predictable and sustained release, leading to a better therapeutic response.
- Localized Effects: targets the area where applied, minimizing systemic exposure and reducing the risk of systemic toxicity.
- Reduced Exposure to Non-Desired Sites: limits drug exposure to unintended areas, enhancing safety (24).

This passage discusses the various routes through which drugs can pass into or through the skin, as well as a contemporary preference for semisolid formulations in dermatological applications. The transcellular route is related to the transport of drugs through the cells of the skin, specifically the SC. The SC is the outermost layer of the epidermis and consists of flattened dead cells called corneocytes embedded in a lipid matrix, in which the drug is transported through the hair follicles, sebaceous glands, or sweat glands. Today, semisolid formulations are preferred for dermatological use (25, 26). The intercellular route involves the diffusion of drugs between the cells of the skin. More precisely, it refers to the drug moving between the lipid layers and corneocytes without actually passing through the cells themselves. This makes them particularly effective for topical treatments. Powders and solutions show important disadvantages for dermal drug delivery, such as low retention time on the skin, thus leading to a transient drug release and therapeutic effect. All semisolid formulations include creams, ointments, gels, and lotions. They are advantageous because they can adhere well to the skin, allowing for sustained drug release, and they are easy to apply and spread. Additionally, they can provide a protective barrier while delivering the active ingredient (27, 28).

The challenges in delivering active ingredients through the skin. The SC, being the outermost layer of the skin, acts as a formidable barrier. To effectively diffuse through the skin, molecules must meet specific criteria such as small molecules (approximately 500, typically about 500 Daltons or less), an adequate partition coefficient (log 1 to 3), and an ionization degree (29). Unfortunately, these criteria pose a challenge for delivering certain pharmaceutically interesting molecules like peptides, proteins, and vaccines through the skin. Due to their larger size, they may struggle to pass through the SC effectively. Moreover, many of these molecules tend to have high molecular weights, which can further hinder their skin permeation (29).

Due to these difficulties, scientists have investigated numerous methods and tools to improve the delivery of bigger and more complex molecules via the skin. There are already a variety of 3D-printing technologies available for use in the pharmaceutical industry. Numerous distinctive characteristics of the various 3D-printing processes, including resolution, output, cost-effectiveness, and biocompatibility of the active molecule, among others, might have an impact on the printing goal (30).

Therefore, 3D-printing techniques can be divided into nine categories.

However, in the pharmaceutical field, only a few technologies and subcategories are currently used (31):

- Binder jetting (BJ)
- Material extrusion (ME)
- Material jetting (MJ)
- Direct powder extrusion (DPE)
- Semi-solid extrusion (SSE)
- SLS
- Photo-polymerization (PP)
- DLP
- CLIP

SSE is also widely known as PAM printing (31), cold extrusion-based printing thermal extrusion robocasting or robotic material extrusion, soft-material extrusion, hydrogel-forming extrusion, melting extrusion, melting solidification printing process, direct ink writing, hot-melt ram extrusion, hot-melt pneumatic extrusion, and micro-extrusion (32). Figure 4.4 presents various possible products developed using 3D-printing technology.

Independent of these techniques used, the first step in CAD software involves designing the object to be printed using specialized software known as CAD software. This digital model serves as the blueprint for the physical object (30).

- Layer-by-Layer Slicing: The 3D model is then divided into a series of thin horizontal layers. This process is often referred to as slicing. Each layer represents a cross section of the final object.
- File Export: The sliced 3D model is exported in a format that the 3D printer can understand. Common file formats for 3D printing include STL (stereolithography) and OBJ (object).
- Fabrication in Layers: The 3D printer reads the file and uses it as instructions to build the object layer by layer. Each layer is deposited or solidified according to the specific technique used (31, 32).

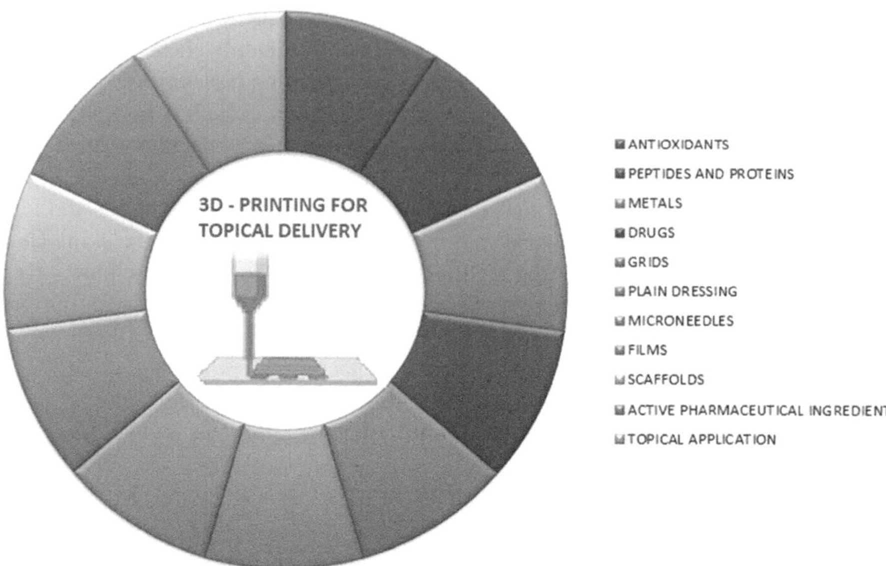

FIGURE 4.4 Possible products using 3D-printing technology and different types of active molecules proposed for dermal delivery (29).

By following these steps, 3D printing enables the creation of highly customized and complex objects with precise shapes and sizes. This technology has found applications in various industries, from manufacturing and health care to aerospace and design. As a result, an individualized object of the desired shape and size can be created (33).

4.5 PHARMACEUTICAL APPLICATIONS OF 3D PRINTING IN DERMAL DELIVERY

4.5.1 Active Ingredient (Drug) Substance

In a study by Maver et al. (2018), a novel approach to pain relief in wound dressings was introduced. This method involved the integration of 3D-printing technology with electrospinning. The researchers incorporated diclofenac sodium, a nonsteroidal anti-inflammatory drug, and lidocaine, a local anesthetic, into the dressings. These drug-loaded dressings were manufactured using SSE in combination with alginate and carboxymethylcellulose (34).

In a study conducted by Long and colleagues (2019), a novel wound dressing was developed utilizing 3D-printing technology. The dressing consisted of a chitosan-pectin hydrogel infused with lidocaine (35). Chitosan, chosen for its favorable attributes in skin applications, possesses bioadhesive, biocompatible, biodegradable, and nontoxic properties. Additionally, it exhibits antimicrobial, antioxidant, hemocompatible, and hemostatic characteristics. The research team utilized SSE in conjunction with lyophilization to fabricate the hydrogel scaffolds. These scaffolds demonstrated excellent properties for an optimal wound-healing environment. They exhibited a high swelling ratio and water absorption capacity, showcasing their proficiency in absorbing exudates and maintaining wound moisture. Moreover, their notable bioadhesive strength ensured secure adherence to the skin. The study also addressed the critical aspect of painless removal, emphasizing the importance of self-adhesiveness in wound dressings (36).

In a study by Long et al. (2019), an innovative wound dressing was developed through the integration of 3D-printing technology, utilizing a chitosan-pectin hydrogel infused with lidocaine. Chitosan boasts a range of advantageous characteristics for skin applications, including bioadhesives, biocompatibility, biodegradability, and nontoxicity, as well as antimicrobial, antioxidant, hemocompatible, and hemostatic properties. The researchers employed a combination of SSE and lyophilization techniques in the fabrication of hydrogel scaffolds. These scaffolds exhibited exceptional attributes conducive to an optimal wound-healing environment (37). They demonstrated a notable swelling ratio and water absorption capacity, underscoring their proficiency in exudate absorption and wound moisture retention. Moreover, the robust bioadhesion strength indicated strong self-adherence to the skin. The study emphasized the importance of wound dressings being both self-adhesive and easy to remove without causing discomfort. The investigation encompassed the evaluation of various drug concentrations, all of which exhibited a rapid initial drug release within the first hour, followed by a sustained release pattern. This controlled release mechanism was attributed to the effective entrapment of lidocaine within the polymer matrix. This research breakthrough represents a significant advancement in wound dressing technology, offering potential benefits for improved wound healing outcomes and enhanced patient comfort (38).

In a study conducted by Navarro et al. (2020), a keratin-based scaffold was effectively engineered to carry halofuginone for the treatment of burn wound healing. Halofuginone, a Food and Drug Administration–approved compound, functions as an inhibitor of collagen I synthesis. This property is pivotal in impeding the buildup of aberrant fibrillar collagen, a phenomenon linked to fibrosis and wound contracture (39).

During the wound-healing process, infections can pose significant challenges, potentially leading to delays in recovery and adversely affecting pain levels and overall quality of life. In a study by Singh and colleagues (2021), a solution was proposed. They designed and assessed neomycin-loaded poly lactic acid (PLA) mats using FDM 3D-printing technology, aiming to serve as both wound coverings and a means for antibiotic delivery. The process involved printing the PLA mats and subsequently immersing them, either in molten polyethylene glycol (PEG) or in molten PEG containing neomycin, to facilitate drug incorporation into the mats (40).

A compelling approach in dermal treatments involves the utilization of stimulus-responsive systems for therapeutic drug delivery. Niziol et al. (2021) introduced a noteworthy concept involving a thermoresponsive hydrogel containing Octenisept®. This antimicrobial agent is constituted of octenidine dihydrochloride and 2-phenoxyethanol, and it holds promise for wound-healing applications. The authors utilized SSE in the production of these hydrogel-based dressings, which are formulated with poly(N-isopropylacrylamide) precursors, sodium alginate, and methylcellulose (41).

Bom and colleagues (2020) pioneered the creation of a dermal drug delivery system utilizing alginate–pre-gelatinized starch as its foundation. The team opted for SSE as the chosen 3D printing method, and they meticulously assessed the process parameters through a quality design approach. The incorporation of starch resulted in an augmentation of both the size and the quantity of open pores, potentially influencing drug release characteristics. During in vitro testing, the alginate-starch patches exhibited a more pronounced burst effect compared to those comprised solely of alginate. This phenomenon was attributed to the swelling properties inherent to starch (42).

The 3D-printed hydrogels, including the blank hydrogel, camptothecin (CPT)-loaded hydrogel, and CPT niosomal-loaded hydrogel, exhibited commendable bio-adhesion, gel strength, and extrusion properties. Additionally, the in vitro release studies indicated that the CPT niosomes loaded with hydrogel demonstrated a notable ability to regulate drug release, extending up to 96 hours. This formulation displayed a lower release rate (61.5%) in contrast to the CPT-loaded hydrogel, which released at a rate of 78.6% (43).

4.5.2 PEPTIDES AND PROTEINS

Indeed, in recent years, there has been a significant surge in research concerning the dermal application of proteins and peptides for treating skin disorders. These large molecules hold substantial relevance for locally addressing various skin ailments. Enhancing their targeted delivery to specific sites on the skin stands as a crucial objective in this field of study (44).

Acetyl-hexapeptide-3 (AHP-3) is a compact peptide employed in dermal applications for its noteworthy anti-wrinkle properties. Despite its effectiveness and safety profile, its ability to permeate the skin is restricted by its relatively high molecular weight and hydrophilic nature. Addressing this, Lim et al. (2020) introduced a personalized 3D-printed microneedle patch, employing a "poke to patch" strategy for the delivery of the AHP-3 solution. While the authors mentioned transdermal delivery, their primary focus was on dermal application (45, 46).

In a study by Derakhshandeh et al. (2020), the FDM technique was employed to create miniature hollow needles capable of administering vascular endothelial growth factor (VEGF) to the deeper layers of the wound bed. The researchers introduced a drug solution into these miniature needles through a wireless stimulus (47).

Healing wounds in diabetic patients remains a significant challenge for both medical practitioners and formulation experts, primarily due to prolonged and persistent inflammation. Addressing this issue, Wan et al. (2019) introduced a bilayered skin substitute. The top layer was constructed using a gelatin cryogel infused with silver, serving as a protective barrier against bacterial infections. Silver is known for its potent antimicrobial properties. The bottom layer, by comparison, incorporated platelet-derived growth factor-BB, a growth factor widely applied in diabetic wound healing (47, 48).

4.5.3 METALS METAL COMPOUNDS

Metals and metal compounds play a crucial role in both wound healing and scar formation. They serve as catalysts for vital enzymes, constitute structural elements in proteins and transcription factors, and can even influence their activity by inducing conformational changes. Metals have the capacity to regulate various stages of the healing process, including hemostasis, inflammation, proliferation, and maturation. When used in conjunction with conventional medical treatments, they have the potential to enhance and optimize these processes (48).

In terms of its properties, zinc plays a critical role in various physiological processes, including growth, immune function, and wound healing. Additionally, it has been proposed that zinc disrupts bacterial cell membranes and promotes skin regeneration through cell proliferation. Copper is known to impact membrane integrity and essential functions of microbial cells, facilitating angiogenesis in the wound area by inducing VEGF. The antimicrobial properties of silver result in the lysis of bacterial cells and the potential modification of vital functions like energy production, although concerns persist about its toxicity (49). Manganese, a significant metal, can influence collagen contraction when bound to the enzyme superoxide dismutase. Moreover, it is linked to protection against UV-induced photoaging and the acceleration of wound healing. Potassium permanganate, recognized for its potent oxidase properties, finds widespread use in wound treatment, disinfection, and managing inflammatory skin conditions, such as contact dermatitis and psoriasis (50).

Muwaffak et al. (2017) engineered 3D-printed wound dressings with antimicrobial properties, enriched with zinc, copper, and silver ions. The filament was created through hot-melt extrusion utilizing Polycaprolactone (PCL). Subsequently, metal ions were integrated into the polymer, followed by the FDM printing process. It was observed that reinforcing the dressings with additional shells resulted in greater strength. However, this augmentation also led to a compromise in structural quality and prolonged the printing duration (51, 52).

Afghah and colleagues developed 3D-printed scaffolds utilizing copolymers of polycaprolactone-block-poly(1,3-propylene succinate) that were enriched with silver nitrate. The incorporation of silver nitrate was achieved through polymer impregnation prior to extrusion. The utilization of copolymers in this study aimed to enhance the physical and mechanical attributes of the filaments, all while requiring a lower processing temperature in comparison to pure PCL. This feature holds significant importance for integrating thermolabile active agents. The resulting 3D-printed scaffold exhibited heightened hydrolytic and enzymatic degradation behavior, along with improved hydrophobicity. The scaffold was meticulously designed to possess a porous structure with interconnected pores, ensuring optimal oxygenation within the wound environment (53).

Shi and colleagues (2019) investigated the potential of employing a 3D-printed dressing membrane that was infused with silver nanoparticles (AgNPs) and oil for treating infected wounds. In this research, polydimethylsiloxane (PMDS) served as the primary polymer matrix for SSE printing, chosen for its biocompatibility and nontoxic characteristics. The incorporation of silicone oil aimed to enhance the nonfouling properties of PMDS and create a smooth surface. Importantly, the release of silver from the membranes was sustained, which is a desirable feature for effective wound treatment (54).

Wu and colleagues (2019) employed FDM to create porous PLA templates. Hydrogel precursors were then cast within these templates, followed by the subsequent removal of the templates. This process yielded a highly porous polyacrylamide/HPMC hydrogel dressing containing cross-linked AgNPs within the hydrogel matrix. This innovative dressing demonstrated commendable cytocompatibility, potent antibacterial activity, and rapid water absorption capacity (54, 55).

4.5.4 Natural Compounds

Exploring natural compounds as a potential alternative for combating infections has been widely documented. Traditional practices across diverse cultures have historically utilized plants as rudimentary wound dressings, while contemporary researchers have subsequently investigated and confirmed the antibacterial, antioxidant, and antifungal properties of specific compounds, among other notable activities (55).

Aranci et al. (2020) found out the functional properties of three printing scaffolds loaded with plant propolis extract. Propolis is a type of plant resin synthesized by bees for hive protection, with well-described effects of antifungal, antibacterial, anti-inflammatory, antiviral, and antioxidant (56).

Andriotis and colleagues (2020) innovated by developing 3D-printed patches composed of a naturally derived compound, such as pectin and manuka honey, and a complex structure of chitosan, beta-cyclodextrin, and propolis extract, which were prepared using SSE. Propolis was chosen as the main ingredient, and the primary objective of their research was to utilize these patches to retain wound moisture and shield it against potential infections and contaminants (57).

Aloe Vera has also been widely studied in wound healing due to its outstanding anti-inflammatory, antioxidant, and antimicrobial effects. Furthermore, certain essential oils, such as eucalyptus essential oil, have garnered attention in the pharmaceutical sector. They have been the subjects of research for their potential in wound healing, attributed to the analgesic, anti-inflammatory, antioxidant, antifungal, and antiradical properties of their terpenes. Karavasili fabricated 3D-printed scaffolds incorporating three distinct natural substances: manuka honey, aloe vera, and eucalyptus essential oil. The polymers employed were alginate and methylcellulose, with the active ingredients being blended with the polymers prior to SSE 3D printing. Nano-indentation and finite element analysis were conducted for mechanical assessment (58). These studies revealed that varying concentrations of the bioactive elements had an impact on the tensile strengths of the scaffolds, notably affecting their elastic moduli. Specifically, an increase in manuka honey and aloe vera content correlated with a decrease in these mechanical properties. Notably, all the printed scaffolds exhibited notable antibacterial and anti-biofilm activity against both gram-positive and gram-negative bacteria (59, 60).

4.6 CONCLUSION

The application of 3D printing in dermal drug delivery holds significant promise for revolutionizing the field of dermatology and personalized medicine. By leveraging this technology, we can enhance the effectiveness of dermal treatments while minimizing adverse effects, ultimately improving patient outcomes. Three-dimensional printing has emerged as a groundbreaking technology with immense promise in the realm of dermal drug delivery. Its ability to customize dosage forms and tailor them to individual patients' needs marks a significant advancement in pharmaceutical manufacturing. The exponential growth of 3D printing in recent years underscores its potential to revolutionize the development of dermal products. This innovative approach allows for precise control over critical dosage form parameters such as size, dose, and drug release profile. Additionally, the versatility of 3D printing enables the incorporation of a wide range of materials, including drugs, metals, proteins, and natural compounds. This opens up new possibilities for creating advanced and multifunctional dermal products. Furthermore, the cost-effective production of high-complexity devices through 3D printing holds the promise of improving accessibility to specialized dermal treatments. Customized dressings, tailored to individual wound shapes and requirements, represent a significant leap forward in wound care. The undeniable advantages that arise from the convergence of 3D printing and dermal drugs, including enhanced patient quality of life and treatment efficacy, signal a transformative shift in health care practices. This review serves as a cornerstone for further studies, encouraging continued exploration of 3D printing's potential in developing advanced dermal drug delivery systems. In summary, the integration of 3D printing technology in dermal drug delivery presents a remarkable leap forward in personalized medicine. Its potential to optimize therapy, improve patient outcomes, and advance wound care demonstrates a bright future for this innovative approach in the pharmaceutical industry.

ACKNOWLEDGMENTS

The authors express their sincere gratitude to the host institutions for generously providing all the necessary facilities throughout the course of this study.

FUNDING

None.

CONFLICT OF INTEREST

None.

REFERENCES

1. Machado AC, Lopes PS, Raffier CP, Haridass IN, Roberts M, Grice J, Leite-Silva VR. Skin Penetration. In: Sakamoto K, Lochhead H, Maibach H, Yamashita Y, editors. *Cosmetic Science and Technology.* Elsevier; Amsterdam, The Netherlands: 2017:741–755.

2. Seth D, Cheldize K, Brown D, Freeman EE. Global burden of skin disease: Inequities and innovations. *Curr. Dermatol. Rep.* 2017;6:204–210.

3. Dąbrowska AK, Spano F, Derler S, Adlhart C, Spencer ND, Rossi RM. The relationship between skin function, barrier properties, and body-dependent factors. *Skin Res. Technol.* 2018;24:165–174.

4. Benson HAE, Grice JE, Mohammed Y, Namjoshi S, Roberts MS. Topical and transdermal drug delivery: From simple potions to smart technologies. *Curr. Drug Deliv.* 2019;16:444–460.

5. Flohr C, Hay R. Putting the burden of skin diseases on the global map. *Br. J. Dermatol.* 2021;184:189–190.

6. Lim HW, Collins SAB, Resneck JS, Bolognia JL, Hodge JA, Rohrer TA, Van Beek MJ, Margolis DJ, Sober AJ, Weinstock MA, et al. The burden of skin disease in the United States. *J. Am. Acad. Dermatol.* 2017;76:958–972.

7. Fonder MA, Lazarus G, Cowan DA, Aronson-Cook B, Kohli AR, Mamelak AJ. Treating the chronic wound: A practical approach to the care of nonhealing wounds and wound care dressings. *J. Am. Acad. Dermatol.* 2008;58:185–206.

8. dos Santos J, Oliveira RS, Oliveira TV, Velho MC, Konrad MV, da Silva GS, Deon M, Beck RCR. 3D printing and nanotechnology: A multiscale alliance in personalized medicine. *Adv. Funct. Mater.* 2021;31:2009691.

9. Maver T, Smrke DM, Kurečič M, Gradišnik L, Maver U, Kleinschek KS. Combining 3D printing and electrospinning for preparation of pain-relieving wound-dressing materials. *J. Sol-Gel Sci. Technol.* 2018;88:33–48.

10. Seoane-Viaño I, Januskaite P, Alvarez-Lorenzo C, Basit AW, Goyanes A. Semi-solid extrusion 3D printing in drug delivery and biomedicine: Personalised solutions for healthcare challenges. *J. Control. Release* 2021;332:367–389.

11. de Oliveira RS, Fantanus SS. Food and drug administration (FDA) approval letter-spritam. accessed on 28 July 2021. https://www.accessdata.fda.gov/drugsatfda_docs/nda/2015/207958Orig1s000Approv.pdf

12. Jamróz W, Szafraniec J, Kurek M, Jachowicz R. 3D printing in pharmaceutical and medical applications–recent achievements and challenges. *Pharm. Res.* 2018;35:1–22.

13. Wang J, Goyanes A, Gaisford S, Basit AW. Stereolithographic (SLA) 3D printing of oral modified-release dosage forms. *Int. J. Pharm.* 2016;35:176.

14. Li Q, Guan X, Cui M, Zhu Z, Chen K, Wen H, Jia D, Hou J, Xu W, Yang X. Preparation and investigation of novel gastro-floating tablets with 3D extrusion-based printing. *Int. J. Pharm.* 2018;503:207–212.

15. Fina F, Madla CM, Goyanes A, Zhang J, Gaisford S, Basit AW. Fabricating 3D printed orally disintegrating printlets using selective laser sintering. *Int. J. Pharm.* 2018;541:101–107.

16. Khaled SA, Burley JC, Alexander MR, Yang J, Roberts CJ. 3D printing of tablets containing multiple drugs with defined release profiles. *Int. J. Pharm.* 2015;494:643–650.

17. Madni A, Kousar R, Naeem N, Wahid F. Recent advancements in applications of chitosan-based biomaterials for skin tissue engineering. *J. Bioresour. Bioprod.* 2021;6:11–25.

18. Manita PG, Garcia-Orue I, Santos-Vizcaino E, Hernandez RM, Igartua M. 3D bioprinting of functional skin substitutes: From current achievements to future goals. *Pharmaceuticals* 2021;14:362.

19. van Kogelenberg S, Yue Z, Dinoro JN, Baker CS, Wallace GG. Three-dimensional printing and cell therapy for wound repair. *Adv. Wound Care* 2018;7:145–156.

20. Chen G, Xu Y, Chi Lip Kwok P, Kang L. Pharmaceutical applications of 3D printing: A review *Addit. Manuf.* 2020;593:120106.

21. Yang Q, Zhong W, Xu L, Li H, Yan Q, She Y, Yang G. Recent progress of 3D-printed microneedles for transdermal drug delivery. *Int. J. Pharm.* 2021;25:593.

22. Tan SH, Ngo ZH, Leavesley D, Liang K. Recent advances in the design of three-dimensional and bioprinted scaffolds for full-thickness wound healing. *Tissue Eng. Part B Rev.* 2021;28:160–181.

23. Economidou SN, Lamprou DA, Douroumis D. 3D printing applications for transdermal drug delivery. *Int. J. Pharm.* 2018;544:415–424.

24. Fayyazbakhsh F, Leu MC. A brief review on 3D bioprinted skin substitutes. *Procedia Manuf.* 2020;48:790–796.

25. Singh Malik D, Mital N, Kaur G. Topical drug delivery systems: A patent review. *Expert Opin. Ther. Pat.* 2016;26:213–228.

26. Chen Y, Feng X, Meng S Site-specific drug delivery in the skin for the localized treatment of skin diseases. *Expert Opin. Drug Deliv.* 2019;16:847–867.

27. Leite-Silva VR, De Almeida MM, Fradin A, Grice JE, Roberts MS. Delivery of drugs applied topically to the skin. *Expert Rev. Dermatol.* 2012;7:383–397.

28. Koppa Raghu P, Bansal KK, Thakor P, Bhavana V, Madan J, Rosenholm JM, Mehra NK. Evolution of nanotechnology in delivering drugs to eyes, skin and wounds via topical route. *Pharmaceuticals* 2020;13:167.

29. Javadzadeh Y, Bahari LA. Therapeutic Nanostructures for Dermal and Transdermal Drug Delivery. In: Grumezescu AM, editor. *Nano- and Microscale Drug Delivery Systems.* Elsevier Inc.; Amsterdam, The Netherlands: 2017:131–146.

30. Wiedersberg S, Leopold CS, Guy RH. Bioavailability and bioequivalence of topical glucocorticoids. *Eur. J. Pharm. Biopharm.* 2008;(68):453–466.

31. Mishra DK, Pandey V, Maheshwari R, Ghode P, Tekade RK. Cutaneous and Transdermal Drug Delivery: Techniques and Delivery Systems Dinesh. In: Tekade RK, editor. *Basic Fundamentals of Drug Delivery.* Elsevier; Amsterdam, The Netherlands: 2019;7:383–397.

32. Namjoshi S, Dabbaghi M, Roberts MS, Grice JE, Mohammed Y. Quality by design: Development of the quality target product profile (QTPP) for semisolid topical products. *Pharmaceutics* 2020;12:131–146.

33. Mayba JN, Gooderham MJ. A guide to topical vehicle formulations. *J. Cutan. Med. Surg.* 2018;22:207–212.

34. Trenfield SJ, Awad A, Goyanes A, et al. 3D printing pharmaceuticals: Drug development to frontline care. *Trends Pharmacol. Sci.* 2018;39:440–451.

35. Maher RL, Hanlon J, Hajjar ER. Clinical consequences of polypharmacy in elderly. *Expert Opin. Drug Saf.* 2013;13:57–65.

36. Alomari M, Vuddanda PR, Trenfield SJ, et al. Printing T3 and T4 oral drug combinations as a novel strategy for hypothyroidism. *Int. J. Pharm.* 2018;549:363–369.

37. Awad A, Yao A, Trenfield SJ, Goyanes A, Gaisford S, Basit AW. 3D printed tablets (printlets) with braille and moon patterns for visually impaired patients. *Pharmaceutics* 2020; 12(2):172.

38. Long J, Gholizadeh H, Lu J, Bunt C, Seyfoddin A. Application of fused deposition modelling (FDM) method of 33D printing in drug delivery. *Curr. Pharm. Des.* Dec 2017;23:433–439.

39. Navarro J, Clohessy RM, Holder RC, Gabard AR, Herendeen GJ, Christy RJ, Burnett LR, Fisher JP. In vivo evaluation of three-dimensional printed, keratin-based hydrogels in a porcine thermal burn model. *Tissue Eng. Part A* 2020;26:265–278.

40. Singh M, Jonnalagadda S. Design and characterization of 3D printed, neomycin-eluting poly-L-lactide mats for wound-healing applications. *J. Mater. Sci. Mater. Med.* 2021;32:44.

41. Nizioł M, Paleczny J, Junka A, Shavandi A, Dawiec-Liśniewska A, Podstawczyk D. 3D printing of thermoresponsive hydrogel laden with an antimicrobial agent towards wound Alomari M, Vuddanda PR, Trenfield SJ, et al. Printing T3 and T4 oral drug combinations as a novel strategy for hypothyroidism. *Int. J. Pharm.* 2018;549:363–369.

42. Bom S, Santos C, Barros R, Martins AM, Paradiso P, Cláudio R, Pinto PC, Ribeiro HM, Marto J Effects of starch incorporation on the physicochemical properties and release kinetics of alginate-based 3D hydrogel patches for topical delivery. *Pharmaceutics* 2020;12:719.

43. Goyanes A, Madla, CM, Umerji A, Duran Pineiro G, Giraldez Montero JM,Lamas Diaz MJ, Gonzalez Barcia M, Taherali F, Sanchez-Pintos P, Couce ML,Gaisford S, Basit AW. Automated therapy preparation of isoleucine formulationsusing 3D printing for the treatment of MSUD: First single-centre, prospective,crossover study in patients. *Int. J. Pharm.* Jul 2019;567:118497.

44. Trenfield SJ, Madla CM, Basit AW, Gaisford S. The shape of things to come: Emerging applications of 3D printing in healthcare, AAPS *Adv. Pharm. Sci. Ser.* 2018;31:1–19.

45. Lim SH, Ng JY, Kang L. Three-dimensional printing of a microneedle array on personalized curved surfaces for dual-pronged treatment of trigger finger. *Biofabrication* Jan 10 2017;9(1):015010.

46. Tagami T, Ando M, Nagata N, Goto E, Yoshimura N, Takeuchi T, Noda T,Ozeki T. Fabrication of naftopidil-loaded tablets using a semisolid extrusion-type3D printer and the characteristics of the printed hydrogel and resulting tablets. *J.Pharm. Sci.* 2019;108(2):907–913.

47. Derakhshandeh H, Aghabaglou F, McCarthy A, Mostafavi A, Wiseman C, Bonick Z, Ghanavati I, Harris S, Kreikemeier-Bower C, Moosavi Basri SM, et al. A wirelessly controlled smart bandage with 3D-printed miniaturized needle arrays. *Adv. Funct. Mater.* Feb 2020, 30(13):1905544.

48. Wang X, Qi J, Zhang W, Pu Y, Yang R, Wang P, Liu S, Tan X, Chi B. 3D-printed antioxidant antibacterial carboxymethyl cellulose/ε-polylysine hydrogel promoted skin wound repair. *Int. J. Biol. Macromol.* 2021;187:91–104.

49. Jyothi SL, Krishna KL, Ameena Shirin VK, Sankar R, Pramod K, Gangadharappa HV. Drug delivery systems for the treatment of psoriasis: Current status and prospects. *J. Drug Deliv. Sci. Technol* 2021;62:102364.

50. Pavithran K. Psoriasis: Topical treatment. *Indian J. Dermatol. Venereol. Leprol.* 2001;67 :85.

51. Muwaffak Z, Goyanes A, Clark V, Basit AW, Hilton ST, Gaisford S. Patient-specific 3D scanned and 3D printed antimicrobial polycaprolactone wound dressings. *Int. J. Pharm.* 2017;527:161–170.

52 Afghah F, Ullah M, Seyyed Monfared Zanjani J, Akkus Sut P, Sen O, Emanet M, .Saner Okan B, Culha M, Menceloglu Y, Yildiz M, Koc B. 3D printing of silver-doped polycaprolactone-poly (propylene succinate) composite scaffolds for skin tissue engineering. *Biomed. Mater.* Apr 15 2020;15:035015.

53. Hu Y, Wu B, Xiong Y, Tao R, Panayi AC, Chen L, Tian W, Xue H, Shi L, Zhang X, et al. Cryogenic 3D printed hydrogel scaffolds loading exosomes accelerate diabetic wound healing. *Chem. Eng. J.* 2021;426:130634.

54. Shi L, Hu Y, Ullah MW, Ullah I, Ou H, Zhang W, Xiong L, Zhang X. Cryogenic free-form extrusion bioprinting of decellularized small intestinal submucosa for potential applications in skin tissue engineering. *Biofabrication* 2019;11:035023.

55. Wu Y. Electrohydrodynamic jet 3D printing in biomedical applications. *Acta Biomater.* 2021;128:21–41.

56. Tian Y, Orlu M, Woerdenbag HJ, Scarpa M, Kiefer O, Kottke D, Sjöholm E, Öblom H, Sandler N, Hinrichs WLJ, et al. Oromucosal films: From patient centricity to production by printing techniques. *Expert Opin. Drug Deliv.* 2019;16:981–993.

57. Aranci K, Uzun M, Su S, Cesur S, Ulag S, Amin A, Guncu MM, Aksu B, Kolayli S, Ustundag CB, et al. 3D propolis-sodium alginate scaffolds: influence on structural parameters, release mechanisms, cell cytotoxicity and antibacterial activity. *Molecules* 2020;25:5082.

58. Karavasili C, Tsongas K, Andreadis II, Andriotis EG, Papachristou ET, Papi RM, Tzetzis D, Fatouros DG. Physico-mechanical and finite element analysis evaluation of 3D printable alginate-methylcellulose inks for wound healing applications. *Carbohydrate Polymer* 2020;247:116666.

59. Xu X, Robles-Martinez P, Madla CM, Joubert F, Goyanes A, Basit AW, Gaisford S. Stereolithography (SLA) 3D printing of an antihypertensive polyprintlet: Case study of an unexpected photopolymer-drug reaction. *Addit. Manuf.* 2020;33:101071.

60. Surjushe A, Vasani R, Saple D. Aloe vera: A short review. *Indian J. Dermatol.* 2008;53:163.

5 3D Printing for *In Vitro* and *In Vivo* Skin Disease Models

Monika Bhairam, Bina Gidwani, Ravindra Kumar Pandey, and Shiv Shankar Shukla
Columbia Institute of Pharmacy, Raipur, India

5.1 INTRODUCTION

Biomedical research predominantly focuses on the advancement of novel and more efficient tools and technologies, such as biosensors, biomaterials, image processing, and artificial intelligence. These innovations aim to enhance disease diagnosis, prevention, and therapeutic strategies. In order to anticipate treatment responses prior to human clinical trials, medical researchers must possess a comprehensive understanding of the intricate biological mechanisms associated with a particular ailment. This understanding encompasses physiological, cellular, molecular, and genetic aspects (1). To achieve this, it is imperative to employ modeling systems that can faithfully replicate the microenvironment within the human body. Both *in vitro* and *in vivo* disease models are integral components of scientific inquiry, offering invaluable insights into health-related concerns and driving progress in the realm of biomedical research (2). Conventional disease models have played pivotal roles in augmenting our comprehension of various medical conditions. These models find applications in diverse areas such as disease diagnostics, therapeutic development, surgical research, toxicological assessments, and drug screening. In order to successfully address health issues, biomedical research is a discipline that is continually seeking to create cutting-edge techniques and technology (3). These developments are crucial for increasing the precision and effectiveness of disease diagnosis, identifying improved methods of disease prevention, and developing more focused and effective therapeutic strategies. For example, biosensors are essential for identifying and quantifying particular proteins that may be used as disease indicators. Medical implants, drug delivery systems, and tissue engineering all heavily rely on biomaterials. The interpretation of medical images has been revolutionized by image processing and artificial intelligence, enabling quicker and more accurate diagnosis and treatment planning. Researchers rely on modeling systems that can accurately reproduce the intricate milieu of organs and tissues for the accuracy of these predictions. In order to test therapies on humans before conducting studies in a controlled environment, these modeling systems are created to simulate the conditions encountered in the human body (4).

DOI: 10.1201/9781032690926-5

Medical researchers need a solid grasp of the underlying molecular mechanisms of a disease in order to create effective remedies. This entails researching the malfunctioning physiological systems, cellular reactions, molecular interactions, and genetic elements that contribute to the onset and development of the disease. Before beginning human clinical trials, such thorough knowledge is necessary to foresee how new medicines would function as well as any potential adverse effects or restrictions. *In vitro* and *in vivo* models are the two main categories of disease models used in biomedical research. Studying cells or tissues outside of a living creature, usually in a laboratory dish, is known as *in vitro* modelling. Understanding cellular behavior and interactions in a controlled environment is made possible by these models. *In vivo* models, by comparison, involve examining illnesses in living things, such as animals, to see how the illness develops in a more intricate biological setting (2). Conventional illness models have been useful in expanding medical understanding and applicability among the numerous disease models. These models are well known and frequently employed in research. They have significantly advanced our understanding of illnesses, paving the way for the development of effective surgical, medicinal, and diagnostic procedures. Before advancing to human clinical trials, these models are essential for evaluating the effectiveness and safety of new drugs and treatment modalities. While traditional skin disease models (SDMs) have been very helpful, current research is looking toward more sophisticated and personalized models that more accurately mimic the human microenvironment and reflect diseases even more accurately. Improved patient outcomes are the ultimate goal of this endeavor, which strives to increase the effectiveness and efficiency of biomedical research (5).

In this chapter, we have covered several important topics related to 3D printing's pivotal roles in the field of medicine and healthcare. These include exploring the significance of 3D printing in advanced skin tissue engineering through techniques like 3D cell printing. Furthermore, we delve into the fundamental concepts of 3D printing for both *in vitro* and *in vivo* SDMs, addressing the pressing need for such technology. The process of generating personalized models for clinical trials is elaborated, followed by an overview of diverse 3D-printed disease models. We showcase the convergence of 3D printing and microfluidics in dermatology for innovative drug delivery solutions. Additionally, we highlight recent research endeavors in this field and conclude by envisioning the prospective horizons and pathways for further advancements (6).

5.2 THE CRUCIAL ROLES OF 3DPRINTING IN HEALTH CARE

Three-dimensional printing, often referred to as additive manufacturing, represents a groundbreaking manufacturing technique that constructs 3D objects by incrementally adding material layer on layer. This stands in stark contrast to conventional subtractive manufacturing processes, where the material is removed from a larger block to shape the final product. Three-dimensional printing has found applications in various industries, including rapid prototyping, and allows for quick and cost-effective testing of product designs before mass production (7). It is used in small-scale production of customized or low-volume parts and products. This is also used in medical and healthcare sectors for creating patient-specific implants, prosthetics, surgical models, and drug delivery systems. Three-dimensional printing is valuable in educational settings for creating models and prototypes and facilitating research. Three-dimensional printing is a revolutionary technology with remarkable versatility, speed, and customization capabilities. Its transformative potential extends across diverse industries. As the technology continues to advance, its impact is anticipated to deepen further, revolutionizing manufacturing, healthcare, and various other fields in profound ways (8).

Three-dimensional printing has a significant role in medicine and the healthcare sector, revolutionizing various aspects of medical design, patient care, and research. Its versatility, speed, and customization capabilities make it a valuable tool in improving medical treatments and advancing healthcare as illustrated in Figure 5.1. Here are some significant contributions of 3D printing to the field of medicine.

5.2.1 Medical Device Customization

This technology facilitates the manufacturing of medical devices customized for individual patients, including implants, prosthetics, and surgical instruments. Customizing these devices to match each individual's unique anatomy results in superior outcomes and enhanced patient comfort (2).

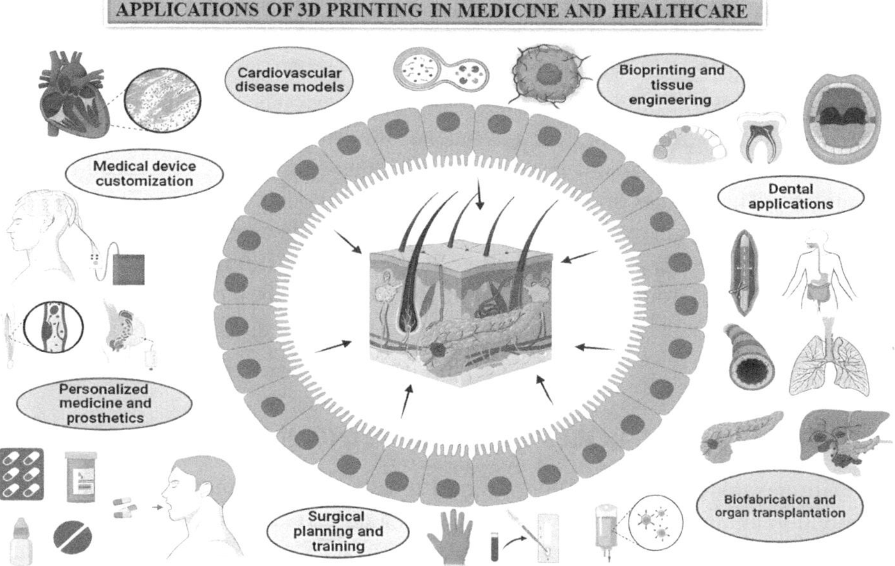

FIGURE 5.1 The manifold applications of 3D printing in the medical and healthcare industries.

[Note: All the diagrammatic illustration are taken from biorender website and arranged after modification (60)].

5.2.2 Personalized Medicine and Prosthetics

Three-dimensional printing enables the production of patient-specific medications, tailoring the drug dose and release profile to individual patients based on their unique characteristics and needs. Patient-specific dosage forms can be particularly useful for individuals with difficulty swallowing pills, pediatric patients, or patients with specific medical conditions. Three-dimensional printing enables the production of custom-fit prosthetic limbs and orthotic devices for patients with amputations or musculoskeletal disorders. This technology allows for a more precise fit and enhances mobility and quality of life for the patients (9).

5.2.3 Surgical Planning and Training

The utilization of 3D-printed anatomical models, generated from a patient's medical imaging data, empowers surgeons to efficiently plan intricate surgeries. This valuable tool aids in comprehending the patient's anatomy and facilitates preoperative rehearsals, ultimately contributing to improved surgical outcomes and reduced operating time.

5.2.4 Patient-Specific Drug Delivery

Through 3D printing, personalized drug delivery systems like implants or microneedles can be crafted to precisely release medications at specific rates and targeted locations within the body. This tailored approach enhances treatment adherence and effectiveness while minimizing the occurrence of side effects.

5.2.5 Bioprinting and Tissue Engineering

A specialized application of 3D printing, known as 3D bioprinting, allows for the fabrication of biological tissues and structures using living cells and biomaterials. This advanced technology holds significant potential in the fields of tissue engineering, regenerative medicine, and the creation of organ-on-a-chip models, offering greater precision in drug testing and research (10).

5.2.6 Education and Medical Training

Medical professionals and medical students have access to useful instructional resources thanks to 3D printing. It enables the development of surgical simulators and anatomical models, boosting learning and training in surgery.

5.2.7 Pharmaceutical Manufacturing

Three-dimensional printing is employed in pharmaceuticals to create personalized medications, particularly for patients with specific dosing requirements or difficulty swallowing traditional pills. It also aids in the rapid prototyping of drug formulations and drug delivery systems.

5.2.8 DENTAL APPLICATIONS

Dental models, surgical guides, and individualized dental restorations like crowns and dentures are all made possible by 3D printing in the area of dentistry. This cutting-edge technology simplifies the dentist office process and improves treatment precision, resulting in more effective and accurate dental care (11).

5.2.9 DRUG DEVELOPMENT AND FORMULATION

Pharmaceutical businesses can more quickly test different medication formulations and dosage forms thanks to 3D printing, which enables fast prototyping of drug formulations. It makes it easier to create sophisticated medication delivery systems, such as multilayered tablets or custom drug formulations, to address the unique requirements of each patient (12).

5.2.10 ON-DEMAND MANUFACTURING

Drug production may be decentralized via 3D printing, which has major benefits for isolated or underserved locations by reducing reliance on complex delivery systems. On-demand medicine manufacture is also made possible by this innovative technology, which lowers waste and lessens the likelihood of drug shortages while improving medication accessibility and availability.

5.2.11 BIOFABRICATION AND ORGAN TRANSPLANTATION

Despite the fact that they are still in their infancy, 3D printing and bioprinting hold enormous promise for producing complex organs and tissues that are safe for transplant. With the potential to save many lives in the future, this groundbreaking technique provides promise for tackling organ scarcity and revolutionizing the field of organ transplantation.

5.2.12 PREOPERATIVE PLANNING AND SURGICAL MODELS

Using 3D-printed anatomical models developed from a patient's medical imaging data gives surgeons the capability to more effectively plan difficult operations. This groundbreaking device helps save operating times and enhance surgical results, which ultimately improves patient care and healing (11).

5.2.13 DRUG COUNTERFEITING PREVENTION

Pharmaceutical companies can produce unique, hard-to-replicate medication components using 3D printing, thereby thwarting drug fraud and preserving patient safety. This technique is essential for preserving the validity of medications and improving their general safety and efficacy (13).

5.2.14 CUSTOMIZED MEDICAL DEVICES

Customized health care items such as implants, surgical tools, and prosthetics, which can better match each patient's demands and anatomy, are produced thanks in large part to 3D printing. With the use of this technology, patient-specific medical equipment may be produced more quickly and affordably (8).

5.2.15 Drug Delivery Systems

Three-dimensional printing enables the development and production of intricate drug delivery devices, such as implants, microspheres, and microneedles. The regulated and targeted medicine delivery provided by these devices improves patient compliance and treatment efficacy while reducing the risk of adverse effects. A promising method to improve patient outcomes in medical treatments is to customize medication delivery systems (14).

5.2.16 Clinical Trials and Drug Testing

Prior to mass manufacturing, 3D-printed medication formulations are useful tools in preclinical investigations and clinical trials to assess their safety, effectiveness, and pharmacokinetic characteristics. Additionally, this technology makes it possible to perform medication trials with patient-specific drug formulations, opening the door to more individualized and successful treatment modalities (1).

The utilization of 3D printing in medicine and healthcare is experiencing a rapid ascent, leading to enhanced patient care with personalized and precise therapeutic approaches. Additionally, it has created exciting opportunities for advancements in pharmaceutical and medical research. Three-dimensional printing had a favorable influence on a variety of medical specialties, resulting in improved treatment outcomes. Nevertheless, it is imperative to prioritize rigorous regulation and implement robust quality control procedures to safeguard patient safety and maintain the effectiveness of 3D printing in medical applications. Three-dimensional printing for SDMs refers to the use of 3D-printing technology to create realistic and customized models of human skin affected by various dermatological conditions. These models can be utilized for research, testing, and educational purposes, both *in vitro* (outside the living organism) and *in vivo* (within living organisms) (15).

5.3 3D CELL PRINTING – A STEP TOWARD ADVANCED SKIN TISSUE ENGINEERING

In the realm of medical applications, artificial skin substitutes have traditionally been found useful in cases involving significant wounds. This is because the skin, being the body's largest organ, plays a crucial role in survival by acting as a protective barrier against the external environment. Three-dimensional human skin models have gained popularity recently, and their uses are becoming more widespread in both the scientific and cosmetic industries. A new, more rapid, automatic, and economical fabrication method is therefore urgently needed. Furthermore, the 2013 outright ban on animal testing in the cosmetic industry has made it even more urgent to find novel ways to make complex skin analogues (16).

The exact capacity of the 3D cell printing approach to arrange living cells in preset spatial locations has attracted much attention as a possible biofabrication platform. This special ability enables the construction of complex microenvironments and architectural frameworks that nearly resemble natural skin tissue (9). However, one of the primary challenges in this field is the search for a suitable bioink capable of effectively supporting the functionality of printed cells and promoting the generation of the extracellular matrix (ECM) required for tissue formation.

Bioinks, used in 3D cell printing, differ from traditional biomaterials, posing challenges for certain materials in skin tissue engineering. In typical skin cell printing, dermal fibroblasts and epidermal keratinocytes are printed together in a compatible bioink like alginate, collagen, or fibrin. The ECM heterogeneity present in native skin cannot be perfectly replicated by these purified materials, though (17).

The quest for a more suitable bioink has been ongoing, with researchers exploring various biomaterial formulations to achieve enhanced ECM mimicry and functional support for the printed cells. Finding the right balance between mechanical properties, cell viability, and ECM-inducing capabilities remains a key focus to create skin tissue constructs that more accurately emulate the complexity and functionality of natural skin. With further advancements in bioink technology, 3D cell printing holds tremendous potential to revolutionize skin tissue engineering and open new horizons in regenerative medicine and personalized healthcare (18).

5.4 ADVANCES IN SKIN DISEASE MODELING: 3D PRINTING *IN VITRO* AND *IN VIVO* SCENARIOS

This technology has revolutionized many industries, including medicine and healthcare. In the context of SDMs, 3D printing offers exciting opportunities for creating more realistic and tailored models for both *in vitro* (in the laboratory) and *in vivo* (within living organisms) applications (19).

5.4.1 *IN VITRO* SDMs

In vitro models focus on cultivating and studying skin cells in a controlled laboratory environment. However, conventional 2D cell cultures have shortcomings in accurately replicating the complex structure and behavior of human skin. To overcome this challenge, 3D bioprinting emerges as a specialized application of 3D printing technology, enabling the creation of 3D tissue-like structures using living cells and biomaterials (15). *In vitro* models are employed to study skin diseases in a controlled laboratory environment outside of the living organism. Nevertheless, traditional 2D cell cultures struggle to mimic the intricate 3D structure of human skin. Addressing this limitation, 3D bioprinting offers a groundbreaking solution that empowers researchers to create more lifelike tissue models, bringing us closer to understanding and potentially treating skin diseases more effectively (20).

5.4.1.1 Exploring the Functionality of *in vitro* SDMs

In 3D bioprinting, skin cells, growth factors, and biomaterials are combined to create bioinks, which are loaded into a 3D printer. The printer then deposits these bioinks layer by layer to form a 3D structure that mimics the architecture of human skin.

5.4.1.2 Advantages

Three-dimensional-bioprinted SDMs more accurately replicate the intricate structure and organization of human skin compared to traditional 2D cell cultures. Patient-specific cells can be used to create disease models, allowing researchers to study the unique characteristics of individual patients' skin conditions. Three-dimensional bioprinting can use patient-specific cells to create personalized disease models. This offers the potential to study disease mechanisms and test treatments on a patient-specific basis (9). Three-dimensional-bioprinted models enable the evaluation of the effectiveness and safety of drugs on diseased skin tissues, potentially aiding in drug development. Using 3D-bioprinted models can reduce the need for animal testing in skin disease research. It enables the accurate arrangement of different cell types and ECM components, accurately mimicking the cellular organization and architecture of human skin (3). With 3D-printed SDMs, researchers can more accurately assess the effects of drugs on diseased tissues and potentially accelerate drug development processes. Three-dimensional bioprinting offers a viable alternative to traditional animal testing in skin disease research, diminishing the reliance on animal models (21). Figure 5.2 illustrates all the benefits of *in vitro* SDMs.

5.4.2 *In vivo* SDMs

In vivo models revolve around the study of skin diseases within living organisms, often using animals as test subjects. While 3D bioprinting is not directly used to create

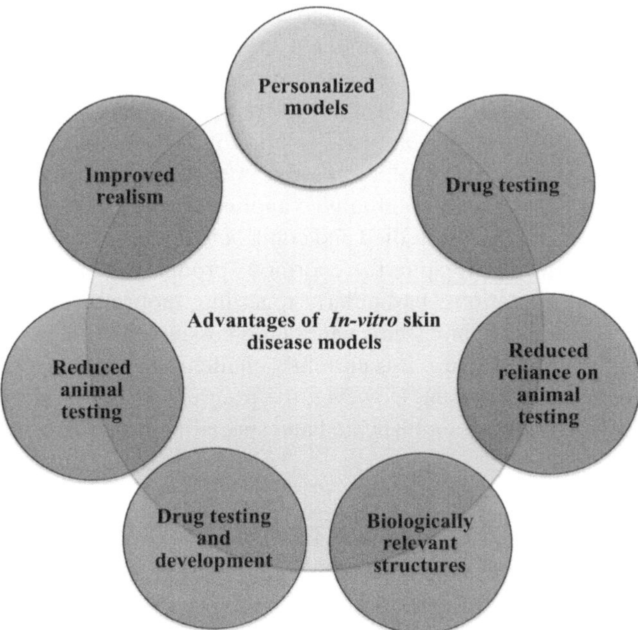

FIGURE 5.2 Various advantages of *in vitro* SDMs.

in vivo models, 3D-printing technology still contributes to this field by enabling the fabrication of personalized devices and implants used in disease research and treatment. *In vivo* models entail the examination of skin diseases within living organisms, commonly utilizing animal subjects for experimentation. Additionally, the development of custom implants, scaffolds, and microdevices for use in *in vivo* environments has found utility for 3D-printing technology. We have come a long way in understanding skin illnesses and investigating new therapeutic approaches thanks to these creative 3D-printed solutions (22).

5.4.2.1 Exploring the Functionality of *in vivo* SDMs

Customized surgical implants, scaffolds, or microdevices can be made via 3D printing and can be utilized to treat skin diseases in animal models. These implants can be used to research *in vivo* medication delivery, tissue regeneration, and wound healing.

5.4.2.2 Advantages

Three-dimensional printing allows the creation of personalized implants that can be tailored to fit individual animals' needs in preclinical research. To treat various skin disorders like severe burns, persistent wounds, or deformities brought on by operations or traumas, 3D printing makes it possible to create scaffolds or implants that are particular to the patient (19). Three-dimensional-printed devices can be designed to deliver drugs or therapeutic agents directly to affected skin areas, enhancing treatment efficiency. Three-dimensional printing can be used to create specialized drug delivery devices that can release medications directly to affected skin areas, offering a more targeted and efficient treatment approach. In cases in which a patient requires skin transplantation, 3D bioprinting can help create custom skin grafts, minimize the risk of refusal, and achieve better graft integration (23). Various advantages of *in vivo* SDMs are represented in Figure 5.3.

Researchers and physicians can use 3D-printing technology to investigate skin illnesses, test treatments, and explore possible medicines in a more individualized and precise way in both *in vitro* and *in vivo* applications (12). It has the potential to change how skin problems are studied and contribute to the eventual development of more effective treatments. Despite the enormous promise of 3D printing, there are still problems and limitations, particularly regarding bioprinting, which should be taken into consideration. Many studies are being conducted to improve the technology and its applications because it is currently challenging to create completely vascularized, functional skin tissue. However, the progress made so far is encouraging and opens the door for more sophisticated and specialized ways to research and treat skin conditions (24).

5.5 SIGNIFICANCE OF 3D PRINTING FOR *IN VITRO* AND *IN VIVO* SDMS

Over the course of numerous years, biologists have heavily relied on a combination of cell culture and mouse models to explore the fundamental cellular mechanisms responsible for human diseases. Despite their limitations, these models have played a crucial role in making significant discoveries and enhancing our comprehension

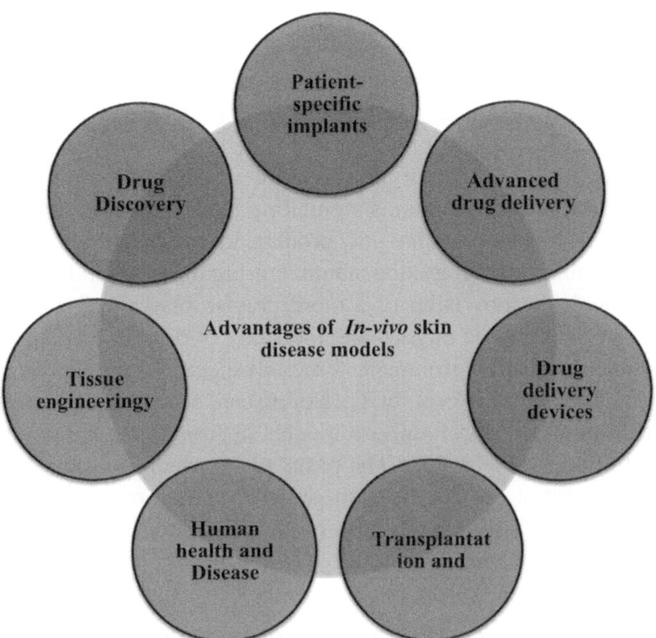

FIGURE 5.3 Various advantages of *in vivo* SDMs.

of various diseases. Although the syntax in this introductory sentence seems to be appropriate, we can expand the content to include more background and examples (25). For many years, biologists have used mice and cell culture models to research the underlying causes of human diseases. Researchers have gained a crucial understanding of how many diseases function by growing cells in a controlled setting or examining animals with disease-like circumstances. These models have been useful resources for understanding biological pathways, locating prospective therapeutic targets, and assessing the effectiveness of treatments. Nevertheless, these traditional cell culture and mouse models fall short in effectively reproducing the intricate tissue microenvironment (µEN). Consequently, the importance of the physical and cellular characteristics of the µEN on the development of illness is being more understood (23). Researchers have recently begun to understand more and more how important a function the physical and biological characteristics of the EN play in the development of illness. The EN can change immunological responses, signaling pathways, and cellular behavior, which has an impact on how diseases begin and progress. For instance, certain molecular alterations and interactions between immune cells and cancer cells inside the tumor microenvironment may encourage the development and metastasis of the primary tumor. Therefore, in order to create more specialized and efficient treatments, it is crucial to comprehend these dynamic interactions within the µEN (26).

This recognition has sparked research into cutting-edge strategies for advancing the complexity 3D *in vitro* models, enabling a deeper understanding of disease causes. The grammar here is correct as well, but we can expand on the significance of developing sophisticated 3D *in vitro* models. The increasing recognition of the µEN's significance has driven researchers to seek alternative approaches that better mimic the complexities of living tissues. There has been a rise in interest in creating sophisticated 3D *in vitro* models as a result, which can better replicate the natural microenvironment. The spatial organization of cells, the connections between various cell types, and the function of the ECM are all captured in these contemporary 3D models with the goal of accurately simulating the intricate details of tissues in the human body (19). Researchers may now produce more physiologically accurate disease models by utilizing cutting-edge manufacturing methods and tissue engineering strategies. Through the provision of a more precise platform for drug testing, the discovery of new therapeutic targets, and the study of disease mechanisms in a controlled yet representative environment, these advanced 3D *in vitro* models have the potential to completely transform the field of disease research. To summaries, biologists have used mouse and cell culture models to investigate human diseases for a long time, with remarkable results. The tissue µEN, which is crucial to the development of disease, cannot be accurately modelled by these models. So, scientists are currently investigating novel 3D *in vitro* models to better understand the causes of diseases and improve treatment approaches (27).

5.6 CRAFTING PERSONALISED 3D-PRINTED HUMAN TISSUE MODELS: THE STEP-BY-STEP PROCEDURE

This section delves into the intricacies of crafting personalized models. This process represents a significant advancement in biomedical engineering, enabling the creation of anatomically accurate and personalized tissue constructs that closely mimic the structure and properties of actual human tissues (28). Various steps are represented here.

5.6.1 CREATING PATIENT

Specific 3D-printed human tissue models are a multistep process that combines medical imaging, computer-aided design (CAD), and 3D-printing technology.

5.6.2 MEDICAL IMAGING

The procedure begins with high-resolution medical pictures of the patient's target tissue or organ obtained by procedures such as CT scans, MRI scans, or ultrasound. These photos give precise information regarding the tissue's architecture, shape, and size (13).

5.6.3 IMAGE SEGMENTATION

The obtained medical pictures are processed in this stage using specialized software to segment and isolate the target tissue or organ. This segmentation results in the creation of a computerized 3D model of the tissue (25).

5.6.4   CAD

The process involves several key stages. First, the segmented 3D model is imported into CAD software. This stage allows for virtual reconstruction and any necessary adjustments to ensure model accuracy before proceeding to 3D printing. Depending on the model's intended purpose, additional modifications can be incorporated to simulate specific scenarios, pathologies, or variations. For instance, a cardiac model might be customized to replicate a particular heart condition. Subsequently, the CAD program generates a 3D-printable file, often in STL format, that represents the tissue model. This file is further processed using slicing software, which divides it into thin layers and generates instructions for the 3D printer to create each layer sequentially (29).

5.6.5   MATERIAL SELECTION

A biocompatible material is selected based on the required use. Biodegradable polymers, hydrogels, and biomaterials that replicate the characteristics of the target tissue are popular options. In multi-material printing of certain circumstances, several materials, such as soft and hard tissues of an organ, can be employed to simulate the diverse components of the tissue (7).

5.6.6   3D PRINTING

The subsequent stage involves the actual 3D printing of the physical model using a suitable bioprinter. Printing parameters: Configure printing settings including layer thickness, print speed, and temperature. These parameters have an impact on the final model's accuracy and quality. Printing technology: Depending on the material and resolution required, choose a suitable 3D-printing method. Fused deposition modelling (FDM), stereolithography (SLA), and selective laser sintering (SLS) are all possibilities. Bioprinting methods utilize controlled 3D spatial manipulation to deposit printing materials, employing modules like inkjet, microextrusion, or laser-assisted techniques (13).

5.6.6.1   Inkjet Bioprinters

Inkjet printers have emerged as the preferred choice for 3D-printing applications in bioprinting. In a groundbreaking demonstration, Robert J. Klebe employed readily available 2D inkjet printers to deposit biological materials, specifically cell adhesion proteins and monoclonal antibodies, onto a flexible substrate. This marked a significant milestone in the field. This was a watershed moment in the field. Subsequent developments involved the enhancement of inkjet printers by integrating an elevating platform, allowing vertical movement. Moreover, traditional ink has been replaced with biologically sourced materials, including cells, proteins, growth factors, and ECM components. Modern inkjet bioprinters now offer high-resolution printing of cell-laden droplets at speeds of approximately 10,000 per second. These printers accurately dispense precise volumes of materials to predefined positions using thermal or piezoelectric actuators (12).

Thermal inkjet printers produce pressure pulses that forcefully expel droplets from the nozzle. This method offers advantages such as rapid printing, cost-effectiveness, and widespread availability. However, it presents a potential drawback—exposing cells and materials to heat and pressure, which might induce damage. Moreover, these printers are susceptible to issues like uneven droplet sizes, limited droplet directionality, and frequent nozzle clogging. Consequently, their suitability for bioprinting applications is restricted (7). In contrast, acoustic inkjet printers use piezoelectric crystals, creating consistent acoustic waves upon voltage application. This breaks down the printing liquid into uniform droplets, ensuring size and directionality. However, inkjet bioprinters face challenges with highly viscous materials, requiring significant force for solutions exceeding 10 cP (4).

5.6.6.2 Microextrusion Bioprinters

In contrast to inkjet printers that release liquid droplets, microextrusion employs a microextrusion head to deposit small beads of the printing material. This deposition transpires in two dimensions, with vertical movement of the stage directed by computer-aided design and manufacturing (CAD-CAM) software for precise layering (16). Microextrusion printing is compatible with a range of materials, including hydrogels, copolymers, and cell spheroids. It can handle highly viscous materials and those with shear-thinning properties. Various curing techniques like ionic cross-linking, photo-crosslinking, and thermal solidification create complex, functional tissues. However, using viscous ink and encapsulating cells may reduce cell viability. Compared to inkjet and laser-assisted methods, microextrusion bioprinters have slower printing speeds (21).

5.6.6.3 Laser-Assisted Bioprinters

Laser-assisted bioprinters create a laser beam that is a high-pressure bubble within the energy-absorbing layer, causing a droplet of bioink to be expelled toward the substrate. The absence of nozzles and reduced mechanical stress contribute to heightened cell viability. These printers enable the printing of materials with a broader viscosity range (1–300 mPas). Remarkably, they possess the capability to encapsulate a single cell within a droplet, facilitating the deposition of diverse cell types (11).

Nevertheless, it is crucial to highlight the substantial effort required in preparing ribbons for this procedure. The subsequent steps encompass post-processing intricacies. Initially, the removal of support structures, which were introduced during the printing process, is imperative. This task involves both manual techniques and automated methods to ensure the final model's integrity. Depending on the chosen printing technique and materials, additional steps such as curing, solidification, or crosslinking might be essential to achieve the desired characteristics of the model. Moreover, a stringent quality control protocol is executed, involving a meticulous inspection of the 3D-printed model. This evaluation is conducted by medical experts and researchers to verify the model's accuracy in representing the patient's tissue and any distinct anatomical or pathological features (20).

5.7 EXPLORING DIVERSE 3D-PRINTED DISEASE MODELS: AN ARRAY OF MEDICAL APPLICATIONS

Although still in its early stages, 3D bioprinting has captured significant attention from medical researchers due to its potential in the development of various tissues. Recent studies focused on creating 3D-printed tissues, including cardiovascular, hepatic, and neural tissues, have sparked interest in utilizing this technology for disease modeling and research (10).

5.7.1 CARDIOVASCULAR DISEASE MODELS

A set of diseases known as cardiovascular disorders damage the heart and blood vessels. Researchers can gain a better understanding of the physiological and molecular mechanisms behind these diseases by using 3D-printed disease models. In an important piece of work, Mosadegh and colleagues developed a paper-based 3D culture model to mimic myocardial ischemia. Cardiac cells were printed onto paper sheets and placed within a hydrogel to create a layered 3D heart tissue model. Cardiovascular disorders harm the heart and blood vessels. 3D-printed disease models provide insights into these conditions. For instance, Mosadegh and colleagues developed a paper-based 3D heart tissue model mimicking myocardial ischemia. They placed cardiac cells on paper sheets within a hydrogel, creating stress like ischemia. Stressed cells release chemokines, prompting cell migration. Ma and colleagues produced a patient-specific 3D cardiac model using laser-based filamentous matrices, incorporating cells from both healthy donors and individuals with specific cardiac conditions like long QT syndrome type 3 (7).

The model investigated medication reactions and contractility issues. Varying matrix stiffness produced different contractile anomalies and drug sensitivities. Bioprinting simplified vascular tissue production, generating endothelial networks in mice post-implantation and *in vitro* lumen-like structures using encapsulated cells in hydrogels. Three-dimensional bioprinting replicated calcific aortic valve conditions, assessing pathogenesis through microcalcification induced with an osteogenic medium. These applications underscore bioprinting's cardiovascular research potential (19).

5.7.2 NEURAL DISEASE MODELS

Globally impacting over a billion people, neurological diseases suffer from limited therapeutic solutions due to the intricate nature of the nervous system and a lack of fitting disease models. Recent years have witnessed 3D bioprinting's potential in generating controlled neural disease models. Nanosheets created from pluripotent NT2 cells displayed neural migration and proliferation responses to time-released growth factors (GFs) (3). Murine neural stem cells, encased in collagen and fibrin hydrogels, demonstrated migration toward the latter and morphological shifts due to GFs. Bioprinted neural constructs showcased neural injury recovery. Neural stem cell-laden hydrogels repaired zebrafish embryo neural injuries. Another group created brain-like structures using modified hydrogels and primary cortical neurons. Bioprinted artificial axons simulated biological counterparts, demonstrating axonal myelination dependency on stiffness, surface chemistry, and diameter (9).

5.7.3 HEPATIC DISEASE MODELS

Hepatic tissue models have been produced using bioprinting. A 3D hepatic tissue model, consisting of 30 gelatin hydrogel layers with hepatocytes, exhibited cell viability and functionality for over two months. Zhong et al. developed hepatic cells within hydrogel scaffolds, with better survival rates for hepatocyte-containing 3D hydrogel scaffolds in mice. Functional 3D mini-livers were used for drug metabolism studies. A microscale device mimicking drug metabolism was created with hepatic tissue using syringe-based cell writing with micropatterning. Patient-specific hepatic models, replicating native cellular architecture, were generated from human-induced pluripotent stem cell–derived hepatic and supporting cells in a hydrogel. This led to enhanced cytochrome P450 activation, increased metabolic product secretion, improved organization, and higher gene expression, promising personalized drug testing possibilities (15).

5.7.4 MUSCULOSKELETAL DISEASE MODELS

Microextrusion bioprinting yielded organized bone tissue using cell-laden hydrogel, maintaining cell viability akin to conventional culturing methods. The study proposed the potential for co-depositing diverse cell types using a single scaffold via microsyringe exchange. Droplet printing enabled a 3D bladder tissue model, with smooth muscle–cell bioprinted blocks showcasing consistent proliferation. These blocks were assembled into a 51-day cultured construct patch mimicking the rat bladder's native structure. Bioprinting holds promise for intricate musculoskeletal and organ tissue engineering (26).

5.7.5 CANCER DISEASE MODELS

Cancer remains a significant global health issue despite medical advancements. Understanding cancer progression and metastasis is limited. A 3D polyethylene glycol (PEG) scaffold compared breast epithelial cells' migration. Cancer cell migration patterns in 3D varied from 2D models, including displacement, velocity, and direction differences. A hydrogel-printed 3D microchip mimicked blood vessels, revealing varying cancerous cell behavior based on channel size. Customized bioprinting produced cellular spheroids. Gelatin arrays printed with breast cancer cells facilitated tumor spheroid development with high viability (6). Scaffold-free 3D neural tissue culture studied glioma cell invasion. Three-dimensional spheroids are valuable for drug testing. Cervical tumor and glioma stem cell models were also developed. Interaction studies between cancer and healthy cells were conducted through bioprinted ovarian cancer and fibroblast models, revealing distance-dependent nodule formation. Alginate fiber-constructed 3D cancer models explored adenocarcinoma-macrophage interactions, elucidating migration effects (26).

5.7.6 OTHER DISEASE MODELS

Various other disease models have been created using 3D bioprinting. A gelatin, elastin, and sodium hyaluronate blend formed a 3D-printed membrane for conjunctival reconstruction. Mechanical and physical characteristics were evaluated *in vitro* (epithelial cell viability, proliferation, and adhesion) and *in vivo* (rabbit healing capability) and compared to those of the amniotic membrane. Intestinal villi epithelium was simulated using a 3D-printed model. Collagen bioink with tannic acid crosslinking achieved a viable, differentiated 3D collagen villus structure. To investigate host–pathogen interactions in communicable illnesses, Rong Lu's team used 3D printing. In line with *in vivo* findings, a human intestinal epithelial model infected with salmonella showed increased inflammatory regulator gene expression. These diverse applications illustrate 3D bioprinting's potential for disease modelling and research (11).

5.8 REVOLUTIONIZING DERMATOLOGY: 3D PRINTING AND MICROFLUIDICS FOR NOVEL DRUG DELIVERY

In the realm of dermatology, the fusion of 3D printing and microfluidics stands as a beacon of innovation, particularly in the domain of drug delivery. This convergence holds immense promise, propelling the field toward the development of groundbreaking solutions. The synergy of 3D printing's precision and microfluidics' intricate manipulation of fluids offers a platform for tailored drug delivery systems. By seamlessly integrating these technologies, novel therapeutic strategies are on the horizon, poised to revolutionize how medications are administered and absorbed through the skin. The journey ahead involves the exploration of complex formulations, optimized dosages, and personalized treatment regimens, ushering in a new era of targeted and effective dermatological interventions (2).

The amalgamation of 3D printing and microfluidics is reshaping drug delivery in dermatology. This cutting-edge approach combines precision fabrication and fluid manipulation to revolutionize therapeutic administration. By leveraging the strengths of both technologies, customized drug delivery systems are emerging, offering unprecedented control over dosage and application. This convergence opens the door to customized therapies that maximize efficacy while minimizing negative effects. As the landscape of dermatological treatments advances, the collaboration of 3D printing and microfluidics has the potential to reshape how pharmaceuticals are administered to the skin, ushering in a new age of sophisticated and patient-centered therapy (19).

5.9 EXPLORING LATEST 3D-PRINTING ADVANCES IN SDMs: *IN VITRO* AND *IN VIVO*

The utilization of 3D-printing technology in the realm of SDMs has garnered significant attention in recent times, signifying an innovative approach poised to propel our comprehension of skin-related ailments forward. This novel method bears the potential to not only refine our understanding of these conditions but also to facilitate the testing of therapeutic interventions and, in a promising trajectory, even offer personalized treatment strategies. The latest strides and perspectives in harnessing

3D printing for SDMs, encompassing both *in vitro* and *in vivo* applications, paint a remarkable picture of progress (16). In the realm of *in vitro* SDMs, the precision and customization afforded by 3D printing are noteworthy. Researchers can fashion remarkably accurate and tailored models that emulate the intricate anatomy and features of human skin. This extends to replicating complex structures like hair follicles, sweat glands, and blood vessels. Moreover, the development of disease-specific models using patient-derived data is a tangible possibility, particularly significant for delving into rare or genetically driven skin disorders. Three-dimensional-printed SDMs serve as platforms for efficacious and safety assessments of drugs within a context that is more pertinent and prognostic. This has the potential to expedite drug development processes while curbing the reliance on animal testing. Furthermore, the true-to-life microenvironment replication enabled by these models offers invaluable insights into disease mechanisms, cellular responses, and tissue interactions that conventional approaches often struggle to unveil. This newfound tool also elevates dermatological research by probing into wound healing, inflammatory responses, and assorted skin conditions (12).

Transitioning to *in vivo* SDMs, the realm of patient-specific implants takes center stage. In this arena, 3D printing emerges as a means to fabricate implants or grafts customized to individual patients, with applications ranging from burn victim recovery to addressing specific skin defects. The union of 3D printing with regenerative medicine materializes in the form of 3D-printed scaffolds housing patient-derived cells, fostering tissue regeneration and wound healing. This innovation holds the potential to revolutionize the treatment of chronic wounds and severe skin injuries (10). A notable stride is the creation of 3D-printed skin grafts, an advancement with implications for enhancing the viability and functionality of traditional grafts. The ability to fashion intricate geometries and incorporate diverse cell types contributes to graft integration and survival. Furthering this exploration, the integration of 3D-printed sensors within living tissue enables real-time monitoring of disease progression and treatment responses, heralding transformative prospects for managing chronic skin conditions. Harnessing patient-specific data in tandem with 3D printing's prowess yields tailored treatment strategies, such as bespoke implants or drug delivery systems, catering to the unique needs of individuals with specific skin diseases (6).

In vitro and *in vivo* 3D-bioprinting models are becoming increasingly important in the contemporary era of biomedical research. This state-of-the-art technology has enormous potential for improving our knowledge of illnesses, enabling more precise testing of prospective therapies, and laying the groundwork for personalized medicine. The incorporation of 3D bioprinting is becoming increasingly important in both *in vitro* and *in vivo* models in the present era of biomedical research (5). By enhancing biomimicry in 3D tissue architectures for *in vitro* models, this cutting-edge technique enables more precise disease modelling and medication testing. Three-dimensional printing helps create customized implants and gadgets for *in vivo* models, bridging the gap between laboratory discoveries and clinical applications. Overall, it increases precision medicine, decreases animal testing, and speeds up medication development. With the help of this innovative instrument, biomedical research might undergo a revolution that will enhance healthcare outcomes and provide a better knowledge of human health and illness (30). Here's recent 3D-printing research for SDMs for both *in vitro* and *in vivo* in Table 5.1 (31, 32).

TABLE 5.1

Recent Advancements in 3DPrinting for *in vitro* and *in vivo* SDMs

S.no	Focus	Methodology	Key Findings	Year	References
1	Customizable Dosage and Timing	Microfluidic-Assisted Printing	Microfluidics-integrated 3D printing allowed precise dosages and timing control for tailored treatments.	2017	(33)
2	Customizable Dosage and Timing	3D-Printed Dissolvable Microcarriers	Dissolvable microcarriers allowed controlled and time-released drug delivery to the skin.	2018	(34)
3	On-Demand Drug Synthesis	Microreactors within 3D-Printed Skin Models	Integrated microfluidic systems within 3D skin models enabled in situ drug synthesis.	2018	(35)
4	Skin Wound Healing	3D-Printed Microreactors	Microfluidic-assisted 3D-printed microreactors enabled real-time synthesis of therapeutic compounds.	2020	(36)
5	Skin-on-a-Chip Models	Development and Production of *in vitro* Human Skin Models	3D printing is a highly potent and promising technology poised to revolutionize the biomedical realm, particularly in the domains of drug discovery and testing	2021	(37)
6	3D-Printed Microneedles	Microfluidic Mixing	Microfluidic-guided fabrication of 3D-printed microneedles enhanced drug penetration through skin.	2021	(38)
7	Enhanced Topical Delivery	3D-Printed Hydrogel Patches	3D-printed hydrogel patches demonstrated improved drug permeation and sustained release for enhanced efficacy.	2021	(39)
8	Microfluidic Skin-on-a-Chip Model	Integrated 3D Printing and Microfluidics	3D-printed microfluidic skin model allowed real-time drug penetration and toxicity studies.	2022	(40)
9	Innovative Drug Delivery Methods Utilizing 3D Printing	Combined 3D Printing and Microfluidics	Multilayered structures facilitated precise drug release profiles for extended efficacy.	2022	(41)

(*Continued*)

**TABLE 5.1
(Continued)**

S.no	Focus	Methodology	Key Findings	Year	References
10	3D Printed Microneedles	Microfluidic Dispensing	Combination of 3D-printed microneedles and microfluidics enhanced drug delivery efficiency.	2022	(42)
11	Microfluidic-Printed Patch	3D Printing of Microneedles	Microfluidic-assisted patch enhanced microneedle drug delivery efficiency and patient comfort.	2022	(43)
12	Personalized Formulations Lipid-Based Nanomedicines	Microfluidic Mixing	Microfluidics enabled tailored topical formulations for individual patient needs.	2022	(44)
13	Microfluidic-Assisted 3D Printed Skin Model	3D Printing and Microfluidic Integration	Integrated system simulated skin microenvironment, aiding drug permeation studies.	2022	(45)
14	Enhanced Topical Delivery	3D Printing of Microneedles	Microneedle patches improved transdermal drug delivery with controlled release.	2022	(46)
15	Microfluidic Chip-Based Skin Mode	3D Printing of Microfluidic Channels	Microfluidic skin model enabled drug penetration studies with enhanced physiological relevance	2022	(47)
16	Microfluidic-Printed Hydrogel	3D Printing and Microfluidic Combination	Combined technology enabled creation of complex drug-loaded hydrogel structures for improved drug release profiles.	2023	(48)
17	Microfluidic-Assisted Wound Dressing	3D Printing and Microfluidic Integration	Microfluidic-driven fabrication of 3D-printed wound dressings optimized drug release profiles.	2023	(49)
18	3D-Printed Skin Model	Microfluidic Integration	Integration of microfluidics with 3D-printed skin model allowed dynamic drug permeation studies.	2023	(50)
19	Hybrid Hydrogel-3D-Printed Patches	Microfluidic Dispensing	Microfluidics guided 3D-printed patch fabrication, offering precise drug dosage control.	2023	(51)

(Continued)

TABLE 5.1
(Continued)

S.no	Focus	Methodology	Key Findings	Year	References
20	Personalized Treatmentin Metabolic Syndrome	3D-Printed Pharmaceutical Systems	Multilayered matrices facilitated sequential drug release profiles, optimizing treatment outcomes.	2023	(52)
21	Nanostructured 3D Printed Scaffolds	Microfluidic Encapsulation	Microfluidic encapsulation of drug-loaded nanoparticles within 3D scaffolds enhanced drug delivery efficiency.	2023	(53)
22	Personalized Formulations	Microfluidic-Printed Gels	Microfluidic-printed gels enabled customization of topical formulations for diverse patient needs.	2023	(54)
23	3D-Printed Skin-Nanofiber Scaffolds	Microfluidic Encapsulation	3D-printed scaffold with encapsulated nanoparticles showed improved drug release kinetics.	2023	(55)
24	3D-Printed Patch for Psoriasis	Microfluidic Mixing	Microfluidics-driven fabrication of 3D patches improved drug delivery for psoriasis treatment.	2023	(56)
25	Microfluidic Skin-on-a-Chip Model	3D Printing and Microfluidic Integration	Integrated system replicated skin microenvironment, aiding drug testing and evaluation.	2023	(57)

5.10　REGULATORY GUIDELINES FOR 3D PRINTING

The Food and Drug Administration (FDA) of the United States has released guidelines for the regulation of medical devices made using 3D printing. This advice covers a wide variety of important factors. To guarantee the security and effectiveness of 3D-printed medical equipment, manufacturers are obliged to follow recognized quality standards, such as the FDA's Quality System Regulation (28). The FDA emphasizes the need for choosing materials that are appropriate for their intended use and adhere to biocompatibility criteria. To ensure that 3D-printed medical devices achieve their intended performance and safety requirements, adequate design controls must be put in place. To evaluate possible dangers to patients, biocompatibility testing may be required depending on the technology and materials utilized. Additionally, software validation is essential to guaranteeing the precision and dependability of devices developed or produced using software. Once 3D-printed medical devices are on the market, manufacturers are also required to set up procedures for monitoring and reporting adverse occurrences connected to those products (13). To enable appropriate device application by medical professionals and patients, proper labelling and clear usage instructions are crucial. Regulatory rules are currently being developed regarding 3D-printed medications and dosage forms. Key factors to consider include the compatibility of materials used for 3D-printing pharmaceuticals with the drug substance, ensuring that stability and efficacy are unaffected. Rigorous quality control measures are imperative to guarantee that 3D-printed dosage forms conform to stipulated standards for drug content, uniformity, and release (11).

The validation of the 3D-printing process is paramount to ensure consistent and reproducible drug products. Manufacturers must collaborate closely with regulatory agencies to establish suitable pathways for submitting 3D-printed pharmaceuticals for approval. It is crucial to note that regulations can differ between countries. Entities involved in 3D printing, especially within regulated sectors like healthcare, should remain current with the latest guidelines issued by relevant regulatory authorities. Given that regulations can undergo changes and evolution, consulting official regulatory bodies and seeking advice from legal and regulatory experts is recommended for the most up-to-date information (58, 59).

5.11 CONCLUSION AND FUTURE PERSPECTIVES

Recent advances in 3D-printing technology have enabled researchers to create models that mimic physiological cell composition, material qualities, and complicated designs replete with correct vascularization. Nonetheless, bioprinting is still in its early phases, and its potential is dependent on ongoing research and innovation, with the long-term objective of perhaps replacing animal or human clinical trials. Pivotal innovations to consider encompass technologies facilitating the integration of printed constructs for *in vivo* safety and efficacy studies, refining post-printing culture platforms, boosting the capacity to print and manipulate substantial material volumes, synergizing with technologies like microfluidics, and advancing imaging systems and analytical tools. This progression holds the promise of revolutionizing research methodologies and accelerating the journey toward comprehensive bioprinted solutions. In the realm of *in vitro* SDMs, 3D printing's precision and adaptability enable the replication of intricate human skin traits, offering insight into disease mechanisms, drug testing, and dermatological understanding. The amalgamation of patient-specific data and 3D printing fosters novel paths in studying rare disorders, accelerating drug development, and refining *in vitro* models' role in dermatology research. These models are pivotal tools for delving into wound healing, inflammation, and skin conditions. Similar to this, *in vivo* 3D printing has the potential to revolutionize personalized regenerative medicine. Severe skin injuries and ongoing wounds may benefit from customized implants, grafts, and scaffolds. Real-time monitoring sensors and functional 3D-printed skin grafts represent breakthrough advancements in the treatment of skin diseases. By combining personalized data with 3D printing, we can treat skin diseases more effectively and move toward more focused therapies. In conclusion, the use of 3D-bioprinting technology has shown to have considerable potential for increasing both our *in vitro* and *in vivo* understanding of skin disorders. The development of bioprinted SDMs successfully mimics the complex structure of skin, with its numerous layers and complicated relationships. These models give researchers cutting-edge platforms to examine disease causes, evaluate prospective treatments, and decipher complex biological reactions. Three-dimensional bioprinting is a great tool to investigate disease development, pharmacological effectiveness, and individualized treatment approaches by simulating the microenvironment of skin diseases. The use of 3D printing to create models of skin diseases has a bright future. The precision and complexity of these models will be improved by ongoing developments in bioprinting methods, materials, and the incorporation of other cell types. Drug research and development procedures will be accelerated by the creation of increasingly complex *in vitro* models that enable high-throughput screening of substances and therapies. Additionally, by transferring these models to *in vivo* settings, the gap between laboratory research and clinical results will be closed, resulting in new insights into disease responses that may revolutionize personalized treatment. As 3D bioprinting develops, it has the potential to transform the field of dermatological research and eventually improve our capacity to successfully treat skin conditions.

ACKNOWLEDGMENTS

The authors express their sincere gratitude to the host institution, Columbia Institute of Pharmacy, Raipur, for generously providing all the necessary facilities throughout the course of this study. Additionally, the authors would like to extend their appreciation to the institution's library and e-library services. Furthermore, the research received valuable support from the Department of Science and Technology (DST), Government of India, for which the authors are deeply thankful. This DST-FIST fund granted to Dr. Ravindra Kumar Pandey.

FUNDING

The authors are thankful to the DST/FIST/(Department of Science and Technology)/ SR/FST/college/418/2018, the Department of Science and Technology, New Delhi, for financial assistance for the institutional research work.

REFERENCES

1. Sachdev A, Raj R, Matai I. 3D printing for *In vitro* and *In vivo* disease models. *3D Printing Technology in Nanomedicine*.2019. 129–142.
2. Kim BS, Kwon YW, Kong JS, Park GT, Gao G, Han W, et al.3D cell printing of *in vitro* stabilized skin model and *in vivo* pre-vascularized skin patch using tissue-specific extracellular matrix bioink: A step towards advanced skin tissue engineering. *Biomaterials*. 2018;168:38–53.
3. Joseph V, Julie AS, Scott AG. 3D printing of tissue engineered constructs for *in vitro* modeling of disease progression and drug screening. *Ann Biomed Eng*. January 2017;45(1): 164–179.
4. Rousi E, Malheiro A, Harichandan A, Mohren R, Lourenço AF, Mota C, et al. An innervated skin 3D *in vitro* model for dermatological research. *Vitr Model*. 2022;2(3):10–2.
5. Choudhury A, Deka H, Dey BK, Bhairam M, Sengupta K. Nanostructured materials for tissue engineering 15 - Nanomaterials for skin repair and regeneration. 2023;(0):8–9.

6. Lee H, Han W, Kim H, Ha DH, Jang J, Kim BS, et al. Development of liver decellularized extracellular matrix bioink for three-dimensional cell printing-based liver tissue engineering. *Biomacromolecules*. 2017;18(4):1229–37.

7. Randall MJ, Jüngel A, Rimann M, Wuertz-Kozak K. Advances in the biofabrication of 3D skin *in vitro*: Healthy and pathological models. *Front Bioeng Biotechnol*. 2018;6(Oct).

8. Verma Atul D. d M us pt. Certain distance degree based Topol indices Zeolite LTA Fram. 2018;(December 2016):11–4.

9. Bahadur S, Baghel P. Nanostructured materials for tissue engineering 4 - Application of nanorange self-assembly in tissue engineering. 2023:8–9.

10. Mandrycky C, Wang Z, Kim K, Kim DH. 3D bioprinting for engineering complex tissues. *Biotechnol Adv*. 2016;34(4):422–34.

11. Tarassoli SP, Jessop ZM, Al-Sabah A, Gao N, Whitaker S, Doak S, et al. Skin tissue engineering using 3D bioprinting: An evolving research field. *J Plast Reconstr Aesthetic Surg*. 2018;71(5):615–23.

12. Matai I, Kaur G, Seyedsalehi A, McClinton A, Laurencin CT. Progress in 3D bioprinting technology for tissue/organ regenerative engineering. *Biomaterials*. 2020;226:119536.

13. Mofazzal Jahromi MA, Sahandi Zangabad P, Moosavi Basri SM, Sahandi Zangabad K, Ghamarypour A, Aref AR, et al. Nanomedicine and advanced technologies for burns: Preventing infection and facilitating wound healing. *Adv Drug Deliv Rev*. 2018;123:33–64.

14. Schuler M, Tomlinson L, Homiski M, Cheung J, Zhan Y, Coffing S, et al. Experiments in the EpiDerm 3D Skin *in Vitro* model and minipigs *in Vivo* indicate comparatively lower *in Vivo* skin sensitivity of topically applied aneugenic compounds. *Toxicol Sci*. 2021;180(1):103–21.

15. Kim BS, Lee J-S, Gao G, Cho D-W, Cubo N, Garcia M, et al. Direct 3D cell-printing of human skin with functional transwell system 3D bioprinting of functional human skin: production and *in vivo* analysis. *Biofabrication*. 2017;9(2):1–12.

16. Assad H, Assad A, Kumar A. Recent Developments in 3D Bio-Printing and Its Biomedical Applications. *Pharmaceutics*. 2023;15(1):9–10.

17. Bainier M, Su A, Redondo RL. 3D printed rodent skin-skull-brain model: A novel animal-free approach for neurosurgical training. *PLoS One*. 2021;16:9–10.

18. Olejnik A, Semba JA, Kulpa A, Dańczak-Pazdrowska A, Rybka JD, Gornowicz-Porowska J. 3D bioprinting in skin related research: recent achievements and application perspectives. *ACS Synth Biol*. 2022;11(1):26–38.

19. Economidou SN, Lamprou DA, Douroumis D. 3D printing applications for transdermal drug delivery. *Int J Pharm*. 2018;544(2):415–24.

20. López de Andrés J, Ruiz-Toranzo M, Antich C, Chocarro-Wrona C, López-Ruíz E, Jiménez G, et al. Biofabrication of a tri-layered 3D-bioprinted CSC-based malignant melanoma model for personalized cancer treatment. *Biofabrication*. 2023;15(3):36041423.

21. Kang MS, Kwon M, Lee SH, Kim WH, Lee GW, Jo HJ, et al. 3D printing of skin equivalents with hair follicle structures and epidermal-papillary-dermal layers using gelatin/hyaluronic acid hydrogels. *Chem - An Asian J*. 2022;17:35866189.

22. Kim BS, Lee JS, Gao G, Cho DW. Direct 3D cell-printing of human skin with functional transwell system. *Biofabrication*. 2017;9(2):28586316.

23. Kang MS, Jang J, Jo HJ, Kim WH, Kim B, Chun HJ, et al. Advances and Innovations of 3D Bioprinting Skin. *Biomolecules*. 2023;13(1):9–10.

24. Choi KY, Ajiteru O, Hong H, Suh YJ, Sultan MT, Lee H, et al. A digital light processing 3D-printed artificial skin model and full-thickness wound models using silk fibroin bioink. *Acta Biomater*. 2023;164:159–74.

25. Kim BS, Ahn M, Cho WW, Gao G, Jang J, Cho DW. Engineering of diseased human skin equivalent using 3D cell printing for representing pathophysiological hallmarks of type 2 diabetes *in vitro*. *Biomaterials*. 2021;272(March):120776.

26. Arenas M, Sabater S, Sintas A, Arguís M, Hernández V, Árquez M, et al. Individualized 3D scanning and printing for non-melanoma skin cancer brachytherapy: A financial study for its integration into clinical workflow. *J Contemp Brachytherapy*. 2017;9(3):270–6.

27. Vrana NE, Gupta S, Mitra K, Rizvanov AA, Solovyeva VV, Antmen E, et al. From 3D printing to 3D bioprinting: the material properties of polymeric material and its derived bioink for achieving tissue specific architectures. *Cell Tissue Bank* 2022;23(3):417–40.

28. de Souza A, Martignago CC, Santo GD, Sousa KD, Cruz MA, Amaral GO, et al. 3D printed wound constructs for skin tissue engineering: A systematic review in experimental animal models. *J Biomed Mater Res - Part B Appl Biomater*. 2023;111(7):1419–33.

29. Tan SH, Chua DAC, Tang JRJ, Bonnard C, Leavesley D, Liang K. Design of hydrogel-based scaffolds for *in vitro* three-dimensional human skin model reconstruction. Acta Biomater.2022;153:13–37.

30. Kim BS, Gao G, Kim JY, Cho DW. 3D cell printing of perfusable vascularized human skin equivalent composed of epidermis, dermis, and hypodermis for better structural recapitulation of native skin. *Adv Healthc Mater*. 2019;8(7):1–11.

31. Bhairam M, Pandey RK, Shukla SS, Gidwani B. Preparation, optimization, and evaluation of dolutegravir nanosuspension: *In Vitro* and *In Vivo* characterization. *J Pharm Innov*. 2023;18:0123456789.

32. Bhairam M, Prasad J, Verma K, Jain P, Gidwani B. Formulation of transdermal patch of Losartan Potassium & Glipizide for the treatment of hypertension & diabetes. *Mater Today Proc*. 2023 Jan 1;83:59–68.

33. Van den Broek LJ, Bergers LIJC, Reijnders CMA, Gibbs S. Progress and future prospectives in skin-on-chip development with emphasis on the use of different cell types and technical challenges. *Stem Cell Rev Reports*. 2017;13(3):418–29.

34. Farias C, Lyman R, Hemingway C, Chau H, Mahacek A, Bouzos E, et al. Three-dimensional (3D) printed microneedles for microencapsulated cell extrusion. *Bioengineering*. 2018;5(3).

35. Damiati S, Kompella UB, Damiati SA, Kodzius R. Microfluidic devices for drug delivery systems and drug screening. *Genes (Basel)*. 2018;9(2).

36. Tottoli EM, Dorati R, Genta I, Chiesa E, Pisani S, Conti B. Skin wound healing process and new emerging technologies for skin wound care and regeneration. *Pharmaceutics*. 2020;12(8):1–30.

37. Risueño I, Valencia L, Jorcano JL, Velasco D. Skin-on-a-chip models: General overview and future perspectives. *APL Bioeng*. 2021;5(3):1–12.

38. Dabbagh SR, Sarabi MR, Rahbarghazi R, Sokullu E, Yetisen AK, Tasoglu S. 3D-printed microneedles in biomedical applications. *iScience*. 2021;24(1):102012.

39. De Oliveira RS, Fantaus SS, Guillot AJ, Melero A, Beck RCR. 3d-printed products for topical skin applications: From personalized dressings to drug delivery. *Pharmaceutics*. 2021;13(11).

40. Fernandez-Carro E, Angenent M, Gracia-Cazaña T, Gilaberte Y, Alcaine C, Ciriza J. Modeling an Optimal 3D Skin-on-Chip within Microfluidic Devices for Pharmacological Studies. *Pharmaceutics*. 2022;14(7).

41. Mohapatra S, Kar RK, Biswal PK, Bindhani S. Approaches of 3D printing in current drug delivery. *Sensors Int*. 2022;3(August 2021):100146.

42. Detamornrat U, McAlister E, Hutton ARJ, Larrañeta E, Donnelly RF. The role of 3D printing technology in microengineering of microneedles. *Small*. 2022;18(18).

43. Rajesh NU, Coates I, Driskill MM, Dulay MT, Hsiao K, Ilyin D, et al. 3D-printed microarray patches for transdermal applications. *JACS Au*. 2022;2(11):2426–45.

44. Osouli-Bostanabad K, Puliga S, Serrano DR, Bucchi A, Halbert G, Lalatsa A. Microfluidic manufacture of lipid-based nanomedicines. *Pharmaceutics*. 2022;14(9).

45. Heuer C, Preuß JA, Habib T, Enders A, Bahnemann J. 3D printing in biotechnology—An insight into miniaturized and microfluidic systems for applications from cell culture to bioanalytics. *Eng Life Sci*. 2022;22(12):744–59.

46. Olowe M, Parupelli SK, Desai S. A review of 3D-printing of microneedles. *Pharmaceutics*. 2022;14(12):9–12.

47. Jia F, Gao Y, Wang H. Recent advances in drug delivery system fabricated by microfluidics for disease therapy. *Bioengineering*. 2022;9(11):1–23.

48. Engineering T, Mechanobiology SC, Lo JF. Emerging Advances in Microfluidic Hydrogel Droplets for tissue engineering and STEM cell mechanobiology. *Gels* 2023;9(10):790.

49. Uchida DT, Bruschi ML. 3D printing as a technological strategy for the personalized treatment of wound healing. *AAPS PharmSciTech*. 2023;24(1).

50. Su R, Wang F, McAlpine MC. 3D printed microfluidics: Advances in strategies, integration, and applications. *Lab Chip*. 2023;23(5):1279–99.

51. Bhattacharjee G, Gohil N, Shukla M, Sharma S, Mani I, Pandya A, et al. Exploring the potential of microfluidics for next-generation drug delivery systems. *OpenNano*. 2023;12(January):100150.

52. Alqahtani AA, Ahmed MM, Mohammed AA, Ahmad J. 3D printed pharmaceutical systems for personalized treatment in metabolic syndrome. *Pharmaceutics*. 2023;15(4):1–23.

53. Jiang Z, Zheng Z, Yu S, Gao Y, Ma J, Huang L, et al. Nanofiber scaffolds as drug delivery systems promoting wound healing. *Pharmaceutics*. 2023;15.

54. Serrano DR, Kara A, Yuste I, Luciano FC, Ongoren B, Anaya BJ, et al. 3D printing technologies in personalized medicine, nanomedicines, and biopharmaceuticals. *Pharmaceutics*. 2023;15(2).

55. Soares F, Ribeiro N, Baião A, Torres PMC, Sarmento B, Olhero SM. Sustained drug release from sintering-free calcium phosphate-based scaffolds. *J Drug Deliv Sci Technol*. 2023;88(February):1–7.

56. Ren Y, Li J, Chen Y, Wang J, Chen Y, Wang Z, et al. Customized flexible hollow microneedles for psoriasis treatment with reduced-dose drug. *Bioeng Transl Med*. 2023;8(4):1–11.

57. Cao UMN, Zhang Y, Chen J, Sayson D, Pillai S, Tran SD. Microfluidic organ-on-a-chip: A guide to biomaterial choice and fabrication. *Int J Mol Sci*. 2023;24(4).

58. Bhairam M, Shukla SS, Gidwani B, Pandey RK. Solid dispersion of dolutegravir: Formulation development, characterization, and pharmacokinetic assessment. *Int J Pharm Qual Assur*. 2022;13(4):496–503.

59. Monika B, Amit R, Sanjib B, Alisha B, Mihir P. Transdermal drug delivery system with formulation and evaluation aspects: Overview. *Res J Pharm Technol*. 2012;5(September):1168–76.

60. Images are sorced from this website and arraged as aper our illustration. https://www.biorender.com

6 3D Bioprinting for Skin and Tissue Engineering

Sachin Gupta
Agra Public College of Higher Education and Research
Centre, Agra, India

Ganesh Kumar
SLT Institute of Pharmacy, Bilaspur, India

Swati Dubey, Geetika Sharma, Shalini Singh, and Sunita Minz
Indira Gandhi National Tribal University, Amarkantak, India

6.1 INTRODUCTION

Three-dimensional (3D) bioprinting is defined as the utilization of computer-assisted transfer techniques for the purpose of patterning and assembling both nonliving and living materials in a predetermined 3D or 2D arrangement, with the aim of creating bioengineered structures that contribute to the process of regeneration. The advancements in the field of 3D printing for inanimate objects have motivated researchers to explore the possibilities of 3D bioprinting technology (1). In the process of 3D printing, the fundamental procedure entails the utilization of 3D software to construct a model. Three-dimensional printing, commonly referred to as rapid prototyping or additive manufacturing, is of great significance in tissue engineering, specifically in the production of scaffolds that are crucial for the repair or replacement of injured tissues and organs (2). Recent years have witnessed remarkable progress in the field of 3D printing, largely driven by the progress made in fabrication technologies and computer-aided design (CAD). Three-dimensional printing has influenced various fields such as medicine, manufacturing, and engineering (3). Bioprinting technology enables the production of precise tissue constructs and the creation of porous structures with tissue models and controlled architecture in a highly efficient manner. The attainment of bioprinting technology is dependent on the efficiency and effectiveness of 3D bioprinters, as well as the availability of bioink, a comprehensive understanding of its physicochemical, thermal, mechanical, and biological characteristics. The introduction of 3D bioprinting presents innovative methods for producing heterogeneous biomaterials with meticulous mechanical attributes and high-resolution scaffolds (4). Three-dimensional printing has emerged

DOI: 10.1201/9781032690926-6

as a remarkable technology that is thriving across various domains within the health care sector. The concept of 3D printing, initially introduced as stereolithography in the late 1980s, rapidly gained momentum (5). Three-dimensional bioprinting has the capacity to address a wide range of demands in medical research, such as the replacement of functional organs, delivery of drugs, and regenerative medicine, thereby offering significant potential for advancement (6). A significant portion of the overall benefits of 3D printing can be attributed to its remarkable capacity for device customization and expedited delivery time (7). With its advanced functionality, the 3D printer is capable of generating 3D structures of orientations, cross sections, various shapes and sizes, and meticulously arranged fibers. With its potential, 3D printers can manufacture organs that exhibit equivalent biological functionalities. In the realm of tissue engineering, the focus lies on the creation and enhancement of tissues and organs, aiming to facilitate the healing, reintroduction, and reconstruction of afflicted regions. In order to be suitable for tissue engineering, biomaterials must possess the qualities of being degradable, cost-effective, and capable of maintaining their structure for a predictable duration (8). The fundamental goal of tissue engineering is to establish approaches that enable the restoration of compromised tissues and organs, specifically targeting those that have been historically classified as non-regenerative (9). Tissues are complex structures composed of different cell types, an extracellular matrix (ECM), and a wide array of signaling molecules. The ECM is the fundamental element of the cellular microenvironment, establishing a sophisticated 3D framework (2). Depending on the severity and circumstances of organ damage, patients have the options of organ repair, replacement, or transplantation. The objective of tissue engineering is to employ the principles of biology and engineering to produce viable substitutes for damaged tissue (10). The utilization of bioprinting technology results in the fabrication of highly precise tissue constructs and the development of porous structures with controlled architecture and tissue models in a streamlined and efficient process (4). The application of hard-tissue engineering is utilized in the restoration and substitution of bones and teeth that have been damaged due to fractures, trauma, and cancer. The application of a 3D printer in tissue engineering stands as one of the most extensively employed disciplines, wherein biological elements, scaffolds, and cells are meticulously arranged in layers to generate native body tissues. In the initial stage of processing, the CAD system receives and evaluates the structure, details, and images derived from the target tissue. This assessment takes place before the printing process, which is utilized to construct the intended tissue (11). Before attempting to repair any tissue or organ, it is essential to comprehend its anatomical structure and biogenesis. This understanding empowers users to regulate the conditions that could potentially influence the development of new tissue. To realize the skin, it is essential to have a fundamental understanding of the structure and functional relationship between normal and pathological tissue. Consisting of three layers, the skin is the largest organ in human beings and each of these layers has significant roles to fulfill (12). While skin exhibits a superior ability to regenerate compared to other tissues, the primary mechanism for healing deep injuries, such as severe burns, is achieved predominantly through the formation of scars. The issue of regenerating skin requires immediate attention in the realm of regenerative medicine and tissue engineering. Tissue-engineered skin (TES) is predominantly composed of biomaterials, cells, and bioactive factors. Its application results in comprehensive coverage of skin wounds, leading to an accelerated wound-healing process with reduced scarring and enhanced vascularization of dermal substitutes. A range of TES options have been established, including PELNAC, Derma Graf, and Integra (13). Currently, autotransplantation has emerged as the optimal clinical choice for treating cutaneous injuries, yet its effectiveness is limited by the scarcity of autologous donors. The primary aim of skin tissue engineering is to facilitate the growth of a living organ that can fully perform biological functions, with the purpose of permanently replacing damaged or diseased skin. An optimal tissue-engineered skin substitute should effectively inhibit microbial contamination and water loss while also facilitating the delivery of bioactive components and promoting cell proliferation, differentiation, and migration (14). For the advancement of this technology, a more comprehensive 3D bioprinting is imperative for its effective implementation in engineering human skin and other tissues.

6.2   BIOMATERIAL USED FOR SKIN AND TISSUE ENGINEERING

As the largest organ in the human body, the skin plays a vital role in shielding other tissues destructed from external stimuli. The occurrence of skin injuries due to infection or other genetic or physical conditions can result in the exposure of adjacent tissues to the external environment, thereby facilitating the entry of bacteria and viruses (15). The restoration of lost skin can be achieved through the implementation of tissue engineering constructs fabricated via 3D printing. The 3D-printed skin model exhibits exceptional maintenance of its shape and structure during the culture period. The outcomes of the study provide compelling evidence for the potential of 3D bioprinting in the treatment of skin diseases (11). The significance of utilizing naturally sourced materials cannot be overstated in the field of tissue engineering, as they play a pivotal role in the advancement of technologies and the refinement of methodologies. Natural polymers are widely recognized as suitable materials for tissue engineering applications due to their biocompatibility (16). Natural polymers have a significant impact on regenerative medicine and tissue engineering due to their diverse chemical and physical properties (17). The process of chemically modifying natural polymers can be seen as a highly effective and influential approach to enhancing the physicochemical, mechanical, and biological attributes of these polymers. The engineering of copolymers enables the modification of surface properties in natural polymers. Natural polymers have been extensively studied and it has been consistently observed that they outperform semisynthetic or synthetic polymers in terms of mimicking the ECM and interacting with tissues. This can be attributed to their remarkable similarity with the surrounding tissue environment (18).

6.2.1   COLLAGEN

The utilization of collagen has been widespread in the domain of tissue engineering and to a certain extent in delivery systems. In the realm of skin tissue engineering, these forms serve as valuable tools for guiding the intricate process of skin regeneration. Currently, there are several collagen-based scaffolds that have been developed for clinical purposes. Despite being biocompatible, collagen, like other natural polymers, possesses mechanical fragility and undergoes rapid degradation upon implantation. The implementation of the crosslinking process would prove to be extremely beneficial in enhancing the various characteristics of collagen, such as its water uptake capabilities, degradation resistance, and mechanical strength. Collagen is primarily obtained from animal tissues, and there is a possibility of viral and prior contamination in collagen derived from animal sources, which raises concerns about its safety (16). Collagen-based scaffolds are widely regarded as the optimal choice for tissue engineering due to the significant presence of fibrous collagenous material in the ECM. The market offers a wide array of collagen scaffolds that are specifically designed for tissue engineering purposes. The efficiency of collagen in various tissue engineering applications has been proven due to its structural integrity and fibrous nature (17). Growth factors and other active agents have the potential to be combined well with collagen-based systems, such as gels and scaffolds, in order to extend the release rate of factors and enhance their therapeutic efficacy (16). Although collagen type I has been widely utilized in the field of 3D bioprinting, it is crucial to recognize the constraints it presents. At low temperatures, it maintains its liquid state and undergoes a transition to a fibrous structure as the temperature rises. The process of complete gelation may require up to 30 minutes at a temperature of 37 °C (6).

6.2.2 Gelatin

Gelatin is a highly recognized biomaterial that finds extensive use in a wide array of applications in tissue engineering. The derivation of gelatin involves the partial hydrolysis of collagen and denaturation. With its presence in cartilage, skin, connective tissues, and bone, it demonstrates a reduced immunogenicity when compared to collagen (17). During the fabrication process, it is possible to alter the isoelectric point of gelatin, resulting in the production of an acidic gelatin with a negative charge or a basic gelatin with a positive charge at physiological pH. The degradation rate of gelatin is impacted by the density of its crosslinking and a similar pattern is seen in the release rate of growth factors from gelatin vehicles. This implies that the enzymatic degradation of the vehicle leads to the release of complex fragments comprising gelatin and growth factors. In the realm of tissue engineering, gelatin has proven to be a valuable tool for the controlled release of growth factors and efficient delivery of cells. This has been particularly beneficial in targeting various tissues, with a special focus on the skin. Gelatin, being denatured, possesses a relatively low degree of antigenicity, unlike collagen, which is derived from animals and is known to have antigenic properties. Gelatin shares similarities with synthetic high polymers, as it possesses a wide distribution of molecular weights (16). Gelatin, which is derived from hydrolyzed collagen, serves as the principal constituent. It occurs naturally in the ECM, allowing for the suspension of cells within the gel under low-temperature conditions (19). The enhancement of cell adhesion by gelatin is instrumental in promoting cellular growth and facilitating the suspension of cells at low temperatures. (8). For regenerative purposes, gelatin derived from mammals has been employed as a biomaterial. Gelatin is characterized by its ability to enhance cell adhesion, low immunogenicity, water solubility, noncytotoxic nature, biodegradability, and biocompatibility (6). In the context of a study, the preparation of a gelatin-sulfonated silk composite scaffold was carried out, followed by its incorporation with fibroblast growth factor 2. It was observed that the adhesion, migration, and cell proliferation experienced an upward trend in child foreskin fibroblasts, as evidenced by the results. The scaffold facilitated the enhancement of skin-like tissue regeneration and promoted dermal vascularization. The incorporation of fibroblast growth factor 2 into the gelatin-sulfonated silk composite scaffold makes it a highly promising candidate for skin tissue engineering (11).

6.2.3 CHITOSAN

Chitosan, which is derived from chitin, is a polysaccharide that is naturally present in the tough exoskeletons of shellfish, including shrimp and crab. Derived from chitin through the process of deacetylation, chitosan is a polysaccharide that is widely available in nature and is recognized for its affordability. Chitosan has gained significant recognition in the field of wound-dressing applications, primarily due to its strong antibacterial properties and minimal risk of foreign body rejection. Bandages with appropriate characteristics can be created by combining them with other natural or synthetic polymers. A notable attribute of chitosan lies in its structural similarity to glycosaminoglycans, resulting in an improved capacity for cell adhesion when compared to other synthetic polymers (17). In the presence of acid, chitosan readily dissolves, but it generally remains insoluble in neutral conditions and organic solvents. This behavior can be attributed to the presence of amino groups and the high crystallinity of chitosan. As a result, various chitosan derivatives have been developed to enhance solubility and aid in processing (16). The scaffold that has been prepared exhibits a high level of viability and uniformity in cell spreading, as it is composed of a linear amino-polysaccharide consisting of β (1–4)-linked D-glucosamine residues (8). Due to its antimicrobial attributes and its ability to initiate hemostasis, chitosan is the preferred option for wound healing applications in comparison to collagen (2). The utilization of chitosan and its derivatives-based constructs is set to be of utmost importance in the upcoming era of tissue engineering and skin grafting (20).

6.2.4 BIOINK

Bioink is a pivotal aspect in the domain of the tissue industry and organ bioprinting (6). The inclusion of therapeutic cells has resulted in a remarkable enhancement of biomaterial functionality. Through the application of bioink, cells are strategically printed to form a 3D tissue structure that replicates the properties and behavior of living biological tissue. After cells have attained confluency, they are integrated with a compatible polymer material in order to generate a bioink (8). The characteristics demanded from a bioink are greatly influenced by the chosen printing technique and the type of tissue being printed. When considering the main components of bioink, namely cellular materials and additive factors, it is evident that the selection of scaffolds in tissue engineering strategies tends to differ significantly (3). Polymeric materials possess biocompatibility, degradation resistance, and affordability, rendering them a suitable choice for bioink applications (6).

6.2.5 POLYLACTIC ACID

Polylactic acid (PLA), an aliphatic polyester, exhibits hydrolytic degradability and possesses a range of advantageous properties. These include degradability, biocompatibility, and the capacity to be utilized in printing, all of which contribute to its status as a prominent polymeric bioink. The acidic by-products released during the degradation of PLA have a detrimental effect on its long-term biocompatibility, leading to tissue inflammation and cell demise. PLA serves as the principal polymer in the fused deposition modeling (FDM) technique, acting as a precursor (6). Lactide, which is the cyclic dimer of lactic acid, exhibits two enantiomers: d and l. The naturally occurring isomer is l-lactide, whereas dl-lactide is a synthetic amalgamation of d-lactide and l-lactide (17). Using direct laser writing through ablation, the surface of the thermoplastic material PLA was modified, and thereafter, it was utilized in the production of a scaffold using the 3D technology known as fused filament fabrication. The development of PLA scaffolds was achieved by employing 3D-printing techniques, with the aim of regenerating nucleus pulposus cells and primary articular chondrocytes (8).

6.2.6 POLYLACTIC-CO-GLYCOLIC ACID

The capacity to copolymerize two monomers with the intention of obtaining a fresh polymer composition that possesses the desired properties is an ever-present possibility. Polylactide-co-glycolic acid (PLGA) is synthesized by copolymerizing polyglycolide with either l-lactide or d-lactide. PLGA, being a promising material for cell adhesion and proliferation, served as the foundation for the creation of diverse 3D scaffolds incorporating micro- and nanostructures (17). PLGA, a polymer renowned for its dependable biodegradability and remarkable cytocompatibility, possesses these desirable characteristics. In addition, PLGA finds application in animal models for bone regeneration and various tissue-restoring systems. Additionally, the linear structures of this material result in inadequate mechanical stiffness, and a high degradation rate, and consequently, restrict its application as a scaffold material (6). Its processability and high mechanical strength made it a suitable choice for the fabrication of scaffolds in FDM applications (2).

6.2.7 POLYURETHANES

Polyurethanes (PUs) are polymers that are composed of a sequence of organic units that are connected by carbamate (urethane) links. Carbamic acids give rise to urethanes, which are solely present in the ester configuration. In addition to the repeating urethane groups, PUs may contain other elements such as ether, urea, aromatic moieties, and esters. Due to their diverse structure and properties, PUs are widely recognized as a significant group of polymers in the medical field. With the aim of advancing tissue engineering applications, we utilized a rapid prototyping technique to manufacture 3D scaffolds comprising superimposed square-meshed PU grids. These scaffolds were then subjected to comprehensive in vivo testing (17). In 3D bioprinting, the combination of a high printing resolution and excellent cytocompatibility significantly contributes to the enhancement of characteristic strength. It exhibits a remarkable elastomeric characteristic that can withstand repetitive contraction and relaxation, making it an attractive choice for muscle generation (6). Types of biomaterials used for 3D printing technology used for skin and tissue engineering have been presented in Table 6.1.

6.3 TYPES OF 3D-PRINTING TECHNOLOGY USED FOR SKIN AND TISSUE ENGINEERING

Skin and tissue engineering is a multidisciplinary area that combines medicine, biology, and engineering skills to create biomimetic tissue systems. Tissue engineering inventions are applicable in organ transplantation, diagnostic research, and medical research. Skin and tissue engineering involves fabricating 3D synthetic materials to establish microenvironments characteristic of human tissue composition. Bioprinting

TABLE 6.1

Types of Biomaterials Used for 3D-Printing Technology Used for Skin and Tissue Engineering

Biomaterials	Advantages	Disadvantages	Applications	References
Collagen	High biological relevance, low immunogenicity	Complex process conditions required, difficult to control	Skin and Tissue Engineering	(21)
Chitosan	Good biocompatibility, excellent antibacterial properties, and good biodegradability	Weak mechanical properties	Skin and Tissue Engineering	(21)
Gelatin	Low cost, feasible to use with synthetic and natural polymer	Low rigidity	Tissue Engineering	(6)
PLA	Good biocompatibility, and excellent biodegradability	Due to its inherent brittleness, PLA exhibits a diminished strength when compared to bone.	Skin and Tissue Engineering	(6)
PLGA	Adequate rigidity, excellent strength, impressive mechanical properties	Low proliferation, inferior biological activity	Skin and Tissue Engineering	(21)
PU	Impressive mechanical properties and is known for its exceptional biocompatibility	Need to upgrade in vitro stability	Skin and Tissue Engineering	(21)

employs biomaterials, cells, and/or bioinks to construct scaffolds aimed at replicating the structure, composition, and functionality of the skin. Various bioprinting methods (like inkjet bioprinting, extrusion-based bioprinting, laser-assisted bioprinting, and stereolithography) have been employed in regenerative wound-healing studies. These methods have been assessed in terms of biocompatibility, cellular microenvironment, cell proliferation, viability, and morphological attributes (22). Bioprinting stands as an advanced manufacturing method enabling the precise application of cell-rich hydrogels to craft intricate tissue structures. This technology demonstrates the potential to produce a wide variety of tissues, such as skin and flexible tissues, as well as bone and cartilage (23). Traditionally, skin and tissue engineering has involved the cultivation of cells, their seeding into scaffolds that are biocompatible, and subsequent growth and maturation either in vitro or by using bioreactors. This procedure enables the advancement of specific target tissue. Here several types of bioink are available, offering adaptable and precise application of various biological substances like live cells, nucleic acids, growth factors, and pre-gelatinized solutions, among others that create tissue structure closely resembling the morphology and physiology of natural skin. While 3D bioprinting demonstrates significant potential in the field of skin engineering, as evident from substantial investments made by the cosmetic industry, it is noted that research in this area is still in its early stages (24). Tissue engineering scaffolds have the potential to fully cover skin wounds, expediting the healing process and minimizing scarring while also promoting the vascularization of dermal substitutes (13). The field of bioprinting encompasses three main procedural methodologies: inkjet, extrusion, laser-assisted bioprinting, and stereolithography, each of which is elaborated on in the following in the context of skin and tissues.

6.3.1　INKJET-BASED BIOPRINTING

Various research papers extensively report on the applications of bioprinting technologies and their diverse uses. Commonly, 3D-printing methods encompass scaffold production, investigations into cellular responses, and deployment in tissue regeneration objectives. Inkjet-based bioprinting technology process and the conventional inkjet printing process generally are used and are usually seen in desktop inkjet printers. Among this technology, the inkjet printer distinguishes itself as a non-contact technique that releases ink droplets onto a material surface. This involves the accurate placement of picolitre-sized droplets of "bioink" onto a hydrogel substrate or culture dish, all meticulously regulated by computerized precision (25). In the context of inkjet bioprinting, the bioink is discharged from the printer nozzle in a droplet-by-droplet manner onto a substrate (26). Inkjet printing processes can be classified into two main categories: continuous inkjet (CIJ) and drop-on-demand (DOD). In CIJ printing, the liquid binder is consistently emitted from the nozzle, resulting in the formation of a jet that fragments into droplets owing to Rayleigh instability. By comparison, in DOD printing, distinct droplets are discharged solely when an electric signal is produced, typically through thermal or piezoelectric effects. Nevertheless, DOD printing is the favored choice for constructing biological constructs intended for soft tissue engineering. This preference arises from its minimal risk of contamination and excellent manageability. As previously indicated, DOD printing systems employ either piezoelectric or thermal forces to expel droplets.

Consequently, the existing methods can be additionally divided into thermal and piezoelectric actuation approaches, distinguished by the triggering mechanism employed for the expulsion of droplets. Within thermal technology, ink droplets are generated through a heating process, causing enlarged air bubbles to propel the ink from a narrow nozzle onto the substrate (Figure 6.1). Localized temperatures can rapidly elevate by several hundred degrees within mere microseconds, generating a pulsed pressure. This approach offers comparatively elevated printing speed, excellent cell viability, and cost-effectiveness. However, droplets prepared by thermal techniques are mixed, disordered, and uneven in size. Achieving seamless printing poses challenges due to recurrent nozzle clogs. Additionally, the viability of cell and protein inks can be influenced by shear and thermal stresses.

In piezoelectric inkjet printer technology, droplets come into existence through the transient pressure exerted by a piezoelectric actuator. When an external voltage is applied to a piezoelectric actuator, pressure is generated that ejects droplets from a nozzle. Low-cost, fast-printing, and popular thermal inkjet printers use electrical heating to create pressure pulses that vaporize a liquid. A small water droplet is ejected from the nozzle when an air pressure pulse is applied. Normally, the heating temperatures typically lie within the span of 200 °C–300 °C, a range that could potentially result in the denaturation of either the hydrogel itself or the biocomponents within the hydrogel. Nonetheless, recent research has revealed that the brief heating duration of approximately 2 microseconds during the printing procedure does not have a detrimental impact on the stability of bio components. Like various other 3D-printing methods, predesigned hydrogel scaffolds are constructed layer by layer through inkjet 3D printers, employing evaporative substances. Furthermore, there exists a wide array of materials accessible for use with inkjet 3D printing (3). In contrast to thermal methods, piezoelectric technology operates without heat and eliminates the risk of orifice clogging, ensuring that droplets maintain their uniform size and orientation. Nonetheless, excessive utilization of piezoelectric technology may lead to cell membrane impairment and cell lysis. Conversely, drawbacks of this approach encompass potential harm to the enclosed cells caused by thermal or mechanical stresses and a limited print range; it is not recommended for high cell densities or for printing thick structures (25).

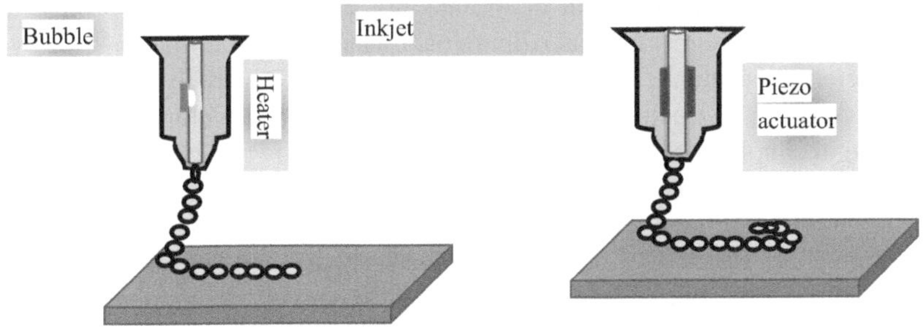

FIGURE 6.1   Illustration showing the process of inkjet bioprinting.

Inkjet printing setups have frequently found application in the bioengineering of skin models or distinct components thereof (26). To illustrate, the dermal layer of a bilayer skin structure was fabricated using inkjet bioprinting techniques by interleaving a layer of primary human dermal fibroblasts with an acellular layer of polyethylene glycol (PEG) based bioink. The bilayer skin structure was established by cultivating primary human epidermal keratinocytes that were placed onto bioprinted dermal equivalents (27). Simultaneously, an epidermal segment of a vascularized skin model was generated by employing inkjet printing to deposit epidermal cells suspended within a cell culture medium (28). The integration of inkjet bioprinting and wound scanning technology was employed for the on-site administration of autologous dermal fibroblasts and epidermal keratinocytes into full-thickness wounds (29). Cells were transferred to a fibrin/collagen hydrogel and delivered in layers based on the wound's depth and topography. The results demonstrated improved healing, marked by increased re-epithelialization, diminished contraction, and extensive formation of collagen fibers. These results were comparable in effectiveness to existing clinical cell spray methods (26). Selected bioinks are the key components of successful bioprinting for optimal results of varying complexity. *Bioink* refers to a biomaterial infused with viable cells, serving as a substrate or framework for 3D bioprinting. Bioink is composed of materials suitable for encapsulating cells and linking biomolecules together. An ideal bioink exhibits minimal toxicity and immunogenicity, and it can degrade at a controlled pace aligned with the physiological demands of the skin tissue. The bioink should provide the necessary support for the cells and tissues specific to a particular tissue structure, thereby generally maintaining adequate mechanical attributes. While there is a wealth of information about bioink and its potential pros and cons, this chapter of the book discusses more broadly the beneficial effects of bioink on human skin. In tissue engineering, bioinks are also referred to as scaffolds. Scaffolds primarily function to provide structural assistance, ensure mechanical stability, maintain cell viability, encourage cell compatibility, and allow for physical expansion (21).

6.3.2 Extrusion-Based Bioprinting

Extrusion-based bioprinting (EBB) has been extensively used in recent years and provides researchers with another scaffold fabrication method so that it often depends on efficient processes that result in the simplicity, versatility, and predictability of the technology. In EBB, biomaterial or bioinks are extruded from the print head via pneumatic or pressure mechanical (Figure 6.2). The extruded bioink is layer by layer in a predetermined manner, from a nozzle in a chain to a freely moving platform to create complex 3D patterns. This represents a highly developed form of inkjet bioprinting technology, which employs either a pneumatic (air-based) or mechanical (screw- or piston-driven) system to facilitate the dispersion of bioink the pneumatic distribution method, the dynamic force is generated by air pressure, whereas in the reciprocating and screw distribution techniques, vertical and field mechanical forces are applied to initiate the dispersion process, respectively. In a pneumatic system, bioink is expelled as a continuous cylindrical filament from a nozzle or needle by maintaining a consistent air pressure, instead of being dispensed as separate droplets. This guarantees a strong structural integrity of the final product (2). The mechanical

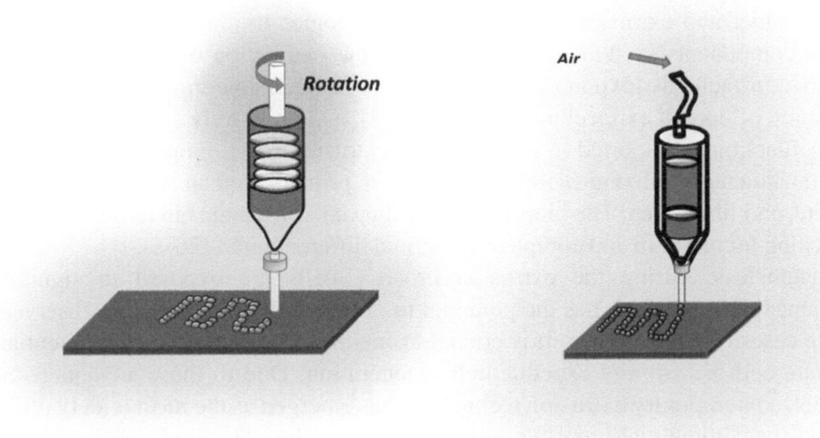

FIGURE 6.2 Illustration showing the process of extrusion-based bioprinting.

arrangement provides enhanced and direct control over the flow of bioink, achieved through the employment of a screw mechanism that facilitates the extrusion of the material. This technology enables precise printing, which is achieved through the implementation of fluid distribution systems and automated mechanical mechanisms and ensures meticulous control over the entire process. Managed by computer guidance, the bioink, composed of cells, is propelled through a micro nozzle in the shape of an uninterrupted filament. This is achieved by utilizing a controlled pneumatic system, a piston or screw mechanism, and following a layer-by-layer printing process, a comprehensive 3D structure is fabricated (13). Utilizing bioink viscosities ranging from $30^{-6} \times 10^7$ mPas has been identified as suitable for extrusion-based printing. Three primary considerations come into play when engaging in extrusion bioprinting. The initial factor involves viscosity adjustment, followed by the state of the bioink before extrusion and, finally, the distinct biomaterial fabrication range. The viscosity of the bioink can be influenced by factors such as temperature or shear thinning and needs to be carefully adjusted based on the specific printing method employed (10).

EBB enables the fabrication of tissues by utilizing a diverse range of bioinks, including hydrogels, carrier cells, microcarriers, and cell aggregates (30). The most common wound skin and tissue care and repair technology in modern regenerative medicine is EBB. These bioprinting methods are applied within the field of skin and tissue engineering and are closely associated with the development of artificial skin and tissue engineering, even various uses of skin and tissue bioprinting discussed in this chapter of this book use different printing technologies. EBB is extensively used to print skin models, especially fibroblasts for creating dermis with a double-layered skin structure (26). A discourse centered on the utilization of an extrusion-based 3D bioprinter for creating and fabricating a two-layer structural model composed of dermal fibroblasts, keratinocytes, and endothelial cells from micro-vessels in humans. Bioprinted skin-like constructs have the capacity to replicate the distinct structure and functionality of skin, encompassing the terminal differentiation of the epidermal layer both in vitro and in vivo. In a current study, researchers employed a hybrid 3D-bioprinting platform that merges inkjet and extrusion bioprinting methodologies to create the epidermal and dermal components of skin structures. During the maturation of the tissue, the bioprinted skin facilitated wound contraction, demonstrated epidermal detachment, and deposition of dermal extracellular matrix (ECM), and effectively simulated the native barrier function; as reported in the study, the extrusion-based bioprinting of skin has been documented utilizing bioink composed of primary human fibroblasts, gelatin, alginate, and fibrinogen. The bioprinted skin showed key features in terms of anatomy mimicking human skin and complete epidermal differentiation (26).

Nonetheless, during the extrusion process, cells are exposed to significant mechanical stress, which has the potential to diminish their viability, as observed in certain cases (23). Moreover, it is crucial to highlight that EBB has the potential to facilitate cell growth and expedite cell regeneration. Due to these advantages and benefits, contemporary extrusion technology has emerged as the most widely utilized method for commercial bioprinters in the market today. The study utilized various cell types including normal human dermal fibroblasts, human dermal microvascular endothelial cells, and normal human epidermal keratinocytes. A 3D bioprinter based on extrusion technology has been customized for research purposes. The bioprinter comprises an integrated control system, a precision motion mechanism, a material feeding system, and a specialized nozzle. Due to its four-axis configuration, the bioprinter has the capability to move independently along distinct orientations. The bioprinter offers a satisfactory printing area spanning 100 mm × 100 mm × 100 mm and achieves a reproducible precision of 0.05 mm. In a mouse model, artificial skin printed with this technique has been shown to have a cell viability of more than 90%. The bioprinted two-layer structure demonstrated an accelerated healing effect on skin wounds and exhibited a notable effect in promoting microvascular regeneration, as observed in the study (21). In contrast to inkjet bioprinting, extrusion bioprinting provides the advantage of higher cell density but comes with the trade-off of lower speed and resolution capabilities, as supported by research findings. Another notable benefit of extrusion bioprinting is the extensive selection of biomaterials and inexpensive equipment for printing.

Furthermore, both inkjet and extrusion bioprinting encounter common challenges, including nozzle clogging caused by cell aggregation, the high viscosity of bioink, and potential issues arising from the drying of materials within the printing nozzle. These issues have been subjects of concern for researchers aiming to enhance the bioprinting process. EBB has the capability to produce a porous mesh structure, enhance the flow of nutrients and metabolites, and attain bioengineering outcomes (25). Modern extrusion bioprinters are equipped with multiple print heads that can simultaneously apply different bioink with minimal cross-contamination. Furthermore, it provides enhanced regulation of porosity, shape, and cellular distribution within the printed framework.

6.3.3 LASER-ASSISTED BIOPRINTING

Laser-assisted bioprinting (LAB) represents an innovative bioprinting system, this process encompasses a pulsed laser source, a donor layer, and a receiving substrate. Initially LA bioprinter was created in 2004 to transfer biological designs to substrates and more precisely print biomaterials (31). The versatility of LAB technology lies in its capacity to generate tissue constructs with exceptional precision, elevated cell density, and viability through a nozzle-free and noncontact methodology is noteworthy. Confines contain high requirements on physical characteristics of bioink, high cost, and labor intensity. The LAB principle is that a bioink is employed under a ribbon containing a thin layer that absorbs energy. The ribbon is aligned in parallel with the receiver. A laser source emitting pulses is directed toward a layer capable of absorbing laser energy, leading to the formation of a vapor bubble. These applied air bubbles create pressure that causes the bioink to deform, resulting in the formation of droplets. These cell-filled droplets of hydrogel run to the receiver, where they are collected and stitched together (Figure 6.3). LAB offers certain benefits, such as no clogging issues occurring as there are no nozzles present in the system, and the noncontact printing approach ensures that there is no mechanical stress exerted on the cells, safeguarding their integrity. These factors collectively contribute to enhanced cell viability. However, LAB systems are costly as compared to other bioprinters (2). The lab uses the effect of laser optical tweezers to absorb trace materials and uses thermal shock to deposit droplets containing cells. LABs rely on laser-induced dynamic forces to impel cell-loaded bioink on collector substrates, containing direct laser-induced writing (LGDW) and direct laser-induced forward transfer (LIFT), along with novel technologies primarily based on LIFT (biological laser processing, absorbing film-assisted LIFT, etc.). Among various LAB bioprinting techniques, LIFT initially found its application in writing on metals but has been effectively adapted for bioprinting DNA and organ cells (31).

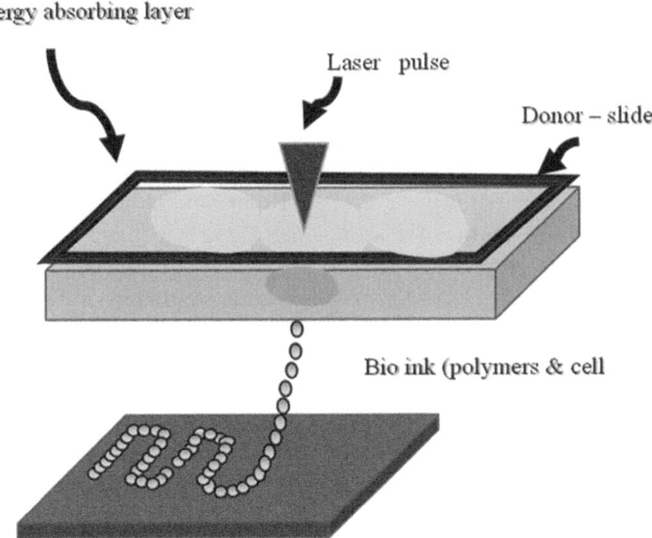

FIGURE 6.3   Illustration showing the process of laser-associated bioprinting.

In this method, two parallel glass slides are used, with the bottom slide serving as a collector to gather the bioink dispensed from the top slide. The upper glass slide can be segregated into two distinct layers: the uppermost layer and the underlying layer. The top layer functions as an energy-absorbing layer, responsible for absorbing the laser-generated energy. The region below the energy-absorbing layer is designated as the bioink storage layer. Once the laser illuminates the energy-absorbing layer, the layer creates high gas pressure that pushes the bioink onto the glass slide below. The size of the bioink droplets is influenced by several factors, including laser energy, laser spot size, and the distance or thickness between the energy-absorbing layer and the bioink storage layer. Cell deposition was monitored with a computerized scanning device containing two mirrors, focusing optics, and a camera on a movable platform (32). The laser beams can have parallel or vertical orientations to generate forces in the direction that cells move in horizontal or vertical directions. When the laser beam intensity surpasses 10 pN and interacts with the cells, they have the capability to move within a range of tens of micrometers to several millimeters and eventually get deposited on the surface of the designated object (33). Biomaterials are built onto materials using lasers as the energy basis for laser bioprinting. This technology offers several advantages, including exceptional resolution and the capability to handle a diverse range of print viscosities. However, because of its high cost, low efficiency, and complexity, laser bioprinting technology can increase cell viability up to 100% with very high cell viability and minimal negative effects on cell proliferation and cell death (31). The high-resolution printing achieved with this technology is comparable to the cell densities observed in living organs. Moreover, it ensures contamination-free bioprinting. However, there is still a need to explore whether this technology can be scaled up effectively for use in larger applications or organizations.

Laser bioprinting can be used to create skin cell structures, showing the potential for bioprinting of therapeutically relevant cell densities in multilayered tissue structures. Future capabilities include the ability to use bioprinting to deliver bioink which can be readily incorporated into patient tissue. Alternatively, the use of the patient's specific cells simplifies the use of these structures by adding structural and functional elements from the tissue (31). Koch and colleagues achieved the successful development of a basic skin substitute by employing laser bioprinting to embed fibroblasts and keratinocytes in a collagen hydrogel. Bioprinted skin substitutes demonstrate precise replication of the natural arrangement and gap junction formation among skin cells, with laser bioprinting facilitating precise cell placement, including fibroblasts, keratinocytes, and mesenchymal stem cells. To understand the process of skin tissue formation, an experiment was conducted on a 3D array of laser-printed cells using existing experimental equipment. Also, the authors discussed the fabricated skin substitutes with laser bioprinting (32).

6.3.4 Stereolithography

Light-curing stereolithography (SLA) technology cures light-sensitive polymers to create tissue structures under precisely controlled light, resulting in more realistic microstructures than other techniques (31). Back in the early 1980s, research was first conducted on Kodama on how to fabricate 3D structures by photo-polymerizing liquid resins using ultraviolet (UV) light. They have introduced two methodologies. One individual uses a mask for individual layers to pass over, and the other uses an optical fiber for selective curing (34). A preestablished design was formed by regulating the movement of the fibers along both the horizontal (x) and vertical (y) axes. In 1986, Hull added to this by creating 3D wireframes in a layer-by-layer approach using UV light with added motion along the z-axis. Photo curing and photo polymerization occur when a liquid polymer is a crosslinked process that occurs by exposing a predesigned pattern to a UV, infrared, or visible laser beam. SLA functions through the utilization of a UV light source, a container holding liquid photopolymer resin, and a three-axis movable platform. Compared to additional bioprinting methods, the SLA has benefits such as high accuracy and high speed. In biology, it is often used to print controlled geometries, as well as porous structured high-accuracy fabric scaffoldings. SLA can attain higher cell viability (more than 85%) without implementing the shear force to the cells and enables rapid bioprinting of high-resolution structures. However, one major drawback of SLA is that it requires the use of clear liquid and material that is not transparent. Alternatively, if the material is not transparent, it can lead to uneven light distribution and consequently produce irregular stitching (Figure 6.4). These requirements limit the bioink's cell density to about 108 cells/ml. In 2014, researchers led by Boland at Clemson University introduced SLA printing that incorporated cells into the printing process (35). Engineered pre-vascular tissues with complex 3D microstructures using microscale continuous optical bioprinting. Currently, SLA technology is extensively employed for scaffold printing, but its application in cell-based printing remains relatively infrequent. A significant limitation of SLA is the high cost of UV sources, which can also have an adverse impact on cell viability. To tackle this issue, researchers have developed visible-light SLA bioprinting. SLA employs an UV laser beam to solidify the material, while digital light processing employs a digital light projector as its illumination source.

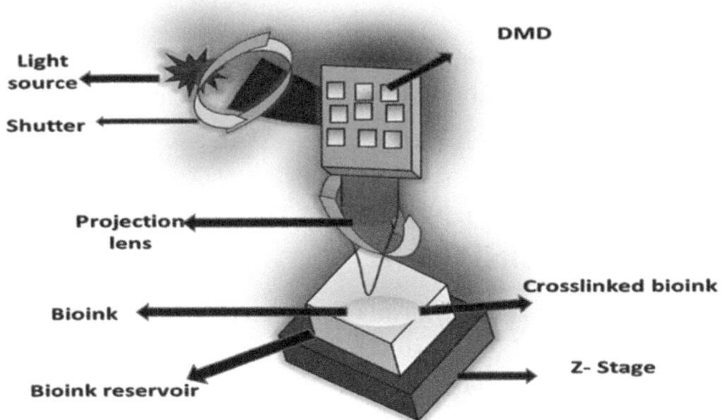

FIGURE 6.4   Illustration showing the process of stereolithography bioprinting.

A micro-mirror device with a user-defined pattern that is sequentially loaded to turn the mirrors reflecting incoming UV light on and off. In this method, the photo-curable bioink is cured selectively in a layer-by-layer process, with precise control provided through a stage moving along the z-axis. Thus, whole layers can be produced concurrently in the same experience step to reduce printing time, in contrast, nozzle-less technology mitigates concerns like cell clogging and excessive shear stress. Both SLA and digital light processing face limitations due to photo initiation and potential cytotoxic effects associated with UV exposure. Furthermore, the variety of bioink materials utilized in SLA and bioprinting through digital light processing is limited by the essential for uncured bioink to freely crosslink under the action of light irradiation to interact with the cured layer (36). Multiscale printing enables the creation of embedded vasculature, which facilitates the development of large-scale hydrogel-engineered tissue models. This vascular network ensures adequate medium perfusion, supporting high cell viability and metabolic function even in the deep core of large models. Nevertheless, their capability to capture the spatial heterogeneity present in mammalian tissues and establish structural and functional relationships is constrained (37). SLA offers many advantages over other methods. First, when printing multiple objects, each layer is printed simultaneously, and the overall printing time depends only on the thickness structure. This greatly reduces printing time (38). In addition, the light source width is very small and carefully controlled, so the external shape and internal framework structure of SLA offer precise control, facilitated by its high-resolution capabilities with an accuracy of 20 μm or more (39). This makes it easy to manufacture even complex frames. The major drawback is that there are only a handful of biocompatible materials available in SLA for tissue engineering scaffold production (7).

SLA-based 3D bioprinting is highly valuable for tissue modeling and regenerative medicine. It is increasingly used to create biomimetic human tissue models and establish co-culture systems with different cell types. Zorlutuna et al. utilized SLA bioprinting to examine interactions between hippocampus neurons and skeletal muscle myoblasts by bioprinting bioink containing myoblasts in a torus form under UV light, followed by the encapsulation of hippocampus neurons. This approach demonstrates the potential of SLA bioprinting in studying cellular interactions and tissue engineering (40).

The four advanced 3D printing methods-inkjet-based, extrusion-based, laser-associated, and SLA-seamlessly work together to create intricate living tissue (Figure 6.5).

6.4 APPLICATION OF 3D-PRINTING TECHNOLOGY FOR SKIN AND TISSUE ENGINEERING

Millions of people require organ transplants to save their lives. Three-dimensional bioprinting has the potential to transform the medical industry by producing more effective, quicker, and specific organs. It permits the researcher to do novel medical research and development. This technique is now accessible for printing a wide range of biomaterials. Biomaterials such as bone particles, cells, chemical compounds, and

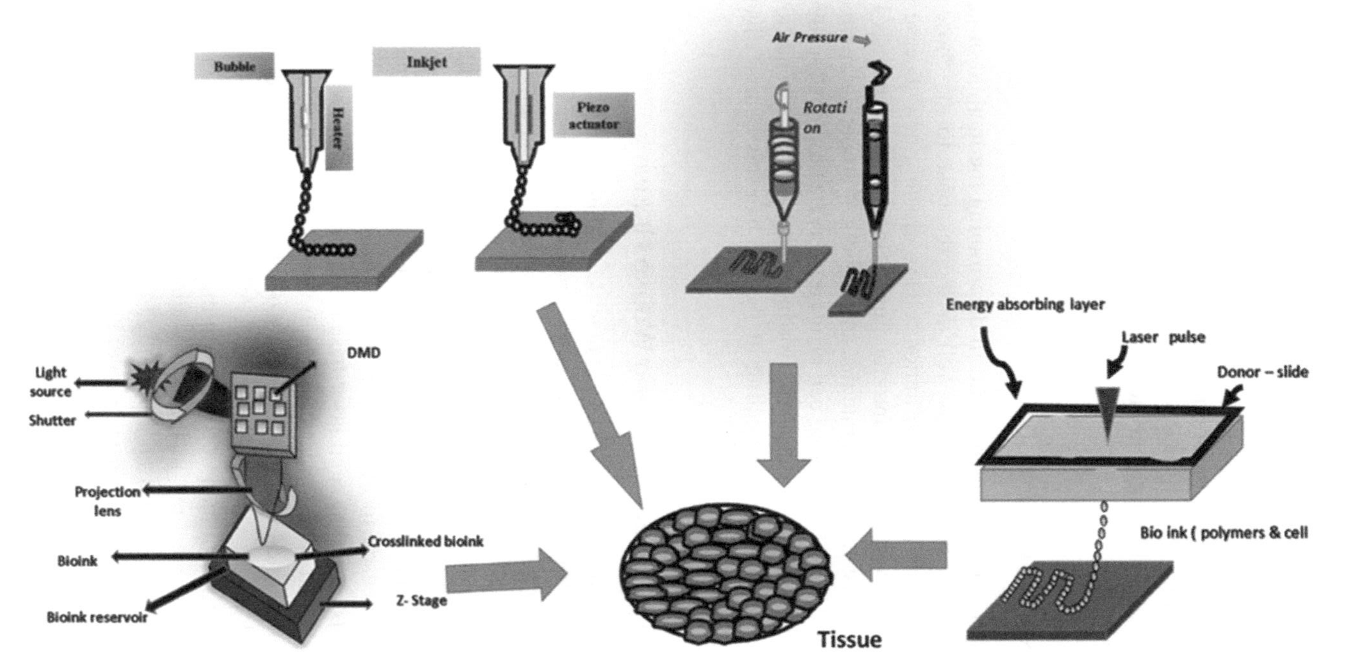

FIGURE 6.5 The four advanced 3D-printing methods—inkjet-based, extrusion-based, laser-associated, and stereolithography—are seamlessly working together to create intricate living tissue. The figure is a work of precision and innovation, as inkjet-based bioprinters delicately deposit layer upon layer of biological material, while extrusion-based bioprinters extrude intricate structures with finesse. The rhythmic movement of laser-associated bioprinting adds an enchanting glow, crafting detailed patterns with laser precision, and the ethereal glow of stereolithography printers completes.

other extracellular matrices are printed using 3D bioprinters. Its applications are now being used successfully to understand the influence of drugs. Tissues and organs manufactured with this technology have improved surgical success rates. Scientists employed 3D bioprinting to construct a skin-like covering with a blood artery, preventing graft tissue rejection in the body (41). Three-dimensional bioprinting has been utilized successfully in reconstructive burns and surgery therapy. This functioning human skin, which is appropriate for transplantation, is manufactured at a lower cost. It is useful for the formation of vascular networks and the appropriate functioning of cells. This revolutionary technology has the potential to reduce donor requirements (42).

6.4.1 Modeling of Skin Diseases

Three-dimensional tumor models may aid in determining the method of action in cancer proliferation and metastasis, as well as the response to the chosen drug. Bioprinted tissues can be mixed with tumor cells to create a new disease model. Melanoma was therefore introduced into the human in vitro skin analog (43). Liu et al. developed skin tissues to generate disease models of atopic dermatitis (AD). This study discovered that bioprinting can be used to create human skin substitutes with varying levels of cellular complexity for modeling a specific condition. This strategy allows for a better understanding of the mechanisms behind diverse illnesses (44).

6.4.2 Treatment of Burn Injuries and Wound Healing

Many people have nonhealing wounds on their skin. Skin injuries have traditionally been treated by transplants from patients' bodies or donors. The key advantage of this cutting-edge technology is that skin analogs may be easily made in less time and at a lower cost. Three-dimensional bioprinting has the potential to revolutionize the way we treat surgeries and injuries. It is especially good for healing burned skin. Three-dimensional bioprinters have been developed, allowing damaged patients to manufacture their skin (45). Ex vivo and in situ bioprinting are two technologies used to create skin for wound-healing treatment. Ex vivo technologies (extrusion, inkjet, and laser-based bioprinting) print a skin construct incorporating the dermis and epidermis, which is then matured in vitro if necessary. It is then transplanted into the patient's wound. Extrusion-based bioprinting is the simplest and quickest ex vivo approach. All of the components required to make the dermis (such as human fibroblasts, human plasma, and calcium chloride) are deposited at the same time in this approach. Human keratinocytes are then put on top of this layer to form an epidermis (43). Lian et al. combined normal human dermal fibroblasts and normal human keratinocytes with hydrogel (including sodium alginate and gelatin methacrylate) to create a skin substitute that was used to decrease scars in naked mice. The bioprinted skin performed far better in wound healing than the bioprinted hydrogel or the untreated wound control. The thickness of the dermis and epidermis was comparable to that of mice, according to histology and immunofluorescence tests done 28 days after transplantation.

Microvascular development in the dermis layer was also discovered (46). Binder et al. developed a computer software and bioprinting tool that included a cartridge delivery system made up of inkjet nozzles and a laser scanner. The 3D model of the wound was re-created using data from the laser. The printing heads then filled the wound dropwise with bioink made of fibroblasts, collagen I, and fibrinogen. Thrombin, which is required to crosslink fibrinogen into a fibrin hydrogel, was also added at the same time. Keratinocytes were printed at the final stage. The trials on nude mice demonstrated that the wound was repaired by printed skin in 3 weeks, which was significantly faster than the controls (5 weeks) This approach is novel and promising, but it is still in its early stages, and further experiments are needed (47).

6.4.3 The Cosmetic and Pharmaceutical Industry

Following the implementation of the EU Cosmetic Regulation (EU/1223/2009), which prohibits the use of animals in cosmetic testing, there is a significant desire to get skin equivalents that could serve as an alternative to animal studies. It should be noted that the use of animal models is prohibited not just for ethical grounds but also due to their insufficient resemblance to human skin. As a result, the research findings are not always apparent (48). The human physiological system differs from that of animals. As a result, around half of the drugs that passed the animal testing proved to be hazardous to people and vice versa. The pharmaceutical and cosmetics industries are both looking for skin models that may be used to test new chemicals and novel topical formulations (49).

As a result, 3D bioprinting has piqued the interest of numerous skin care companies. This new technique is intended to revolutionize cosmetic and topical product testing. Skin, as previously stated, is stratified and comprises a variety of cell types. Three-dimensional bioprinting allows cells to be deposited in this configuration. Both the cosmetic and pharmaceutical industries may benefit from 3D-bioprinted skin. In vitro tests should be performed on each novel substance/drug before clinical trials. Pharmaceutical and chemical businesses may test drugs and chemicals on skin models created with 3D bioprinters, but cosmetic compositions must be evaluated for potentially hazardous and allergic effects before being released to the market (50).

6.4.4 Drug Screening

The development of drug screening methods using 3D bioprinting is a promising new direction. For evaluating and screening the interactions between cells and the tested medications, bioprinting might distribute cells uniformly throughout a microdevice surface as opposed to traditional manual screening procedures (51). Chang et al. constructed an extrusion-based bioprinter that is pneumatically powered to construct a drug testing platform for the liver using alginate-encapsulated immortalized hepatocytes. This method may distinguish the drug metabolism capacity beneficial for screening efficacy and toxicity for the agent of interest and simulate the in vivo microenvironments of various mammalian tissues (52). According to other studies, skin infectious cells can be incorporated into biomaterials to create skin tissue via 3D bioprinting. In this manner, the pathophysiologies of skin diseases could be studied using skin tissue printed with pathogenic cells (53). Current research on electrospun materials is made of natural and synthetic materials that incorporate bioactive and/or antibacterial compounds for skin and tissue engineering has been presented in Table 6.2.

6.4.5 NEURAL TISSUE ENGINEERING

Neurological disorders pose persistent threats to both physical and mental health, often tied to the limited regeneration of neurons within the nervous system (NS). Repairing NS damage remains challenging despite conventional treatments like surgery and medication. This challenge in neurology prompts the exploration of tissue engineering, a discipline merging cell biology and materials science to reconstruct or mend organs and tissues. While tissue engineering has found success in addressing bone, periodontal tissue defects, skin repairs, and corneal transplantation, recent strides in the field have notably advanced its application within neuroscience. Tissue engineering in neuroscience focuses on addressing nerve injuries and neurodegenerative disorders by utilizing bioengineered biomaterials like electrospun nanofibers, electroactive biomaterials, and 2D materials. Electrospun nanofibers imitate the structure of the extracellular matrix, aiding nerve regeneration, but further improvements are sought through combining biochemical factors and cell therapies. Electroactive biomaterials provide electrical cues to modulate cell behavior, while 2D materials like graphene demonstrate promise in scaffold construction for neurological disorders, enhancing nerve regeneration. However, further research is needed to assess the long-term safety and biocompatibility of these materials in vivo. In the future of tissue engineering in neuroscience, overcoming challenges remains crucial. Neurological disorders like Alzheimer's, Parkinson's, and brain stroke, linked to non-regeneration of neurons, lack adequate treatments to fully restore the central nervous system (CNS). Understanding the intricate CNS mechanisms is essential for developing novel medications, hindered by the blood–brain barrier's restrictive nature. Technologies like brain–computer interfaces and optogenetics show promise in bypassing this barrier, impacting the CNS directly. Controlling scaffold biodegradation rates and exploring biodegradable biomaterials via 3D printing could enhance nerve regeneration. Investigating the complex interplay between biomaterials and the body's immune system is also vital for future advancements in tissue engineering for neurological repair.

While skin engineering primarily focuses on developing engineered skin substitutes for repairing skin injuries or disorders, there is no direct application of skin engineering in neural tissue engineering. However, some indirect connections might arise in research methodologies or technological advancements (69).

6.4.6 REGENERATIVE MEDICINE

Discovering new solutions to enhance the healthcare of aging and diseased individuals remains a global challenge. Among various strategies, tissue engineering and

TABLE 6.2

Current Research on Electrospun Materials is Made of Natural and Synthetic Materials That Incorporate Bioactive and/or Antibacterial Compounds for Skin and Tissue Engineering

S.NO.	Solvent	Electrospinning Technique	Antimicrobial agent	Additional Polymer	Cell Lines	References
1.	Dimethyl sulfoxide	Wet	Pullulan	Polyvinylpyrrolidone	L929	(54)
2.	Polyvinylpyrrolidone	Co-axial	Amoxicillin	Polyvinylpyrrolidone	L929	(55)
3.	Methanol	Blend	Irbesartan	–	Ex vivo skin permeation studies	(56)
4.	Acetone	Blend	Graphene oxide	–	L929	(57)
5.	Acetone	Blend	Zwitterionic	–		(58)
6.	Acetone	Blend	Enrofloxacin	–	HDF	(59)
7.	Dimethylformamide	Blend	Spirulina extract	Polycaprolactone	HaCaT	(60)
8	Acetic acid	Blend	Gentamicin		L929	(61)
9.	Hexafluoro-2-propanol; HS-27	Blend	Leaf extract of *Coccinia grandis*	Gelatin	NIH/3T3	(62)
10.	Hexafluoro-2-propanol	Co-axial	Epigallocatechin-3-O-gallate	Hexafluoro-2-propanol	NHDF	(63)
11.	Hexafluoro-2-propanol	Conventional	Polydopamine	Polydopamine	L929	(64)
12.	Trifluoroethanol	Blend	Curcumin	Polyvinyl alcohol	HS-27	(65)
13.	deionized water	Blend	Centellaasiatica	Polyvinyl alcohol	L929	(66)
14.	Formic acid	Blend	Maleinized soybean oil	–	NIH/3T3	(67)
15.	Dichloromethane	Conventional	Silver nanoparticles (Ag NPs)	–	AFSC	(68)

regenerative medicine (TERM) have emerged as a promising approach to address the future healthcare needs of patients. Recent advances in TERM in Asia demonstrate a dynamic landscape of research and application. Across the continent, significant contributions have been made to various aspects of TERM, including biomaterials, cell sources, and bioactive factors, aimed at fostering tissue-specific scaffolds and innovative cell therapies. Scholars have explored diverse biomaterials such as polymers, ceramics, and metals, leveraging cutting-edge technologies like 3D bioprinting and microfluidics to fabricate intricate scaffolds. They have also introduced inventive methods like cell sheet technology and investigated chemical enhancements to improve biomaterial properties. Stem cell research has notably expanded, encompassing a range of sources like embryonic stem cells, bone marrow stem cells, and induced pluripotent stem cells. These studies have shown promising outcomes in various preclinical and clinical trials focused on stem cell therapy for diverse medical conditions. Moreover, efforts to recreate and optimize tissue microenvironments using bioactive factors and stimuli like electrical, mechanical, and magnetic forces have progressed significantly. Breakthroughs such as mineralized collagen for bone regeneration and nerve scaffolds have demonstrated successful clinical translations. The emergence of commercial technologies, including 3D bioprinters, and ongoing clinical trials across multiple regions indicate the growing convergence of TERM with clinical practice. However, while there are promising developments, the clinical application of tissue-engineered products remains limited. Biomaterial-based scaffolds are predominantly utilized, and the integration of stem cells into clinical practice alongside TERM approaches requires further exploration and advancement (70).

Artificial 3D scaffolds have proven to be effective templates for dermal regeneration in treating skin defects resulting from burns, trauma, or chronic diseases within regenerative medicine. However, their application sometimes leads to insufficient angiogenesis, and the formation of new blood vessels, which is crucial for optimal tissue healing and can pose a challenge in this context (71). Skin engineering contributes significantly to regenerative medicine, particularly in skin regeneration for addressing facial aging and cutaneous wound healing. Advanced techniques in regenerative medicine, utilizing stem cells, growth factors, and biomaterial applications, aim to enhance the skin's natural healing process. These approaches offer opportunities to tackle issues like fine lines, wrinkles, skin dryness, and laxity caused by factors such as UVB radiation exposure. Additionally, regenerative medicine presents cell-based and cell-free therapies, including autologous adult stem cells, platelet-rich plasma, and emerging pluripotent stem cell-derived products, offering promising avenues for effective skin regeneration. Regulatory frameworks, as in Japan, oversee these therapies, ensuring safety and efficacy in clinical applications, and paving the way for future skin regeneration treatments (72).

6.4.7 TRANSPLANTATION

The strategy involves the facilitation of in situ tissue regeneration using an instructive scaffold. This scaffold serves as a guide and regulator during the regeneration process within the body (73). It relies on an artificial matrix that, upon implantation, attracts host cells and leverages the body's natural regenerative capabilities. The recruitment of these cells is achieved through signal presentation. For instance, the introduction of PEG–collagen matrices containing enzyme-cleavable matrix metalloproteinases (MMPs) links, releasing bone morphogenic protein-2 (BMP-2), has proven effective in stimulating the regeneration of critical-size bone defects by encouraging the invasion of host cells. Research has shown that the absence of MMP-sensitive linkages and/or BMP-2 impedes the regeneration process, underscoring the significance of using scaffolds equipped with appropriate soluble and insoluble signals (74).

Furthermore, in addressing cartilage defects, the integration of microfracture techniques with 3D-printed scaffolds, specifically functionalized with aggrecan, has demonstrated notable advancements in cartilage tissue regeneration. This approach has exhibited an enhanced expression of type II collagen (75). Therefore, the effectiveness of scaffold transplantation-based approaches predominantly relies on the precise presentation of signals that facilitate host cell mobilization and orchestrate subsequent cellular behaviors, such as adherence, migration, and proliferation.

Cellular scaffolds serve as a platform for cell attachment, proliferation, and the generation of an ECM in a predetermined 3D arrangement. Moreover, contemporary techniques like 3D printing and casting facilitate the direct incorporation of cells into scaffolds. This method often involves integrating cells within the internal structure of the scaffold, reducing their requirement to migrate independently (76). Key challenges associated with this strategy encompass the creation of fully functional tissue, maintaining cell viability and function post-transplantation, achieving both biological and mechanical integration with surrounding tissue, and ensuring adequate oxygen and nutrient supply to transplanted cells. This is particularly pertinent as cells transplanted within significant defects frequently face viability issues, impeding their contribution to the healing process.

Skin engineering plays a pivotal role in transplantation by offering innovative solutions for severe injuries, burns, and reconstructive surgeries. Engineered skin substitutes serve as alternatives to traditional grafts, aiding in the treatment of severe burns by promoting healing, reducing infection risks, and minimizing scarring. In cases of trauma or extensive skin loss, these substitutes provide temporary coverings, safeguarding against infections and creating a conducive environment for healing until permanent solutions are available. Moreover, in reconstructive surgeries requiring extensive skin grafts, engineered skin substitutes contribute to restoring skin integrity and function. Their ability to regenerate complex skin defects, tailored to individual needs, showcases the potential for personalized treatments, potentially reducing rejection risks and improving transplantation outcomes. This multifaceted application of skin engineering offers diverse solutions, revolutionizing the landscape of transplantation procedures involving the skin.

6.4.8 Replacing/Regenerating Target Organs

Tissue engineering focuses on replacing or regenerating organs. Skin regeneration aims to restore function in trauma cases like burns, wounds, and ulcers. Products like Integra use collagen-based dermal grafts for tissue healing. These grafts contain components like collagen, fibrin, hyaluronic acid (HA), and PLGA. They incorporate keratinocytes and fibroblasts, mimicking native skin. Challenges in engineered skin involve issues like scar formation, wound contraction, incomplete healing of deep wounds, and limitations in regenerating skin functions like glands and hair follicles. To achieve effective healing, tissue-engineered skin must attach to the wound bed and avoid rejection by the immune system.

Skin tissue engineering has made strides but faces challenges like scar formation and incomplete regeneration of skin functions. Liver tissue engineering aims to address organ shortages but encounters hurdles in replicating the complex vasculature and ensuring long-term functionality. Heart tissue engineering targets cardiovascular diseases but grapples with replicating the intricate nature of heart tissues. Kidney tissue engineering seeks to restore function but faces complexities due to the kidney's intricate 3D structures and multiple cell types, exploring options like using decellularized ECM for its complexity and biocompatibility. In tissue engineering, challenges persist, including poor in vivo integration, limited endothelialization, immune responses, and uncertainty regarding the ideal cell types. Orthopedic tissues like bone and cartilage have seen advancements in clinical therapies such as MACI, Hyalograft, Bond Apatite, and TruGraft. However, engineering these tissues encounters hurdles due to the complexity of bone architecture and the acellular nature of cartilage, which hampers its regenerative capacity. Finding materials with optimal mechanical properties for bone repair and developing effective, long-term solutions for cartilage defects remain active areas of research, with ongoing clinical trials exploring the potential of mesenchymal stem cells (MSCs)for cartilage regeneration. Despite progress, creating high-quality artificial cartilage remains a challenge (77).

6.4.9 DRUG DELIVERY

Regenerative medicine relies on the controlled delivery of therapeutic agents to achieve precise and lasting effects. Localized delivery of growth factors and small molecules plays a pivotal role in promoting tissue regeneration and healing. For instance, bone regeneration involves distinct stages, each regulated by different growth factors and cytokines, including inflammation, vascularization, scar formation, and mineralization. Effective wound recovery necessitates targeted administration of specific biomolecules, such as recombinant human bone morphogenetic protein-2 on an absorbable collagen sponge carrier, as seen in bone grafts like InFUSE by Medtronic (78).

Considerable research efforts within tissue engineering have focused on devising methods to encapsulate biomolecules and therapeutic compounds within biomaterials. These strategies aim to achieve predefined release rates, offering controlled and sustained delivery. The integration of 3D printing into drug delivery has gained ground, notably with the Food and Drug Administration's approval of Spritam (Aprecia Pharmaceuticals) in 2015, a 3D-printed drug designed for seizures and epilepsy. This technology strategically deposits a bioink in layers, allowing precise control over the release profiles of various biomolecules within the same construct. In tissue-engineered scaffolds, the clinical significance of drug delivery is substantial. Moreover, emerging therapies like RNA delivery, in situ injectables, extended-release oral delivery systems, and biological carriers for drug delivery are pushing the boundaries of regenerative medicine, significantly enhancing patient outcomes (79).

The integration of skin engineering in drug delivery methodologies showcases its multifaceted contributions to dermatological therapeutics. Engineered skin models, central to this field, meticulously replicate human skin properties, facilitating the evaluation and optimization of transdermal drug delivery systems. This technological advancement not only enhances targeted drug delivery but also deepens our understanding of skin barrier functions, revolutionizing drug formulation designs for transdermal applications. Moreover, the innovative scaffold-mediated drug delivery strategies hold significant promise in augmenting cutaneous wound healing. These scaffolds, functioning as protective barriers while delivering specific biochemical cues and drugs, offer a profound avenue for treating wounds. Cell-laden scaffolds, combined with genetic engineering approaches, present potential solutions for personalized wound therapy, aiming to mimic fetal wound healing characteristics for scarless skin regeneration. The synergistic advancements in 3D bioprinting further bolster precision in replicating native skin architecture, promising transformative developments in skin engineering for advanced drug delivery systems. This collective progress signifies a leap towards highly effective and tailored therapeutic interventions in dermatology, underscoring the pivotal role of skin engineering in advancing drug delivery methodologies (80).

6.4.10 MODELING DISEASES AND THERAPEUTIC APPROACHES

Tissue engineering strategies offer unconventional yet crucial applications that prove to be both valuable and significant. Novel applications of tissue engineering extend to advanced drug screening methods. Synthetic tissue microfabrication has enabled the development of in vitro systems mimicking organ-level functions and disease progression, aiding drug assessment before clinical studies. These models encompass various organs, including (81), lung (82), liver (83), and cancer models (84). While 2D cultures have limitations in assessing cancer progression and drug responses, 3D tumor models provide insights into tumor morphology, cell interactions, and drug penetration. Incorporating biological factors and engineering approaches enhances our understanding of cancer progression, paving the way for more personalized treatments for patients.

Skin engineering plays a vital role in modeling diseases and exploring therapeutic approaches. Engineered skin models serve as valuable tools to replicate disease conditions, such as dermatological disorders or skin cancers, offering a controlled environment to study disease progression, drug responses, and potential therapies.

6.4.11 ORGAN-ON-A-CHIP SYSTEMS

Microfluidic chip-based platforms provide a more sophisticated cell culture environment than traditional 2D substrates yet offer higher throughput than complex 3D biomaterial platforms. This approach allows constant nutrient perfusion, facilitated by soft lithography's precise fabrication control over biochemical and biophysical cell culture aspects (85). Each chip system acts as a miniature bioreactor, enabling regulated fluid flow for studying diverse cell responses. Lung-on-a-chip (86), gut-on-a-chip, heart-on-a-chip (87), and liver-on-a-chip (88) models have been developed and continue to evolve. Companies like Emulate Inc., Hesperos Inc., Tissue, and Tara Biosystems, among others, have commercialized on-chip technologies. Multiorgan-on-a-chip systems offer significant advantages for in vitro studies related to absorption, distribution, metabolism, excretion, and toxicity (89). These platforms assess the pharmacokinetics and pharmacodynamics of potential drug candidates, evaluating their safety, efficacy, and dosage. While in vivo animal studies remain the gold standard for preclinical trials, they are costly and time-consuming. Consequently, interconnected multiorgan on-chip platforms (90) using human-derived cell sources provide a rapid, reliable means to screen numerous drugs, aligning more closely with clinical applications.

Organ-on-a-chip systems show great potential in progressing tissue and skin engineering applications by replicating human organs, like skin, on a microscale. They enable accurate studies and simulation of physiological functions. In the realm of skin engineering, these platforms create controlled settings to mimic skin properties, enabling research into drug delivery, wound healing, and diseases. Notably, organ-on-a-chip systems aid in incorporating vascular networks into engineered skin structures, crucial for their sustained function and survival over time. The potential of merging bioprinting with skin-on-a-chip systems to address this challenge. While the specific combination for skin applications is less explored, combining 3D printing with fluid perfusion offers promise for creating detailed and functional vasculature. The study discussed integrating 3D-printed, perfusable vasculature into skin models for drug delivery research. This integration of bioprinting and organ-on-a-chip technology holds potential in advancing skin tissue engineering, aiming to replicate natural skin features in research models for drug delivery and tissue engineering applications (91).

6.5 CONCLUSION AND FUTURE PROSPECTS

Three-dimensional bioprinting exhibits tremendous promise in revolutionizing tissue engineering, offering innovative solutions for therapeutic applications. Notably, skin bioprinting technology emerges as a game-changer, showcasing the potential to construct fully functional skin and significantly reduce healing time and pain for patients with burns and skin lesions.

LAB, with its micron-scale focal size, stands out for its higher resolution, enabling the precise fabrication of complex 3D structures. The use of biomaterials like collagen, chitosan, gelatin, PLA, PLGA, and PU in skin and tissue engineering underscores their advantages in terms of biocompatibility, antibacterial properties, and biodegradability. Overcoming challenges related to speed, printing capability, and the maturation of bioprinted vascular networks is crucial for large-scale tissue production, addressing the high demand in hospitals. The current landscape presents opportunities for further study and development in bioink formulations, innovations in 3D printer units, and novel approaches in 3D printing/bioprinting. Exploring diverse directions, such as stereotactic bioprinting using robotic technology and the development of heterogeneous scaffolds based on tissue anisotropy, unveils exciting prospects for advancing 3D bioprinting in tissue engineering.

Moreover, the integration of natural and synthetic polymers as scaffolding biomaterials opens new avenues for research and application. While synthetic biopolymers offer engineerable mechanical characteristics, the challenge lies in addressing their lack of organic features. Future efforts should focus on creating novel procedures or approaches for modification to enhance the overall performance of synthetic biomaterials in 3D bioprinting. Looking ahead, the field of 3D bioprinting holds the potential to shape the future of regenerative medicine, offering customized solutions and contributing to global medical advancements. Collaborative efforts across disciplines, encompassing manufacturing, material science, biology, and medicine, are essential to overcoming challenges and propelling 3D bioprinting toward greater precision, speed, and expanded applications in tissue engineering, drug delivery, and beyond. As we continue to delve into uncharted territories, the evolving landscape of 3D bioprinting promises a future marked by groundbreaking innovations and transformative impacts on healthcare and regenerative medicine.

ACKNOWLEDGMENTS

We would like to express gratitude to our co-authors, and the institutions—Indira Gandhi National Tribal University Amarkantak, Madhya Pradesh, India and SLT Institute of Pharmacy Guru Ghasidas Vishwavidyalaya, Bilaspur, Chhattishgarh, India-for their support in drafting this chapter on "3D Bioprinting for Skin and Tissue Engineering." Special thanks to Dr. Sunita Minz for her guidance. We also appreciate the contributions of reviewers and mentors.

FUNDING

None.

CONFLICT OF INTEREST

None.

REFERENCES

(1) Fang Y, Guo Y, Liu T, Xu R, Mao S, Mo X, et al. Advances in 3D bioprinting. *Chinese Journal of Mechanical Engineering: Additive Manufacturing Frontiers* 2022 Mar;1(1):100011.

(2) Tamay DG, Dursun Usal T, Alagoz AS, Yucel D, Hasirci N, Hasirci V. 3D and 4D printing of polymers for tissue engineering applications. *Frontiers in Bioengineering and Biotechnology* 2019 Jul 9;7:164.

(3) Bishop ES, Mostafa S, Pakvasa M, Luu HH, Lee MJ, Wolf JM, Ameer GA, He TC, Reid RR. 3-D bioprinting technologies in tissue engineering and regenerative medicine: Current and future trends. *Genes & Diseases* 2017 Dec 1;4(4):185–95.

(4) Roy A, Saxena V, Pandey LM. 3D printing for cardiovascular tissue engineering: a review. *Materials Technology* 2018 May 12;33(6):433–42.

(5) Pavan Kalyan BG, Kumar L. 3D printing: applications in tissue engineering, medical devices, and drug delivery. *AAPS PharmSciTech* 2022 Mar 17;23(4):92.

(6) Vanaei S, Parizi MS, Vanaei S, Salemizadehparizi F, Vanaei HR. An overview on materials and techniques in 3D bioprinting toward biomedical application. *Engineered Regeneration* 2021;2: 1–18.

(7) Colasante C, Sanford Z, Garfein E, Tepper O. Current trends in 3D printing, bioprosthetics, and tissue engineering in plastic and reconstructive surgery. *Current Surgery Reports* 2016 Feb; 4:1–4.

(8) Gupta S, Bissoyi A, Bit A. A review on 3D printable techniques for tissue engineering. *Bio Nanoscience* 2018 Sep 1;8(3):868–83.

(9) Zaszczyńska A, Moczulska-Heljak M, Gradys A, Sajkiewicz P. Advances in 3D printing for tissue engineering. *Materials* 2021 Jun 8;14(12):3149.

(10) Derakhshanfar S, Mbeleck R, Xu K, Zhang X, Zhong W, Xing M. 3D bioprinting for biomedical devices and tissue engineering: A review of recent trends and advances. *Bioactive Materials* 2018 Jun 1;3(2):144–56.

(11) Janmohammadi M, Nourbakhsh MS. Recent advances on 3D printing in hard and soft tissue engineering. *International Journal of Polymeric Materials and Polymeric Biomaterials* 2020 May 2;69(7):449–66.

(12) Singh D, Singh D, Han SS. 3D printing of scaffold for cells delivery: advances in skin tissue engineering. *Polymers* 2016 Jan 16;8(1):19.

(13) Weng T, Zhang W, Xia Y, Wu P, Yang M, Jin R, Xia S, Wang J, You C, Han C, Wang X. 3D bioprinting for skin tissue engineering: Current status and perspectives. *Journal of Tissue Engineering* 2021 Jul; 12:20417314211028574.

(14) Ma J, Wu C. Bioactive inorganic particles-based biomaterials for skin tissue engineering. *Exploration* 2022 Oct;2(5):20210083.

(15) Gu BK, Choi DJ, Park SJ, Kim YJ, Kim CH. 3D bioprinting technologies for tissue engineering applications. *Cutting-Edge Enabling Technologies for Regenerative Medicine* 2018:15–28. https://doi.org/10.1007/978-981-13-0950-2_2

(16) Huang S, Fu X. Naturally derived materials-based cell and drug delivery systems in skin regeneration. *Journal of Controlled Release* 2010 Mar 3;142(2):149–59.

(17) Tang X, Thankappan SK, Lee P, Fard SE, Harmon MD, Tran K, Yu X. Polymeric biomaterials in tissue engineering and regenerative medicine. *Natural and Synthetic Biomedical Polymers* 2014 Jan 1:351–71.

(18) Abbasian M, Massoumi B, Mohammad-Rezaei R, Samadian H, Jaymand M. Scaffolding polymeric biomaterials: Are naturally occurring biological macromolecules more appropriate for tissue engineering? *International Journal of Biological Macromolecules* 2019 Aug 1; 134:673–94.

(19) Poomathi N, Singh S, Prakash C, Subramanian A, Sahay R, Cinappan A, Ramakrishna S. 3D printing in tissue engineering: a state of the art review of technologies and biomaterials. *Rapid Prototyping Journal* 2020 Jun 24;26(7):1313–34.

(20) Pandey AR, Singh US, Momin M, Bhavsar C. Chitosan: Application in tissue engineering and skin grafting. *Journal of Polymer Research* 2017 Aug; 24:1–22.

(21) Cai R, Gimenez-Camino N, Xiao M, Bi S, DiVito KA. Technological advances in three-dimensional skin tissue engineering. *Reviews on Advanced Materials Science* 2023 Feb 2;62(1):20220289.

(22) Ishack S, Lipner SR. A review of 3-dimensional skin bioprinting techniques: Applications, approaches, and trends. *Dermatologic Surgery* 2020 Dec 1;46(12):1500–5.

(23) Mandrycky C, Wang Z, Kim K, Kim DH. 3D bioprinting for engineering complex tissues. *Biotechnology Advances* 2016 Jul 1;34(4):422–34.

(24) Tarassoli SP, Jessop ZM, Al-Sabah A, Gao N, Whitaker S, Doak S, Whitaker IS. Skin tissue engineering using 3D bioprinting: An evolving research field. *Journal of Plastic, Reconstructive & Aesthetic Surgery* 2018 May 1;71(5):615–23.

(25) Li J, Chen M, Fan X, Zhou H. Recent advances in bioprinting techniques: approaches, applications and future prospects. *Journal of Translational Medicine* 2016 Dec;14(1):1–5.

(26) Daikuara LY, Chen X, Yue Z, Skropeta D, Wood FM, Fear MW, Wallace GG. 3D bioprinting constructs to facilitate skin regeneration. *Advanced Functional Materials* 2022 Jan;32(3):2105080.

(27) Rimann M, Bono E, Annaheim H, Bleisch M, Graf-Hausner U. Standardized 3D bioprinting of soft tissue models with human primary cells. *Journal of Laboratory Automation* 2016 Aug;21(4):496–509.

(28) Kim BS, Lee JS, Gao G, Cho DW. Direct 3D cell-printing of human skin with functional transwell system. *Biofabrication* 2017 Jun 7;9(2):025034.

(29) Albanna M, Binder KW, Murphy SV, Kim J, Qasem SA, Zhao W, Tan J, El-Amin IB, Dice DD, Marco J, Green J. In situ bioprinting of autologous skin cells accelerates wound healing of extensive excisional full-thickness wounds. *Scientific Reports* 2019 Feb 12;9(1):1856.

(30) Ozbolat IT, Hospodiuk M. Current advances and future perspectives in extrusion-based bioprinting. *Biomaterials* 2016 Jan 1; 76:321–43.

(31) Assad H, Assad A, Kumar A. Recent developments in 3D bio-printing and its biomedical applications. *Pharmaceutics* 2023 Jan 11;15(1):255.

(32) Gao C, Lu C, Jian Z, Zhang T, Chen Z, Zhu Q, Tai Z, Liu Y. 3D bioprinting for fabricating artificial skin tissue. *Colloids and Surfaces B: Biointerfaces* 2021 Dec 1;208:112041.

(33) Gu Z, Fu J, Lin H, He Y. Development of 3D bioprinting: From printing methods to biomedical applications. *Asian Journal of Pharmaceutical Sciences* 2020 Sep 1;15(5):529–57.

(34) Kodama H. Automatic method for fabricating a three-dimensional plastic model with photo-hardening polymer. *Review of Scientific Instruments* 1981 Nov 1;52(11):1770–3.

(35) Zhu W, Cui H, Boualam B, Masood F, Flynn E, Rao RD, Zhang ZY, Zhang LG. 3D bioprinting mesenchymal stem cell-laden construct with core–shell nanospheres for cartilage tissue engineering. *Nanotechnology* 2018 Mar 8;29(18):185101.

(36) Wu CA, Zhu Y, Woo YJ. Advances in 3D bioprinting: Techniques, applications, and future directions for cardiac tissue engineering. *Bioengineering* 2023 Jul 16;10(7):842.

(37) Xie M, Su J, Zhou S, Li J, Zhang K. Application of hydrogels as three-dimensional bioprinting ink for tissue engineering. *Gels* 2023 Jan 19;9(2):88.

(38) Wang Z, Abdulla R, Parker B, Samanipour R, Ghosh S, Kim K. A simple and high-resolution stereolithography-based 3D bioprinting system using visible light crosslinkable bioinks. *Biofabrication* 2015 Dec 22;7(4):045009.

(39) Ji K, Wang Y, Wei Q, Zhang K, Jiang A, Rao Y, Cai X. Application of 3D printing technology in bone tissue engineering. *Bio-Design and Manufacturing* 2018 Sep; 1:203–10.

(40) Li W, Wang M, Ma H, Chapa-Villarreal FA, Lobo AO, Zhang YS. Stereolithography apparatus and digital light processing-based 3D bioprinting for tissue fabrication. *Iscience* 2023 Jan 24;26.

(41) Javaid M, Haleem A. 3D bioprinting applications for the printing of skin: A brief study. *Sensors International* 2021 Jan 1; 2:100123.

(42) Ng WL, Qi JT, Yeong WY, Naing MW. Proof-of-concept: 3D bioprinting of pigmented human skin constructs. *Biofabrication* 2018 Jan 24;10(2):025005.

(43) Olejnik A, Semba JA, Kulpa A, Danczak-Pazdrowska A, Rybka JD, Gornowicz-Porowska J. 3D bioprinting in skin related research: Recent achievements and application perspectives. *ACS Synthetic Biology* 2021 Dec 30;11(1):26–38.

(44) Liu X, Michael S, Bharti K, Ferrer M, Song MJ. A biofabricated vascularized skin model of atopic dermatitis for preclinical studies. *Biofabrication* 2020 Apr 8;12(3):035002.

(45) Mason J, Visintini S, Quay T. An overview of clinical applications of 3-D printing and bioprinting. 2019 Apr 1. In *CADTH Issues in Emerging Health Technologies. Ottawa (ON): Canadian Agency for Drugs and Technologies in Health*; 2016–2021. 175. PMID: 31211545.

(46) Lian Q, Jiao T, Zhao T, Wang H, Yang S, Li D. 3D bioprinted skin substitutes for accelerated wound healing and reduced scar. *Journal of Bionic Engineering* 2021 Jul;18(4):900–14.

(47) Binder KW, Zhao W, Aboushwareb T, Dice D, Atala A, Yoo JJ. In situ bioprinting of the skin for burns. *Journal of the American College of Surgeons* 2010 Sep 1;211(3): S76.

(48) Garcia M, Escamez MJ, Carretero M, Mirones I, Martinez-Santamaria L, Navarro M, Jorcano JL, Meana A, Del Rio M, Larcher F. Modeling normal and pathological processes through skin tissue engineering. *Molecular Carcinogenesis: Published in cooperation with the University of Texas MD Anderson Cancer Center* 2007 Aug;46(8):741–5.

(49) Hansen K, Khanna C. Spontaneous and genetically engineered animal models: use in preclinical cancer drug development. *European Journal of Cancer* 2004 Apr 1;40(6):858–80.

(50) Millás A, Lago J, Vasquez-Pinto L, Massaguer P, Maria-Engler SS. Approaches to the development of 3D bioprinted skin models: the case of natura cosmetics. *International Journal of Advances in Medical Biotechnology-IJAMB* 2019 Mar 1;2(1):03–13.

(51) Xie Z, Gao M, Lobo AO, Webster TJ. 3D bioprinting in tissue engineering for medical applications: the classic and the hybrid. *Polymers* 2020 Jul 31;12(8):1717.

(52) Chang R, Emami K, Wu H, Sun W. Biofabrication of a three-dimensional liver microorgan as an in vitro drug metabolism model. *Biofabrication* 2010 Nov 15;2(4):045004.

(53) Lee V, Singh G, Trasatti JP, Bjornsson C, Xu X, Tran TN, Yoo SS, Dai G, Karande P. Design and fabrication of human skin by three-dimensional bioprinting. *Tissue Engineering Part C: Methods* 2014 Jun 1;20(6):473–84.

(54) Atila D, Keskin D, Tezcaner et al. Cellulose acetate based 3-dimensional electrospun scaffolds for skin tissue engineering applications. *Carbohydrate Polymers* 2015 Nov 20; 133:251–61.

(55) Castillo-Ortega MM, Nájera-Luna A, Rodríguez-Félix DE, Encinas JC, Rodríguez-Félix F, Romero J, Herrera-Franco PJ, et al. Preparation, characterization and release of amoxicillin from cellulose acetate and poly (vinyl pyrrolidone) coaxial electrospun fibrous membranes. *Materials Science and Engineering* 2011 Nov;31(8):1772–1778.

(56) Kamble RN, Gaikwad S, Maske A, Patil SS et al. Fabrication of electrospunnanofibres of BCS II drug for enhanced dissolution and permeation across skin. *Journal of Advanced Research* 2016 May 1;7(3):483–9.

(57) Jiang S, Wu J, Hang Y, Liu Q, Li D, Chen H, Brash JL et al. Sustained release of a synthetic structurally-tailored glycopolymer modulates endothelial cells for enhanced endothelialization of materials. *Journal of Materials Chemistry B* 2019 Feb; 7(25):4017–29.

(58) Venault A, Lin KH, Tang SH, Dizon GV, Hsu CH, Maggay IV, Chang Y et al. Zwitterionicelectrospun PVDF fibrous membranes with a well-controlled hydration for diabetic wound recovery. *Journal of Membrane Science* 2020 Mar 15; 598:117648.

(59) He T, Wang J, Huang P, Zeng B, Li H, Cao Q, Zhang S, Luo Z, Deng DY, Zhang H, Zhou W et al. Electrospinningpolyvinylidene fluoride fibrous membranes containing anti-bacterial drugs used as wound dressing. *Colloids and Surfaces B: Biointerfaces* 2015 Jun 1; 130:278–86.

(60) Choi JI, Kim MS, Chung GY, Shin HS et al. Spirulina extract-impregnated alginate-PCL nanofiber wound dressing for skin regeneration. *Biotechnology and Bioprocess Engineering* 2017 Nov;22:679–85.

(61) Bakhsheshi-Rad HR, Hadisi Z, Ismail AF, Aziz M, Akbari M, Berto F, Chen XB et al. In vitro and in vivo evaluation of chitosan-alginate/gentamicin wound dressing nanofibrous with high antibacterial performance. *Polymer Testing* 2020 Feb 1;82:106298.

(62) Ramanathan G, Singaravelu S, Raja MD, Nagiah N, Padmapriya P, Ruban K, Kaveri K, Natarajan TS, Sivagnanam UT, Perumal PTet al. Fabrication and characterization of a collagen coated electrospun poly (3-hydroxybutyric acid)–gelatin nanofibrous scaffold as a soft bio-mimetic material for skin tissue engineering applications. *RSC Advances* 2016;6(10):7914–7922.

(63) Shin YC, Shin DM, Lee EJ, Lee JH, Kim JE, Song SH, Hwang DY, Lee JJ, Kim B, Lim D, Hyon SH et al. Hyaluronic acid/PLGA core/shell fiber matrices loaded with EGCG beneficial to diabetic wound healing. *Advanced Healthcare Materials* 2016 Dec;5(23):3035–45.

(64) Yan X, Yu M, Ramakrishna S, Russell SJ, Long YZ et al. Advances in portable electrospinning devices for in situ delivery of personalized wound care. *Nanoscale* 2019;11(41):19166–78.

(65) Dai X, Liu J, Zheng H, Wichmann J, Hopfner U, Sudhop S, Prein C, Shen Y, Machens HG, Schilling AF, et al. Nano-formulated curcumin accelerates acute wound healing through Dkk-1-mediated fibroblast mobilization and MCP-1-mediated anti-inflammation. *NPG Asia Materials* 2017;9(3):e368–e368.

(66) Yao CH, Yeh JY, Chen YS, Li MH, Huang CH et al. Wound-healing effect of electrospun gelatin nanofibres containing Centellaasiatica extract in a rat model. *Journal of Tissue Engineering and Regenerative Medicine* 2017 Mar;11(3):905–15.

(67) Dias FT, Ingracio AR, Nicoletti NF, Menezes FC, Agnol LD, Marinowic DR, Soares RM, da Costa JC, Falavigna A, Bianchi O et al. Soybean-modified polyamide-6 mats as a long-term cutaneous wound covering. *Materials Science and Engineering: C* 2019 Jun 1; 99:957–68.

(68) Groeber F, Holeiter M, Hampel M, Hinderer S, Schenke-Layland K et al. Skin tissue engineering—In vivo and in vitro applications. *Advanced Drug Delivery Reviews* 2011 Apr 30;63(4–5):352–66.

(69) Zhang X, Liu F, Gu Z. Tissue engineering in neuroscience: Applications and perspectives. *BME Frontiers* 2023;4:0007

(70) Han F, Wang J, Ding L, Hu Y, Li W, Yuan Z, … Li B. Tissue engineering and regenerative medicine: Achievements, future, and sustainability in Asia. *Frontiers in Bioengineering and Biotechnology* 2020;8:83.

(71) Nourian Dehkordi A, Mirahmadi Babaheydari F, Chehelgerdi M, Raeisi Dehkordi S. Skin tissue engineering: wound healing based on stem-cell-based therapeutic strategies. *Stem Cell Research & Therapy* 2019;10(1):1–20.

(72) Shimizu Y, Ntege EH, Sunami H. Current regenerative medicine-based approaches for skin regeneration: A review of literature and a report on clinical applications in Japan. *Regenerative Therapy* 2022;21:73–80.

(73) Zhao W, Karp JM, Controlling cell fate in vivo. *ChemBioChem* 2009;10(14):2308–2310.

(74) Lutolf MP, Lauer-Fields JL, Scheckel HG, Metters AT, Weber FE, Fields GB, Hubbell JA. Synthetic matrix metalloproteinase-sensitive hydrogels for the conduction of tissue regeneration: engineering cell-invasion characteristics. *Proceedings of the National Academy of Sciences* 2003;100(9):5413–5418.

(75) Guo T, Noshin M, Baker HB, Taskoy E, Meredith SJ, Tang Q, Ringel JP, Lerman MJ, Chen Y, Packer JD, Fisher JP. 3D printed biofunctionalized scaffolds for microfracture repair of cartilage defects. *Biomaterials* 2018;185:219–231.

(76) Kottamasu P, Herman I. Engineering a microcirculation for perfusion control of ex vivo–assembled organ systems: Challenges and opportunities. *Journal of Tissue Engineering* 2018;9:2041731418772949.

(77) Van Belleghem SM, Mahadik B, Snodderly KL, Fisher JP. Overview of tissue engineering concepts and applications. In *Biomaterials Science* (pp. 1289–1316). Academic Press, 2020.

(78) McKay WF, Peckham SM, Badura JM. A comprehensive clinical review of recombinant human bone morphogenetic protein-2 (INFUSE® Bone Graft). *International Orthopaedics* 2007;31(6):729–734.

(79) Thambi T, Li Y, Lee DS. Injectable hydrogels for sustained release of therapeutic agents. *Journal of Controlled Release* 2017;267:57–66.

(80) Kim HS, Sun X, Lee JH, Kim HW, Fu X, Leong KW. Advanced drug delivery systems and artificial skin grafts for skin wound healing. *Advanced Drug Delivery Reviews* 2019;146:209–239.

(81) Ralphe JC, de Lange WJ. 3D engineered cardiac tissue models of human heart disease: learning more from our mice. *Trends in Cardiovascular Medicine* 2013;23(2):27–32.

(82) Chen YW, Huang SX, De Carvalho ALRT, Ho SH, Islam MN, Volpi S, … Snoeck HW. A three-dimensional model of human lung development and disease from pluripotent stem cells. *Nature Cell Biology* 2017;19(5):542–549.

(83) Broutier L, Mastrogiovanni G, Verstegen MM, Francies HE, Gavarró LM, Bradshaw CR, … Huch M. Human primary liver cancer–derived organoid cultures for disease modeling and drug screening. *Nature Medicine* 2017;23(12):1424–1435.

(84) Benam KH, Dauth S, Hassell B, Herland A, Jain A, Jang KJ, … Ingber DE. Engineered in vitro disease models. *Annual Review of Pathology: Mechanisms of Disease* 2015;10:195–262.

(85) Bhatia SN, Ingber DE. Microfluidic organs-on-chips. *Nature Biotechnology* 2014;32(8):760–772.

(86) Benam KH, Mazur M, Choe Y, Ferrante TC, Novak R, Ingber DE. Human lung small airway-on-a-chip protocol. *3D Cell Culture: Methods and Protocols* 2017:345–365. https://doi.org/10.1007/978-1-4939-7021-6_25

(87) Parsa H, Wang BZ, Vunjak-Novakovic G. A microfluidic platform for the high-throughput study of pathological cardiac hypertrophy. *Lab on a Chip* 2017;17(19):3264–3271.

(88) Bhise NS, Manoharan V, Massa S, Tamayol A, Ghaderi M, Miscuglio M, … Khademhosseini A. A liver-on-a-chip platform with bioprinted hepatic spheroids. *Biofabrication* 2016;8(1):014101.

(89) Ishida S. Organs-on-a-chip: current applications and consideration points for in vitro ADME-Tox studies. *Drug Metabolism and Pharmacokinetics* 2018;33(1):49–54.

(90) Maschmeyer I, Lorenz AK, Schimek K, Hasenberg T, Ramme AP, Hübner J, … Marx U. A four-organ-chip for interconnected long-term co-culture of human intestine, liver, skin and kidney equivalents. *Lab on a Chip* 2015;15(12):2688–2699.

(91) Fetah K, Tebon P, Goudie MJ, Eichenbaum J, Ren L, Barros N, … Khademhosseini A. The emergence of 3D bioprinting in organ-on-chip systems. *Progress in Biomedical Engineering* 2019;1(1):012001.

7 Newer Dimension
4D- and 5D-Printing Opportunities in Drug Delivery to the Skin

S Princely Ebenezer Gnanakani
Parul University, Waghodia, India

R Vijayalakshmi
GIET School of Pharmacy, Rajahmundry, India

7.1 INTRODUCTION

Three-dimensional (3D) printing, an imminent additive manufacturing (AM) technique, has been used in a number of therapeutic contexts, including the production of drug delivery systems (DDSs), organs and tissues, and regenerative medicine (1–4). Amidst the use of computer-aided design (CAD) models and 3D printing, the method integrates magnetic resonance imaging and computed tomography (CT) imaging techniques to collect human-specific data (5–8). The capacity of this technology to 3D-print patient-specific biomedical equipment in accordance with specifications enables the provision of customized biomedical services (9–11). However, the biomedical devices created with this technique are physiologically fixed and not intended for use in dynamic environments (12, 13). Four-dimensional (4D) printing machinery has been cultivated to alleviate this issue. The brainstorm of 4D printing was initially put forth by Professors Tibbits and Jerry in 2013 (2, 9, 14, 15), in which sophisticated materials change their structure over time in a simulated environment. Tibbits introduced the idea of 4D printing as a dynamic material that may change its shape over time (16). The most cutting-edge manufacturing method is 4D printing, which is an improved form of 3D printing (17). Considering the advanced materials' propensity to change function or shape periodically in a specific environment and in reaction to stimuli, 4D printing is defined as having an additional dimension that is defined as "time" in comparison to 3D printing (18). An intelligent choice of smart materials inhabiting a 3D space is necessary to achieve dynamic capabilities (19). To make sure that the numerous materials contained are correctly created and dispersed, mathematical modeling must be applied. The 4D structure ought to include at least two steady states, which alternate between them when the right stimulus is present (20). It is crucial to thoroughly evaluate the material genres and characteristics of

DOI: 10.1201/9781032690926-7

bioprinters (21). Four-dimensional printing is a more sophisticated kind of 3D printing that seems to be able to attain self-repair, self-assembly, and multifunctionality. As an outcome, it may produce items with a variety of functions, dynamic structures, and adaptable shapes (18, 22). These complex materials are transformed into new dimensions when exposed to a variety of external stimuli, such as moisture, light, temperature, pH, magnetic and electric fields, cell traction force, enzymes, and biomolecules via 4D printing (23–26).

Several 4D-printing techniques, such as stereolithography (SLA), inkjet printing (IJP), digital light processing (DLP), fused deposition modeling (FDM), direct ink writing (DIW), selective laser sintering (SLS), and micro-extrusion, are employed in DDSs (27–31). The impact of 4D printing is astounding in the biomedical industry, particularly in the sectors of dentistry, scaffolds, and tissue engineering (TE), which increase our healthcare practices and profoundly assist patients (32–34). Additionally, in the wake of a mishap, the surgical placement of any tissue or organ rejuvenation is also required. The parameters ultimately promote the formation of artificial tissues and organs deploying living cells (35–37). This initiates the implementation of bioprinting technology, which relies on the utilization of bioprinters, specialized devices capable of accurately replicating and printing organs and stem cells (38).

In 4D printing, customization refers to the fabrication of customized drug delivery devices with definite control over the shape, size, and geometry of the device. This customization enables pharmaceutical dosage forms with several drug molecules, varied internal geometries, and drug delivery profiles based on individual patient needs, potentially leading to improved treatment outcomes and patient satisfaction (39, 40). This flexibility allows for the design of a large variety of DDSs like capsules, tablets, multilayered DDSs, nanosuspension, transdermal implants, wound-healing patches, and vaginal or rectal systems with specific features to enhance drug delivery efficiency (40). The aid of 4D printing machinery in the medical area can utilize a self-deforming component on a patient's body to correct any abnormalities, thereby reducing the need for surgery (19, 41). Additionally, because 3D and 4D printing are so flexible, they may be perfect for creating DDSs that can then be customized to give specific treatments. For instance, it would be ubiquitous and simple to print pills and tablets (also known as polypills) with customized doses that contain a variety of therapeutic substances (42). Devices that can be made to deliver individualized medicine have drawn a lot of interest, ranging from simple oral dosage forms to drug-releasing implants. Four-dimensional printing has prospective applications in the advancement of DDSs, hydrogels, microneedles (MNs), personalized dressings and drug dosage forms, drug-eluting implants, and more.

Five-dimensional (5D) printing refers to an advanced version of 3D printing technology that creates objects from five different directions, whereas 4D printing creates objects from just four. In 4D printing, the object gradually changes shape in reaction to outside stimuli; however, in 5D printing, the imprinted object swivels as the printing process continues, with the ability to design a part with a curvaceous layer instead of a flat layer with improved strength (43, 44). 5D printing has inherent applications in the construction of patient-specific customized curved implants, smart DDSs, oral formulations, biomaterials for the release of proteins/oxygen, customized drug-eluting patches, and dosage forms (45–48). Five-dimensional printing machines are programmable, which enables the fabrication of more complicated and anomalous rigid structures compared to 3D and 4D printers (49). Four-dimensional printing has applications in sensors, electronics, aerospace, soft-robotics, medicine, military, textiles, energy, and vehicle manufacturing. However, further research and development are needed to optimize the 4D/5D printing techniques, material formulations, and design considerations for the successful implementation of DDSs in skin drug delivery. This chapter addresses an overview of the concept and principles of 4D and 5D printing, distinct features and capabilities compared to traditional 3D printing, and advancements and applications of 4D printing in skin drug delivery, with special emphasis on targeted and on-demand drug release for localized skin conditions and exploring 5D printing for skin drug delivery with emphasis on its application for personalized medicine.

7.2 MATERIALS

Stimuli-responsive materials are crucial for converting a static 3D object into a dynamic 4D one from a material standpoint. Four-dimensional-printed things may shape morph or shape memory based on stimulus (17, 50, 51). Shape morphing involves irreversible shifts in the object's attributes, whereas shape memory involves switching between enduring and programmed temporary shapes after stimulus exposure (52). Shape memory effect may occur in materials that may be programmed and recovered after susceptibility to a distinct stimulus. Shape memory materials (SMMs) intentionally deform into a transient shape during programming and retain it until a stimulus has been applied. The original/permanent form may be reclaimed after stimulation (50, 53). Shape memory hybrids (SMHs), shape memory polymers (SMPs), shape memory alloys (SMAs), liquid crystal elastomers (LCEs), shape memory ceramics (SMCs), other stimuli-responsive materials, and their combinations have been used in 4D printing for biological purposes.

7.2.1 SMPs

Most SMPs have exceptional inherent biocompatibility, biodegradability, and response to stimuli, making them the utmost common material for biomedical applications (17). Thus, SMPs are distinct and diversified materials that provide exceptional adaptability throughout the production process. Due to their considerable physical and mechanical variability, thermoresponsive SMPs are among the most highly explored external stimuli-responsive SMPs for a broad variety of applications (17, 58, 59). Programming and recovery are needed for SMP shape modification. After printing, thermoresponsive SMP actuators undergo thermomechanical programming (17, 54, 55). Programming and recovery are needed for SMP shape modification. After printing, thermoresponsive SMP actuators undergo thermomechanical programming (50, 53). For programming, a single SMP is first changed at a temperature above its typical transformation temperature, which might be the melting temperature based on the polymer. After cooling below the typical transition temperature (Tg), the SMP's programmed form is fixed. Heat above the typical Tg may restore the SMP to its original form (53). Stretchability at temperatures over the

TABLE 7.1

Choice of Techniques for Printing Smart Materials by 4D and 5D Methods

Material	FDM	SLA	SLS	DLP	Hydrogel Extrusion	PolyJet
Shape Memory Polymers	Y	Y	Y	Y	Y	Y
Smart Polymers	Y	Y	Y	Y	Y	Y
Hydrogels	L	L	L	L	Y	L
Elastomers	Y	Y	Y	Y	L	Y
Metals	L	L	Y	L	L	L
Biodegradable Polymers	Y	Y	L	Y	L	Y
Composites	Y	L	L	L	L	L

Note: Y – yes; L – Limited.

SMP transition point also affects 4D shape transformation (49, 53). For biological 4D printing, a sufficient preliminary evaluation of the SMP's material characteristics is needed (Table 7.1).

Ge et al. described a method for modulating SMP stretchability (56). Particularly, distinctive blending proportions of SMP within a photo-crosslinkable hydrogel caused unique glass Tg, which impacted flexibility and rate of recovery over time. Jin et al. created a programmable polyurethane network–based integrated soft material robot with localized spatial actuation utilizing thermally induced trans-carbamoylation, trans-esterification, and photo-reversible dimer formation of nitro-cinnamate (57). Zarek et al. investigated using methacrylated PCL as the main SMP for DLP-designed shape-changing devices. The methacrylation level is greatly influenced by resin crosslinking density and crystallinity (58).

7.2.2 SMAs

SMAs were discovered earlier in the 1970s using a Ti–Ni alloy at Naval Ordnance Laboratories (59, 60). SMAs have very much attracted the attention of mechanical, material science, and biomedical engineering experts. Thus, SMAs have been created and constructed into thin films and solid objects (60, 61). An SMA, a metal alloy subdivision, is similar to an SMP but distinct. SMA uses thermal or magnetic triggering and needs programming to change phases (61). SMA has three types of shape memory and three crystal structures (17, 61). A naturally derived SMA may be twinned with martensite and detwinned when loaded. When the temperature goes above the austenite transition point, detwinned martensite becomes austenite, restoring the shape (61). The pseudoelasticity phase is independent of thermal stimuli usually associated with SMAs as a type of SMMs. SMAs have been studied for biomedical uses besides the cutting-edge research noted earlier. SMAs made from Ni and Al are not biocompatible, although research is continuing (50). Reversible porous structures are made by 4D-printing Ni–Mn–Ga SMA powder. Despite the various manufacturing phases, the SMA and method combination may be effective for biomedical applications that need complicated designs, such as magnetic-responsive platforms. Controllable robots for operational duties are another SMA priority (62).

7.2.3 Composites and Hydrogels with Shape Memory Properties

SMHs and SMCs are potential 4D-printing candidates. SMHs are a subgroup of SMPs; however, their actuation methods are distinct (63). Hydrogels used in 4D printing alter shape by swelling and de-swelling. Photo, pH change, solution strength, and other stimuli may affect these swelling properties in a smart material (64, 65). To achieve complex shape-morphing activities like unfolding or coiling, hydrogels with different compositions or a single hydrogel with varying swelling behaviors due to anisotropic distribution are needed (64, 66). A swellable medium (cyclopentanone) in the SU-8 matrix and controlled printing settings are needed to produce controllable transformation phases. Various biopolymers are used in 4D printing after the league. However, SMCs increase 4D shape change by combining composite materials with SMPs (67, 68). Miao et al. found that graphene in soybean oil epoxidized acrylate (4D inks) is crucial. Like photoabsorbers, graphene-controlled light diffusion was used to produce laser-incited assorted internal stress, which caused a 4D metamorphosis in printed constructions owing to internal stress release and equilibrium (49). In addition, graphene doping in thermoresponsive materials drastically reduced the shape recovery time. Also, these structures could go through a near-infrared (NIR) light-sensitive 4D transition (69). PLA with Fe_3O_4 nanoparticles makes structures that are thermo- and magneto-responsive (70). Zarek et al. printed CNT inks on methacrylated polycaprolactone (PCL-MA) SMP frameworks to create flexible electronics with electro-thermal shape memory (58). A bilayer built of silicone with silica layers and laterally connected films has been examined for 4D morphing. Thermal stimulation and external stresses caused folding and buckling in these constructions by modifying composite viscoelasticity (71).

7.2.4 LCEs

Due to their unique shape-altering behavior and material properties, LCEs have been widely studied for a decade (72). LCEs are SMPs; however, they have anisotropic transformation activity and rubber-like elasticity (73). Thus, LCEs are the extension of SMPs but not materials. LCEs are mostly liquid crystal chain units, which may start the mesomorphic-to-isotropic phase transition (74). LCEs have temperature- or light-responsive actuation mechanisms like other SMMs (75–77). LCEs' higher reversibility, fast deformation, and dominating amplitude set them apart from other SMMs (73). LCEs are great soft-actuating options for 4D biological applications because of these properties. To regulate LCE shape alteration, mesogen units must be arranged and the crystal-line network crosslinked (78). Current 4D biological investigations use LCEs because of their properties. Recently, He et al. created a synthetic vascular muscle that uses LCE thermal reversibility (79). Although the construction approach is not 3D/4D printing, this study showed that weakly crosslinked LCE films might function like muscle tissue. LCEs are also popular for microscale soft biorobots (80). Also produced are cylindrical/disc microscale photoresponsive soft biorobots (81). LCEs, combined with other materials, may be utilized to create adaptive optical devices. Research by López-Valdeovilas et al. demonstrated a thermosensitive focus lens using integrated LCE and polydimethylsiloxane (PDMS) (82). The construct performed electro-thermal and photothermal actuations by combining liquid metal's electrical conductivity with shape-changing LCEs (83). Another research paper by Kaiser et al. used super-paramagnetic Fe_3O_4 nanoparticles in LCE following contactless electromagnetic stimulation (84). These advances expanded LCEs' 4D biological applications.

7.3 REQUISITES FOR THE PROCESS OF PRINTING IN 4D

To comprehend and examine the physics that controls the capability of 4D-printed items to change the form, Momeni et al. established three laws that regulate the geometry-altering deeds of all 4D-created objects (85). These principles govern the shape-morphing activity of all 4D-printed structures. According to the first rule, "most of the shape-changing phenomena like wrapping, bending, twisting, stretching, etc. of multi-material 4D frameworks emerge from the basic phenomenon referred to as relative dilatation among both active and passive materials." According to the second law, "almost all multi-material 4D-printed materials show shape-morphing traits based on four types of physics: mass diffusion, expansion due to heat, molecular alteration, and organic development," which causes relative expansion between active and passive materials and shape morphing when stimulated (Figure 7.1). According to the third rule, "nearly all multi-material 4D printed constructions' time-dependent shape-morphing behavior is dictated by two 'types' of time constants" (85, 86). These laws sought to comprehend and promote the fourth dimension through extensive quantitative and qualitative studies (86).

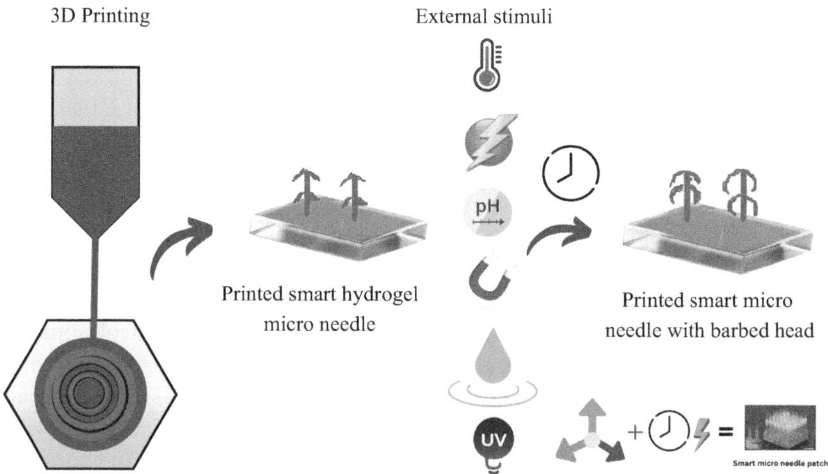

FIGURE 7.1   Transformation of smart materials to 4D-printed drug delivery system on a 3D printer.

7.3.1 Stimuli Sensitive Biomaterials for Use in Bioprinting and 4D Printing

For 4D printing and 4D bioprinting, the application of materials that are sensitive to diverse stimuli is required. When a stimuli-responsive material modifies its physiologic attribute pertaining to a specific stimulus, the printed 3D structure may alter its form over the course of time. The form of SMP may shift from a transitory shape to a permanent, predesigned form because SMP can remember its initial shape and restore its shape when heat stimuli are added or withdrawn (87). All of the SMP materials have a relatively quick reaction time, and either the Tg (glass-transition temperature) or the melting point plays a significant part in the transformation of the structure of temperature-responsive SMP (88). Similarly, the provisional shape of SMP polymers that have been 3D-printed may be maintained by chilling at a temperature that is lower than the Tg, and the printed item can restore its permanent shape by heating it to a temperature that is higher than the Tg (89). Polymers that include polyelectrolyte functional groups are able to respond to an electric field, which results in their capacity to swell and has a direct influence on the structure of printed constructs. In a similar fashion, light-based SMP operates by utilizing the photothermal impact, which results in better spatial and temporal resolutions (90). Likewise, the utilization of material-responsive components and the printing design or patterns have also attracted increased attention as a means of generating 4D-printed structures. The patterns that are utilized for 4D printing also might alter their form spontaneously over the course of time, even if the process does not make use of materials that are sensitive to external stimuli. For instance, hydrophilic polymer-based hydrogels have a swelling characteristic, which refers to the absorption of water. As a consequence of this feature, the structure of the hydrogels changes geometrically as a result of folding, curling, and expanding mechanisms (91). The use of renewable bioink materials that have the property of shape memory is also exploited for 4D printing. An SLA-based printing approach is employed to fabricate a 3D-printed scaffold utilizing an epoxidized acrylate-based substance that is derived from soybean oil. This material is used as a printing material. This polymer's pendant functional groups contribute to its shape memory feature by causing the polymer to freeze at 218 °C in the form of a permanent shape and then to restore its shape at 37 °C via the changeover of functional groups in the polymer (87).

7.3.2 Thermoresponsiveness of SMPs

SMPs (a subset of the soft active material class) are characterized by the fact that it is proficient at experiencing elastic shifts in response to external stimuli. Because SMPs can maintain their temporary shape without deforming permanently and because heating causes them to reform into their original form, temperature-based responsiveness may be achieved (56). According to Mehrpouya et al, the glass Tg of the polymer as well as the melting point profile may be used as design elements to change the temperature sensitivity of SMP. The Tg of the SMP polyurethane, has been identified to be 34 °C. The seeded cells have been subjected to this time-based and temperature-controlled shape modification in order to offer mechanical stretching to the cells and so improve their capacity for regeneration (92). Polylactic acid (PLA), polyurethane, and poly(etheretherketone) are three examples of additional SMPs that, like PLA, have a significant influence on the shape of the cell (71, 93, 94). For the treatment of stenosis, a SMP called VeroClear is available for commercial purchase and utilized to create drug-eluting cardiovascular stents that are equipped with shape memory effects. Presently, Wang Zang and colleagues have printed a structure with the effect of shape memory and the capacity to change color using a method called two-photon polymerization lithography (TPL). This structure is 300 nanometers in size and recovers both its form and its structural color at temperatures greater than Tg. The change in color of the structure is brought on by a modification to the grid height and gridline width, both of which are affected by the form (69). Like SMPs being employed as printing materials in 4D printing, SMAs are additionally used. An example of an SMA is an alloy powder combination that is discovered to display the shape-altering memory as a consequence of the martensitic transfiguration effect when exposed to a heating and cooling cycle. Because of the change in the framework of the crystal, a reversible transition may take place in the structure. Copper–aluminum, nickel–manganese–gallium, nickel–titanium, and other similar alloys are examples of the types of materials that might be used as implants in orthopedics and dentistry (95).

7.3.3 Materials That Can Respond to Light, Magnetic Field, and Electric Field

Amendments in the mechanics of the 3D item can also be devised and employed in 4D bioprinting, in addition to changes in the forms of the object's physical representations. There are several other crosslinking methods, including crosslinking via light, ionic, and chemical methods, which all contribute to the increase in stiffness that occurs in the printed construct (96). It is possible to obtain the appropriate level of stimulus responsiveness in 4D printing of desired constructions by conjugating polymers with materials that quickly respond to external stimuli. For instance, as a result of the interaction between proteins and ions, peptide-conjugated polymers undergo retractable and dimer formation in order to create supramolecular structures. This happens because of the incidence of metal ions (97). When a magnetic field is applied, the magneto-mechanical property of materials causes the active functional groups to move, which enables the movement of planned or printed structures to be controlled (98). It is possible for this kind of device to be effectively included in 4D-printing technology. The magnitude and orientation of the magnetism in the intended or fabricated 3D design exert a significant impact on the velocity and motion, leading the printed structure to respond in a substantial way. In addition to this, combinatorial stimuli-responsive structures based on 4D printing are now in development with the purpose of successfully implementing this approach toward clinical translation.

7.3.4 Materials That Are Sensitive to Moisture for Use in 4D Printing

There is a significant amount of interest in the development of moisture-responsive polymers due to the fact that this kind of stimulation is almost everywhere and might have a wide variety of uses. The dispersal of seeds and spores by plants and fungi, the opening of pine-cone structures, and the crooking and twisting action of wheat awns are all instances of moisture-responsive behaviors that can be seen in nature and serve as excellent models for these processes. When there is an alteration in the relative humidity, an element of the organic system will reversibly either absorb or expel moisture. This will cause a mechanical deformation, which will then result in the desired function. Due to their accessibility and environmental safety, moisture-responsive materials are thereby designated as candidates for several employments (soft robotics, sensors, and actuators). By comparison, the availability of extremely faster sensitive materials beyond the molecular level is limited (99). Polyurethane films and epoxy-crosslinked chitosan are two types of materials that have been used as examples of moisture-responsive materials (100, 101). Polyglycidyl methacrylate has been used as the foundation for the creation of a water-responsive hydrogel that is being used for actuator design (102). Because of their high capacity for water absorption, hydrogels are typically the first type of material that arises when thinking about materials that are responsive to moisture. In addition, hydrogels, which are polymer classes, have great printing capability, yet the reverse process of their reaction (drying and shrinking) is relatively at a slow pace (99, 103). Incorporating anisotropy into the swelling process is mandatory to successfully program the functionality of the hydrogel. Gladman et al. studied the use of an amalgamation of hydrogel ink and cellulose fibrils as a strategy for 4D bioprinting. The hydrogel ink and cellulose fibrils experienced deformation due to the shear pressures encountered throughout the printing process. The scientists also demonstrated that shape-morphing technologies for drug delivery and TE rely on homologous plant organ movements via modification of the internal turgidity in reaction to external stimuli. This is done in order to show that these devices may be used in both applications. The bioinspiration is accomplished by the 4D printing of several mathematically calculated floral models. Anisotropy in the microstructure of the cell wall is responsible for the ensuing dynamism in conformation, which is regulated by the composition of the tissue. This is done so that the ink can be used to print on plant surfaces. The modeling implies an increase in the number of inter-particle polymer chains that could be used for cross-linking when there is more clay present (clay acts as a multifunctional crosslinker). When compared to clay-free hydrogels that have been covalently crosslinked, the gel network that is produced exhibited significantly improved stretchability and strength. This approach yielded printed filaments exhibiting anisotropic stiffness that varied depending on the direction, resulting in longitudinal swelling as dictated by the printing path. This strategy acts as a valuable framework for technology owing to the amalgamation of materials as well as space and time-controlled geometry (19).

Mao et al. 3D-printed a hydrogel and a temperature-responsive SMP, which used the hydrogel swelling to drive the change in shape and govern the rate at which the shape changed over time. Modification between two robust configurations that are each capable of bearing loads is made possible by exercising control over the amount of moisture present as well as the temperature. Specified shape change effects (SCEs) are made possible as a result of the specified interaction with the polymers and the 3D-printed constructions (104). A significant amount of interest has been generated in the production of intelligent materials as a result of the usage of ecological materials in this notion, like cellulose. Cellulose, which is formed of

1,4e-linked anhydroglucose units (AGUs), is the substance that may be found in the greatest abundance on our planet. Researchers have made use of the moisture-responsive properties of shape-memory composites by integrating materials such as cellulose nanowhiskers (CNWs). Zhu et al. presented another design that is influenced by nature: one that takes its architecture and the capacity to mechanically adjust from cellulose whiskers and bases it on the features found in sea cucumbers by means of the linking and dissociation of a 3D nanofiber network. Likewise, the moisture-responsive shape memory effect (SME) is enhanced using a percolation model with carbon nanowires (CNW), and it remains unaffected by fluctuations in temperature. After just 10 minutes of immersion in water, the form could be recovered at room temperature or lower, and there is an increase in the pace at which the shape could be fixed by drying it at 75 °C for 10 minutes. This is an innovative step forward for SMP systems. These kinds of systems are brought to people's attention as having potential applicability as medical devices that are activated by bodily fluid (105, 106). Using cellulose-derived cellulose stearoyl esters (CSEs), Zhang and colleagues are able to create films that could stand on their own, respond to changes in humidity, and be transparent. The moisture responsiveness of these films is determined by the degree of substitution present in the film, with a lesser amount of substitution, which allows for a more immediate and reversible reaction (99).

7.4   DISTINCT FEATURES AND CAPABILITIES OF 4D/5D COMPARED TO TRADITIONAL 3D PRINTING

The distinct features and capabilities of 4D and 5D printing over traditional 3D printing encompass the capability to amend shape over time, the production of objects from five directions, and the creation of curved layers that are tougher than traditional 3D-printed flat layers. These advancements offer more versatility and capabilities in creating complex and robust products in various industries (107). Five-dimensional printing fabricates objects in five directions, with the printer head moving around at three distinct angles while the print bed can spin on two axes, creating curved layers that are more robust than conventional 3D-printed flat layers (108). The essential application of 5D printing lies in the enhanced strength of the printed objects. When curved layers are produced, weaker points more often found in 3D-printed objects can be eliminated, resulting in increased durability compared to traditional 3D printing (107).

Four-dimensional printing affords a notable benefit over 3D printing by enabling the construction of massive objects as discrete components via computational folding. Four-dimensional-printed devices or objects can alter shape through shrinking and/or unfolding, allowing objects to print larger than the printer itself that are initially 3D-printed in a compressed form and then transformed into their final shape (109). With respect to material adaptability, 4D printing is advantageous by enabling the accurate manufacturing of dynamic objects that can respond to an external stimulus (110). Four-dimensional printing offers distinct features and capabilities compared to traditional 3D printing, including shape-shifting, smart materials, precise geometric code, multi-material printing, self-assembling structures, and customization (Table 7.2).

TABLE 7.2

Analogy of 3D Printing with 4D- and 5D-Printing Technology

S.N.	Features	3D Printing	4D Printing	5D Printing	References
1	Process	Creates static objects layer by layer repeating a 2D structure to create a 3D volume	Creates objects with a 3D printer that could change over time in accordance with external stimuli in terms of shape/behavior	5-axis printing, allowing for more complex shapes and curved layers	(111)
2	Material	Metals, ceramics, biomaterials, gels, thermoplastics, nanomaterials, and others	Uses materials such as plant oil, self-assembled materials, biomaterials, smart materials (SMAs and SMPs) and sophisticated materials that can be programmed to change their properties or shape	Uses a range of materials, including smart materials, for more advanced applications	(111)
3	Printer	3D printers use a fixed plateau to create objects (SLS, FDM, SLS)	Multi-material 3D printers with fixed platform.	Five-axis printer with moving platform	(111)
4	Design Concept	Limited to static designs using drawing or scanning	Creating intriguing designs made possible	Designs can include curved layers and more intricate shapes	(111)
5	Flexibility of the product	Not flexible	Flexibility of color, shape, and other functions	Allows for more flexibility in terms of shape and movement due to the use of curved layers and 5-axis printing.	(111, 112)
6	Additive/ subtractive manufacturing	Additive manufacturing	Additive manufacturing	Both additive and subtractive manufacturing	(113)

(Continued)

TABLE 7.2
(Continued)

S.N.	Features	3D Printing	4D Printing	5D Printing	References
7	Applications	In sectors like health care, aviation, automotive, and more	In several industries, including biomedical engineering, machine learning, intelligent fabrics, and building design	Still an emerging technology, but potential applications could include advanced manufacturing, aerospace, and health care.	(111, 114–117)

Four-dimensional printing incorporates a distinct geometric identification code into the process, which allows the printed object to transform into a specific shape or function (118). Four-dimensional printing enables the printing of smart and multi-materials, which can lead to faster growth and more flexible designs (86). Four-dimensional printing allows for customization of printed objects, which can be tailored to specific applications (119). Five-dimensional printing provides structural integrity by incorporating a curved layer, which eliminates the creation of weak places and makes the product up to five times sturdier than if it were originally 3D-printed (120). Five-dimensional printing offers more versatility and capabilities than traditional 3D printing, allowing for the fabrication of incredibly sophisticated and curved structures with the help of five-axis movement (Figure 7.2). Fewer supports are required to print intricate and complex models, which reduces material

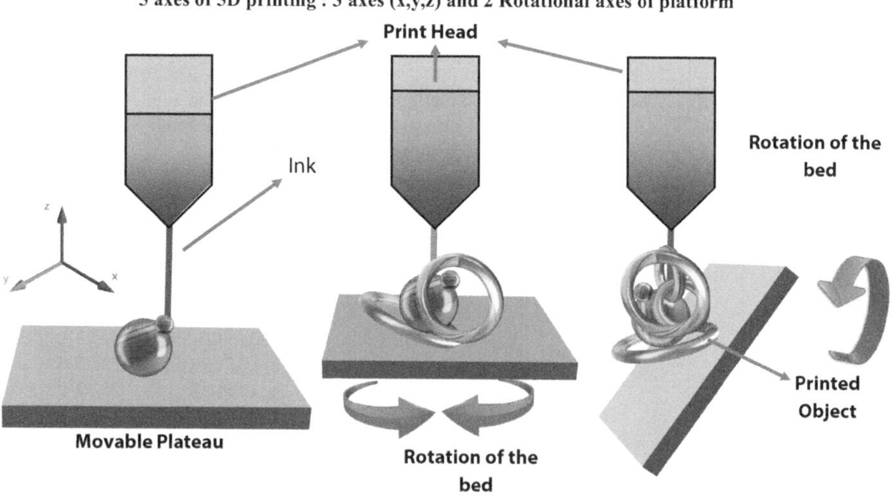

FIGURE 7.2 Complex curved 5D structures printed on 3D printer with two axes rotatable platform.

waste, saves time, and simplifies the process. Five-dimensional printing is a hybrid technology that adds both additive and subtractive manufacturing techniques, enabling the production of fast-growing smart and multi-material that are more flexible and customizable (86).

7.5 CONSTRAINTS OF 4D PRINTING

The disadvantages of 3D printing may also be suitable for 4D printing in the same way that they apply to its benefits. The complexity of 4D design is higher than that of 3D design due to the extra steps that need to be taken to address the shifting behavior of printed items due to their mechanical nature (121). Because its history of invention is so recent, the field of 4D printing does not yet have a significant corpus of published work. In this respect, Wang et al. claimed that shape-memory 4D printing remains in its infancy and has not been developed enough, in contrast to the scaffold technique used in 3D printing (122). In addition, Chu et al. and Cai both mentioned that the exertion of 4D-printing technology has resulted in the expansion of a number of new alternative smart materials (110, 123). In addition, Raghavendra et al. identified a drawback associated with 4D printing, which is the boredom of ensuring its accuracy due to variations in the context of refining attributes to govern the performance of size and form (124).

7.6 APPLICATIONS OF 4D/5D PRINTING IN SKIN DRUG DELIVERY

Drug delivery and TE can use 4D printing to create drug carriers, implants, and tailored medicinal items. A 4D-printing approach can progress 3D-printed materials in reaction to temperature or pH, similar to innate structures. Four-dimensional bioprinting currently remains in its infancy and needs smart materials and more investigation to reach clinical transformation. Several studies have shown that 4D printing can help create tissue-engineered remedial items like bone grafts, heart valves, skin, neural conduits, stents, and DDSs.

7.6.1 TE OF SKIN

Artificial skins are generated in laboratories as natural or synthetic alternatives to human skin. A number of materials, including skin replacements, are used to help close wounds, either permanently or temporarily. An ideal skin accessory should be resilient; low cost; easy to manufacture, store, and use; and able to fight infection, stop water loss, and resist shear forces (125). Skin TE uses both a top-down and a bottom-up strategy as its two main approaches. The bottom-up approach uses cell-laden hydrogels or sheets to create tissue building blocks that are then put together to construct engineered tissues. In order for cells to travel over the scaffold and generate an extracellular matrix while layers of scaffold are subject to biodegradation, the centralized approach demands an impermeable scaffold, allowing for the culture and propagation of cells until completely matured tissue can be acquired. Natural biopolymers, including gelatin, collagen, chitosan, and silk fibroin, are frequently utilized in skin bioengineering, although synthetic biopolymers like polycaprolactone (PCL), polylactic acid (PLA), poly(L-lactide) (PLLA), and poly(lactic-co-glycolic acid) (PLGA) are more frequently used. The process of creating nanocomposite biopolymers by combining a natural and a synthetic polymer is known as electrospinning. Then, for skin TE, these serve as the scaffold. The success of the TE process depends primarily on choosing the right cells for regeneration. Because they can be freely cultivated, multiplied, and maintained under laboratory conditions, keratinocytes are typically utilized for this purpose (126).

7.6.2 Tissue-Engineered Drug-Eluting Implants

Tissue engineered medical products (TEMPs) like cardiac patches, heart valves, and vascular stents need size- or shape-changing materials and should adapt to pH, temperature, and pressure. A SLA-based polyethylene glycol diacrylate and gelatin-methacrylate photo-crosslinked, hydrogel-based, anisotropic myocardial fiber patch is constructed that can change shape to match the native cardiac tissue's ventricular surface curvature. This printed patch can tolerate systolic and diastolic pressure during heart muscle contraction/relaxation, by changing the fiber configuration from mesh to a hexagon/wavy design (50). Significant findings on individual differences in illness effects and progression have led to the development of customized therapies. When establishing therapeutic treatments, personalized medicine considers a person's full biochemical and physiological constitution (127).

A breast cancer 4D-printed implant with carboxymethyl cellulose sodium (CMC) salt and cellulose nanocrystals (CNCs) coated with doxorubicin is examined. The smart device is engineered to shrink under swelling to fit in the tissue cavity, offering customization and aesthetics. The implants examined *in vitro* on human breast cancer cell lines (MDA-MB-231) showed −58% anticancer viability after 72 h of incubation, despite 4 weeks post-printing. The dome-shaped implant is created implementing Thinkercad, a CAD software. The Biox™ 3D bioprinter, with a 22G conical needle and 2 mm/s speed, enables customized implant construction for patient demands. The 4D shape is tested with various infill densities and patterns, and 25% infill is chosen for the best swelling without structural integrity (128). Zhang et al. explored 4D-printed magneto-active soft materials for magnetic actuating transformations. Magneto-active materials are created utilizing magnetic iron oxide nanoparticles and thermoplastic elastomer matrixes that reshape magnetic fields. Multi-material extrusion created multilayered structures like a valve and soft gripper. Fast and reversible magnetic actuation could benefit biomedical devices (129). Liu and colleagues created shape-changing bioinspired tubes by exercising dual-gel extrusion printing, which is used to make tubular constructions with one gel as a structural material and the other as a sacrificial substance. The sacrificial gel is detached to reveal regulated and reversible tube deformation in response to stimuli. The authors suggest using soft robotics–based tubes to build vascular implants and endoscopic applications (130).

Cui et al. created remote and dynamically controlled 4D-printed near-infrared (NIR) light-responsive nanomaterials. The nanomaterial is made from PCL-polyethylene glycol copolymer and black phosphorus quantum dots by TPL.

It displayed efficient proliferation, morphological adaptation, and cell feasibility under NIR light, suggesting cardiac TE potential. Also, they proposed a viable myocardial infarction treatment (131). Wang et al. created a myocardium-regenerating 4D-printed cardiac patch. A specialized 4D printer created a cardiac patch with allied myofibers and a configurable arc. Biodegradable and biocompatible PCL fibers are implemented to print the patch in a stipulated pattern. In an effort to enhance the patch, adipose-originated stem cells and vascular endothelial growth factor (VEGF), a blood vessel–evolving peptide, are introduced. Biocompatible and remote-controlled by NIR light, the cardiac patch possesses great myocardial regeneration potential (69). TE 4D-bioprinted silk hydrogels by Kim et al. used silk fibroin and gelatin to make a biocompatible hydrogel ink and a 3D bioprinter to produce a complex structure. These structures displayed hydrogel formation at different pHs and temperatures. Hydrogel biocompatibility testing showed human mesenchymal stem cell (hMSC) growth and proliferation. Kim et al. found that 4D-bioprinted silk hydrogels might be employed in TE and regenerative medicine (132). A 4D self-morphing culture substrate by Miao and colleagues modified cell differentiation, highlighting the relevance of vibrant microenvironment signals in cell phenotypic organization. A substrate with an SMP and a sacrificial layer that deforms and differentiates cells upon temperature stimulation is used. Stem cells showed that a 4D self-morphing substrate influenced the microenvironment and cell shape, modifying cell development. It improves TE by producing scaffolds for tissue and cell culture regeneration (133).

7.6.3 DDSs

Novel smart materials are being developed to deliver target-site-specific therapeutic medications. The conventional DDSs have drawbacks, such as uncontrolled drug release, nontargeted administration, and low bioavailability, resulting in various side effects. After application of temperature, light, pH, or magnetic field stimuli, smart responsive materials could retain and deliver medicines at tailored rates by folding/unfolding, swelling, and self-assembly/disassembly. Numerous SMMs are created to transport medications to the appropriate spot by changing shape in response to environmental changes (30). Gioumouxouzis et al. created individualized 3D-printed dose-dependent osmotic constructions with cellulose acetate shells and diltiazem-loaded polyvinyl alcohol (PVA) filament cores. The caplet-shaped first preparation lacked a top outer shell layer, the second had one linear chamber in the middle, and the third had two at the top and bottom. The two initial printed formulations had quadratic kinetics *in vitro*, wherein erosion/diffusion accelerates drug release in osmotic pressure. The third preparation with two linear cavities displayed uniform outer shell component dissolution due to continuous drug release, zero-order kinetics, and excess osmotic pressure (134). Using SMP PVA, Melocchi et al. administered medicines into the gastrointestinal tract. When exposed to 0.1N HCl at 37 °C, the conical, cylindrical, S-, and atom-shaped 4D-printed structures turned to supercoiled helical and elliptical structures that dispersed the medicines for nearly a 2-h period (135). Villar et al. printed multisomes in water. Interfacial bilayers formed when water droplets adhered to each other, and the pH or temperature changes the released droplet components (136). The multisome contained aqueous droplets of Ca^{2+} and dextran-conjugated fluo-4 in 1,2-dioleoyl-sn-glycero-3-phosphoethanolami ne (DOPE) and oleic acid. This multicomponent multisome architecture is presented as a small bioreactor for cell delivery or medication. Functionalizing membrane proteins could enable multisomes to communicate quickly electrically. Programming complicated structures with osmolarity gradients and drug encapsulation and release is another option (68).

In analogy to the "bottom-up" mode, researchers created a piezo-based 3D printer to create structures with many water droplets that interact in predetermined patterns and oil droplets in an aqueous medium that generated printed droplet networks, resulting in a lipid bilayer structure. Membrane proteins enable external communication. The structures could alter shape dynamically. When water streamed among the bilayers, the layers of different osmolarity droplets formed a four-petal structure that pleated into a hollow sphere. The resulting "tissue-like" materials can fold or conduct electrical signals. Comparable to living organisms, the structures have many partitions that communicate and could change shape dynamically. These qualities can be extended into full synthetic tissues by executing high-level operations like protein synthesis with sheathed DNA using *in vitro* transcription machinery triggered by light (137). The PCL-MA predecessor bioink conforms to a crystalline state and is generated utilizing a UV-light-emitting diode (LED) SLA printer (SLA DLP) with a tailored heating reservoir based on anatomical data. The printed stent is less intrusive since it deforms into its transitory shape and rearranges to its stable shape as the body temperature rises. The cartilaginous rings' specific fit reduces structural movement (138). Melocchi et al. tested a 4D-printed drug delivery device where the gadget uses a water-impelled shape memory response of PVA to release medications into the bladder over time, employing an FDM printer. The 4D-printed gadget could be stored within the bladder and had a high degree of shape fixity and retrieval. According to the findings, PVA-based retentive gadgets can deliver intravesical drugs and may be a potential bladder disease treatment (135). Engineered living materials (ELMs) that alter shape in response to molecules are printed by Laura et al. using DIW. Genetically engineered yeast that only proliferated with certain macromolecules stimulated ELMs. The yeast cells' proliferation altered the ELM geometry to fit the biomolecule. Bioinks with several yeast strains are co-printed to make ELMs. Regulated cell multiplication caused morphological changes and a 370% volume increase locally. When imperiled to target amino acids and nucleotides comprehensively, the printed structures' volume increased while regions remained unchanged, allowing for programmable form alterations. A reservoir-based drug delivery device prints a model drug to release it exactly when exposed to a biomolecule (83).

Chadwick et al. created 4D cellular culture arrays to instantly assess drug reactions in patient-derived glioblastoma (GBM) models. These arrays are 3D-printed with thermosensitive smart memory polymers. Heat transformed these polymers into histology cartridges. Using high-precision projection micro-SLA, the authors created self-transforming SMPs through 3D printing. The selected SMPs' biocompatibility and 4D printing performance can be confirmed. This scaled-up approach improves 3D pattern inadequacies by increasing screening ability and organoid model preprocessing for high levels of throughput evaluation. The implementation of self-transformation techniques on 3D cell cultures to convert them into histology cartridges offers several advantages. First, it saves time by doing away with the necessity for labor-intensive manual transfer procedures. Additionally, this approach minimizes the risk of causing harm to delicate patient-originated spheres and patient-derived GBM organoids, which are highly sensitive. Maintaining a consistent arrangement of biological samples within cell-culture compartments during transformation expedited the process and enhanced compatibility (139). Additionally, targeted medicinal agents have had low efficacy in clinical trials. The fundamental reason is genetic variation between patients. Four-dimensional-printed SMPs are employed to generate single-cell clonal patient-derived glioblastoma organoids (PDGOs). These PDGOs are utilized for evaluating the efficacy of targeted therapy against the temozolomide (TMZ) pathway as well as investigating the effects of various combinations of molecular entities that target mTOR, DDR, PTEN, NF-1, PI3K, or ATRX (139). The utilization of 4D arrays of PDGOs has proven to be an excellent method for the detection of combinatorial treatments with high efficacy. A study conducted using 3D pancreatic ductal organoids in vitro demonstrated that the efficacy of certain medications targeting specific pathways surpasses that of monotherapy. The research investigation additionally revealed that the combination of the PI3K/mTOR inhibitor BEZ235 with the DDR targeting agent niraparib exhibits synergistic effects. Furthermore, it is seen that BEZ235 may have a protective effect against TZ toxicity. These findings provide support for the utilization of patient-derived gastric organoids in PI3K/mTOR-targeted therapy and offer new possibilities for combination therapy approaches. Four-dimensional printing can identify therapeutic combinations with synergistic action at lower concentrations than predicted, potentially avoiding dosage-limiting toxicities in GBM (140). Finally, 4D-printing systems evaluate on-target activity, validating tailored therapy (139).

7.6.4 Smart MN Transdermal Patches

Since the mid-1990s, high-resolution MN patches with 150–200-µ widths have been a major research topic. The fabrication of entire MN patches is now possible by utilizing a number of 3D/4D-printing techniques, or the patches can be coated with a particular therapeutic formulation. For micron-scale sizes up to 1500 m, arrays of MN patches with up to 2000 pieces are employed. MNs are commonly used in medicine administration, diagnostics, dermatology, cancer, insulin injection, protein delivery, and disease therapy (141–146). MNs bypass the skin barrier and improve transdermal delivery (147). The Dermaroller, Dermapen, Derma-stamp, Hollow Microstructured Transdermal System (HMTS), Macroflux, 3M Soluvia, Candela Exceed, MicronJet600, MicronJet, SkinPen, AdminPen, MicroHyal, and Clearside (CLS) are still in experimental stages despite MNs' success in transdermal applications (148). MNs are made in roller, syringe, pen, patch, lancet, or patch form depending on their usage and can administer medications with little discomfort or intrusion (148, 149). It allows precise MN form, size, and geometry control for drug delivery applications (150). This dynamic characteristic allows MNs to dynamically respond to the epidermal environment, improving drug delivery. Small compounds, biologics, and vaccines can be delivered via them (151). Cosmetic applications include injecting active cosmetic molecules into the skin with MNs (152). A study showed how to 3D and 4D manufacture polymeric MNs. The bioinspired MN array, created using projection micro stereolithography (PμSL) technology, demonstrated remarkable mechanical qualities and potential for biomedical applications (153).

Hollow MNs coupled to a drug repository for transdermal drug delivery via two-photon polymerization (TPP) have gained popularity in recent years (154, 155). Moussi et al. printed hollow MNs with a depot that can fill up and trench fluids at 20–160 L/s using TPP. Because the structures are so small (0.3–3 mm³), they maintained a great resolution. They also evaluated the MNs' ability to carry materials on mouse skin and PDMS and found that fluorescent dye could penetrate 100–180 micrometers. Later cell culture assays showed MN arrays' outstanding cytocompatibility (155). For transdermal administration of insulin, Ross et al. loaded metallic MN assemblies with insulin-carrying polymers (156). In another study, researchers stacked sheets of a copolymer comprising curcumin, 5-fluorouracil, and cisplatin on metallic MNs using similar methods. Drug release in porcine skin increased considerably after coating MNs (157). Pere and colleagues used SLA and UV photopolymerization to generate insulin cone and pyramid MNs. Xylitol, insulin, mannitol, and trehalose are printed using a piezoelectric inkjet printer over a MN. *In vitro* pig skin tests showed a 90–95% release within 30 min (158). A printed fluorescein-containing PLA MNs using FDM showed how 3D printing and chemical etching can change MN length, shape, and array density (159).

7.6.5 HYDROGEL BIOPOLYMER-BASED PATCHES

Hydrogels have been employed in medication delivery, regenerative medicine, and TE in recent years (160). Drug-releasing hydrogels can be prepared from natural polymers like chitosan, alginate, cyclodextrin, and collagen or synthetic polymers like poly-N-isopropylacrylamide (NIPAM), PVA, and PEG. Hydrogel and biopolymer reservoir patches, dissolving tips, and matrixes can contain drugs (161). Natural hydrogel materials from animal and plant extracts are biocompatible and biodegradable, while synthetic hydrogel materials offer precision and control in industrial production and chemical modification. Renewable and readily available biocompatibility-friendly hydrogels and biopolymers are commonly used in medication therapy and their capacity increases with patch size or MN density (162, 163). Four-dimensional printing could help develop engineered and beneficial materials for vascular TE. Hydrogels with embedded cells printed in layers create cylindrical vascular representations. Vascularization follows vascular cell maturation through necessary factors (164). Hong et al. used 4D printing to shape fibroblasts, MSCs, and endothelial cells (ECs) in a hydrogel. Cell culture showed adequate cell movement and accumulation by 16 days, indicating endothelial-specific gene expression for vascular structural integrity (165). Previous studies have shown that microvascular networks can be constructed *in vitro* to create pre-vascularized bioengineered tissues (166). Conversely, viability post-implantation is challenging, as it takes a few days to weeks for adjacent arteries to penetrate the tissue, potentially causing ischemia. This study improved complex tissue design with a graded macro-to-microvascular tree. This technology allowed for certain container diameters and shapes. The spatial resolution of the final construct limits this approach, and a more amalgamated, multilayered tank entails 4D printing (164). Miao et al. worked on photocurable biocompatible liquid resins for stereolithography apparatus (SLA) printing. For multipotent human bone marrow mesenchymal stem cells (MSCs), bio-based, replenishable acrylate scaffolds epoxidized with soybean oil, were created using 3D laser printing. Printed scaffolds outperformed PEGDA in hMSC adhesion and proliferation. This strategy may work for neural and osteochondral TE due to multipotent hMSCs (87). Dai et al. developed a hydrogel composed of pluronic F127 diacrylic polymers that exhibited sensitivity to infrared radiation. The researchers deployed graphene oxide as a photosensitive ingredient in their formulation. The hydrogel, upon exposure to infrared (IR) light for a duration of 240 s, exhibited a reversion to its initial folded shape. The alteration in the surface area acted as the predominant catalyst for the liberation of the drug with reference to superficially induced pressure (167).

7.6.6 4D BIOPRINTING

Biomedicine and healthcare are greatly impacted by 3D and 4D bioprinting. The fabrication of biomedical devices with precise geometry is possible via 3D printing and bioprinting, but the resulting structures are static and do not act in response to physiological changes like pH, temperature, and others (168). Four-dimensional bioprinting has surpassed the constraints of 3D bioprinting by leveraging stimuli-responsive biomaterials to generate 3D tissues that modify their physicochemical attributes gradually. The materials expended in 4D bioprinting usually self-fold, assemble, and disassemble in response to external stimuli and redesign themselves. Furthermore, ECM deposition and cellular self-organization in response to external stimuli, mature 4D-bioprinted tissue structures into functioning tissue constructs. Stimuli-responsive advanced 4D-bioprinted structures may be useful in TE and medication delivery (96). Yang et al. employed myoblast (C2C12) cells and gelatin-methacrylate (GelMA) hydrogel as bioinks to produce perfectly symmetrical skeletal muscle tissue using an external electric field. The electric field aligns printed myoblasts, inducing differentiation, maturation, and organized tubular microbundle creation in cell-laden structures to simulate real skeletal tissues. Cell-laden GelMA film with thicknesses extending from 100 to 500 μm is constructed by photo-crosslinking printed GelMA hydrogels. GelMA's shape-changing nature allowed the film to inflate and fold (169). Researchers generated a cell-compatible bioink for 4D TE shape-changing hydrogels. They made a bioink from poly(ethylene glycol) dimethacrylate (PEGDM), GelMA, photoinitiator, and a photoabsorber. DLP 3D bioprinters formulate bioink with visible light (405 nm). Differential cross-linking from photoabsorber-induced light attenuation gave 3D-printed objects structural anisotropy and quick shape distortion within 30 min after hydration. Angled strands controlled printed build distortion, while sheet thickness affected curvature. Bioprinted 4D gels supported cell growth and viability (170).

7.6.7 5D PRINTING FOR SKIN DRUG DELIVERY

Five-dimensional printing approach endures the creation of personalized nanomedicine for targeted therapy, which merges data to create personalized therapy by combining information exercised to fabricate 3D models with information about physiological activity. This integration of data allows for the development of personalized nanomedicine and targeted therapy. Here is a breakdown of how 5D printing merges data for personalized therapy. The process begins by collecting and integrating data from various sources. This includes patient-specific data, such as medical imaging scans, genetic information, and physiological activity data. The integrated data is used to create 3D models that represent the patient's anatomy or specific target areas. These models serve as the foundation for designing personalized drug delivery systems or medical devices. In addition to the anatomical data, physiological activity data are incorporated into the 3D models. These data provide insights into the specific conditions or responses within the body that need to be addressed. Using the integrated data, the drug delivery systems or medical devices can be tailor-made to match the patient's explicit needs. This customization may involve adjusting the size, shape, or drug release mechanisms to optimize treatment outcomes. Once the personalized design is finalized, the 5D-printing process begins. Five-dimensional-printing technology, which combines additive and subtractive techniques, is used to fabricate personalized drug delivery systems or medical devices. Five-dimensional printing can incorporate smart materials that respond to specific stimuli, enabling on-demand drug release and personalized therapeutic responses. These materials may be programmed to release medications in response to certain physiological states, allowing for very selective and individualized therapy of localized skin disorders and other medical requirements (171). Five-dimensional printing offers increased precision and design flexibility compared to custom manufacturing techniques, considering factors such as dosage, release profiles, and targeted delivery. While specific applications of personalized therapy using 5D printing are still emerging, the technology holds promise in areas such as dermatology, wound healing, MN, transdermal patches, and DDSs for localized skin conditions and optimizing treatment outcomes by combining patient-specific data. Personalized therapy takes into account the individual's anatomy, physiological activity, and specific treatment requirements, aiming to craft complex structures for TE, such as blood vessels and organs. Further research advancements are needed to thoroughly investigate the possibilities of merging data into 5D printing for personalized medicine (172).

7.6.8 5D-Bioprinted Implants

The 5D printing approach combines 3D printing technologies with the confined regulation of biomimetic material characteristics (+1D) and particle dispersion. This approach aims to replicate the reactions of organs during physiology tests, as documented in previous research (173, 174). A computed tomography (CT) scan of the patient is utilized in the construction of the 3D model, and the aerogel is infused with nanoparticles, facilitating rapid dissolution of the nanoparticles. The utilization of bioprinted devices is employed in the development of a 4D simulated biocomposite material intended for both *in vitro* and *in vivo* research purposes. The 4D model is tailored by employing particles that establish communication with the physiological functions of organs, resulting in the creation of a 5D-bioprinted gadget. For sustained release testing of innovative components, the 5D-bioprinted device can execute a coating balloon. Starting with organ restoration, the manufacturing approach prepares for post-printing and the "6D" smart material device for therapy personalization and continual improvement training, to sustained release systems for long-term vascularized scaffold functionalization. Scientists have the potential to develop and utilize customized scaffolds, such as nanoparticles (NPs) or functionalized matrices, for the controlled release of progressive medicine. This advancement in technology could lead to the creation and bioprinting of 5D-tailored medical devices (175, 176). Modifying the composite biological material and fabrication protocols enables the tailoring of the interface between transplanted components and the biological substrate according to the specific requirements of the studies. The research presented findings that demonstrate the feasibility of developing nano-enhanced 5D devices for many uses, including training, pharmacological testing, and in vivo experimentation. The advanced resolution of the fast-freeze prototyping technique, combined with human anatomy, improved drug-eluting balloon therapy. The parts of a human body are twisted and lack sharp edges. Curved parts are needed to make precise implants. The aforementioned implants serve to reinstate the biological framework, while the utilization of 5D-printing technology facilitates the fabrication of implants possessing remarkable structural robustness (177). The assessment of durability and ultimate flexibility holds significant importance in the realm of bioprinting technology, particularly in relation to printed bioinks. The mechanical and structural properties of printed objects are observed to deteriorate when cells are enclosed within bioinks (178). Contrary to 3D printing, 5D-printing technology possesses the capability to fabricate very complex and curved bioprinting structures that exhibit exceptional strength while ensuring excellent reliability and limited side effect products. This characteristic has the potential to facilitate the preservation of their distinctive mechanical properties post-printing with customized, complex shape requirements (179).

In a recent study, scientists successfully developed a specialized nanomedicine for peripheral arterial disease (PAD) utilizing advanced techniques such as 3D and 4D bioprinting. The investigators employed NP distributions and data from 3D printing to generate a plausible organ response while simultaneously collecting physiological data. Rapid freeze bioprinter prototypes created 3D scaffolds with 7%, 9%, or 11% alginate. For the technology employed, the scaffold printed with 11% alginate displayed superior resolution when compared to the 7% and 9% solutions. Using bioprinting, the scientists created a 5D NP-laden hydrogel scaffold for rapid therapeutic release and ethanolic freeze gelation. The utilization of a scanning electron microscope facilitated the observation of notable characteristics in scaffolds, including elevated porosity, a fibrillary microstructure, and a substantial surface area. These attributes have been found to contribute to enhanced interactions with biological tissues. Nevertheless, the process of freeze-gelation resulted in a denser and less permeable scaffold. Vascular smooth muscle cells (VSMCs) are viable during dissolution and gelation in vitro. In stimulation-emission depletion (STED) confocal imaging, NPs are found to be internalized into cells. To validate the viability of these techniques in a living organism, the identical NP-laden structures in the vena cava of rats were introduced and watched as the NPs quickly dissolved, allowing them to be internalized by interstitial tissue and vascular cells. The investigation focused on assessing the impact of several printing processes on the metabolic activity and cellular vitality of a human umbilical vein endothelial cell line with no amendments. The scientists employed the CT scan of the patient to generate a 3D-bioprinted model of the bifurcation of the femoral artery. This model is utilized for the controlled administration of medication. These findings establish a benchmark for tailored therapy employing "5D" smart material devices for controlled-release systems (171).

7.7 CURRENT LIMITATIONS AND FUTURE PERSPECTIVES

First, 4D printing is still a new technology, and printing materials and printers are still being developed. Current printing accuracy and material performance fall short of this criterion. Second, everyone's biological environment is complex and evolving. Biomedicine materials must be biocompatible, noncytotoxic, mechanically durable, and response stimulus durable without impairing tissues, even though several innovative polymers and nanocomposites can modulate their function or shape as they respond to stimulus (87). Thus, some dynamic materials meet the following conditions: A lot of materials merely react to one type of stimulus, and utmost of them are temperature-related, limiting their biological applicability. New materials or improved monomer and polymer integration to make them printable or biocompatible may lead to novel biomedical devices (180). Despite being utilized to create tissues with intricate structures, 4D materials have not yet been fully implemented in therapeutic applications due to the insufficient development of the printed material and the absence of supporting data from clinical trials. In an attempt to optimize the development of the printed tissue bio-objects, post-printing procedures, including cellular coating and cell self-organization, must be used. It turns out that post-tissue maturation offers the chance to produce manufactured tissue bio-objects with functioning features that are similar to those of natural tissue (66). All groundbreaking discoveries and methods are first visible at their exposed edges, while enormous "icebergs" lie concealed below the surface. People only perceive the transition from 4G to 5G in the field of communication as an increase in speed and are not aware of the economic potential it opens up. Contrary to propagation, the preliminary development of individualized medical devices will help address this constraint. As for adapting to the body, items might be made of a variety of dynamic polymers that react to an array of stimuli. The added cost of these two axes limits this 5D technology, and consumers are unaware of this revolutionary innovation. The customized machine needs precise software and hardware, as well as skilled workers for its machine operation and maintenance. In summary, 4D printing is opening up innovative avenues for biomedical therapy, making both inorganic and organic materials more appropriate for usage in living things. Five-dimensional printing figures prominently in pushing the frontiers of additive manufacturing to see a multitude of applications across many industries. High-pressure applications in the manufacturing and medical fields are one potential area. Despite the potentiality for 5D printing to deliver specialized medical solutions that respond to the needs of specific patients, the healthcare sector in particular could experience significant advancement (181).

Metallic compounds and multi-materials are printed only with selective laser melting (SLM) and PolyJet printers. In the field of SLM, lasers are utilized to induce the melting of powders, resulting in the production of things. Conversely, in PolyJet printers, the materials dwell in a liquid state due to the application of UV radiation. This approach has the potential to generate a limited number of smart materials. Prior to the administration of medications within a certain context, it is imperative to possess a comprehensive understanding of the underlying biological system. Patient adherence is an additional concern. The precise immunological response elicited by 4D-printed smart materials remains uncertain. The utilization of this particular technique is deemed inappropriate for the production of cell-laden scaffolds owing to its limited scalability, protracted manufacturing duration, and potential for laser-induced thermal damage. Therapeutic appropriateness is also influenced by patient heterogeneity. The investigation of customized 4D-printable polymeric materials is imperative for the advancement of patient-centered therapies. Ongoing research attempts are being conducted to deal with the constraints pertaining to printing methods, materials, and things with the goal of enhancing their overall efficacy (182).

7.8 CONCLUSION

Future effects of 3D/4D bioprinting on biological research, drug development, and medicine. The rise in pessimism may be due to 2 years of scientific and technological advances in TE, which gave participants a greater understanding of the future. In summary, 3D/4D-bioprinted tissues and organs for human implantation, investigation, and toxicity assessment may be predicted in less than 20 years. If these predictions come true, a bioprinted goods business may solve organ shortages and drug responses. Research, clinical practice, technology management, and public health policymakers must be prepared for the future as technology's impact on the health sector grows. Their narrower scope makes them better for technological analysis, but they lack a participatory method and policy focus. Four-dimensional printing has been widely used in tissue regeneration, implants, medicine administration, and pharmacology. However, bringing 4D-printing applications into health care faces various restrictions and hurdles. Biocompatible and tissue-specific smart materials for use in biomedicine have not yet been developed, despite the fact that several composite or polymeric cantered materials that respond to stimuli have. These materials only react to one stimulus, which may not meet biological requirements since native tissues and cells react to various stimuli. The majority of biological 4D-printed products have not been tested in biomimetic fluid flow and mechanical stress environments. To solve this problem, microfluidic systems and bioreactors can provide native physiological cues to fully functionalize printed constructions. Future preclinical and clinical investigations using 4D-printed structures are needed. To manufacture sophisticated tissue architecture, smart 4D-printable materials require the development of printer elements with enhanced resolution and processability. Overall, 4D printing opens up new possibilities for creating smart inorganic and organic cantered materials that respond to many stimuli, produce and mature complicated individualized tissue characteristics, and lead to clinical translation. Four-dimensional-printing development requires creative, multipurpose ink, which is sought. Unlike artificial tissues and organs made through cell culture or implantation, cell-infused ink may print biological structures with bioactive chemicals and cells. Syringe printing and PolyJet are the most common 4D-bioprinting methods, while 3D-printing platforms hold the most promise for this technology. With 4D-bioprinting, therapeutic chemicals may be administered more quickly and precisely. Precision drug encapsulation and release can be achieved using equipment that folds and unfolds on its own at a specified schedule.

In the context of their improved robustness and proficient design, 5D printing offers 3D- and 4D-printed goods extra advantages. The method can be applied to the preparation of personalized nanomedicine, the production of auto parts, jewelry creation, patient education, and surgical planning. As the field of 4D printing develops, smart materials and morphing structures will become more common. Four-dimensional printing features a self-constructing structure that may alter shape and can save printing time by 70–90%. Additionally, it is more effective and of higher quality than traditional production, but it has a detrimental effect on material strength. Five-dimensional printing helps overcome this problem by creating components with curved surfaces. Research is still being done on the 5D-printing technique, which has the ability to endure pressure up to 3.4 mega Pascals and can be utilized for component production, medical treatment, and so on. This allows for the construction of complex forms and curved layers, reducing material waste by up to 25–30%. Since curved or complex structures require high strength, the 5D, like the 3D and 4D in the near future, may offer up endless alternatives, encourage innovative disruption, and deliver superior healthcare amenities. Five-dimensional printing offers great potential in several industries because of its extreme stress-bearing capacity, five times greater than 3D printing, making it more effective in all sectors. By rehearsing disease and medication physiological processes, 5D printing has saved many lives and is growing rapidly with bioprinting.

In the future, self-assembling materials with greater strength could be printed using 5D printing. The ability to print curved, intelligent medical devices that can change shape over time will become a necessity. In order to provide stronger 3D objects in curved layers with less material waste, 5D printing advances the medical profession and is the most revolutionary technology to date. Therefore, 5D printing has the potential to produce vital devices, tools, implants, and prostheses with increased strength in accordance with patient needs. Accordingly, compared to 3D- and 4D-printing techniques, 5D printing has substantial benefits regarding durability and versatility. Five-dimensional printing has the potentiality to ameliorate the way objects are designed and help researchers expand their comprehension of the method while generating novel approaches. Additionally, research on 4D/5D-printed systems is still in the conceptualization and *in vitro* stages, and it is crucial to move on to the preclinical and clinical stages in order to validate its appropriate relevance with respect to the individualization for improved therapeutic output of this forward-thinking viewpoint to drug delivery and tissue engineering design. This technology has the potential to transform the biomedical and pharma industries in accordance with human growth.

ACKNOWLEDGMENTS

The authors express their sincere gratitude to the host institutions for generously providing all the necessary facilities throughout the course of this study.

FUNDING

None.

REFERENCES

1. Singh N, Singh G. Advances in polymers for bio-additive manufacturing: A state of art review. *J Manuf Process*. 2021;72:439–57. Available from: https://www.sciencedirect.com/science/article/pii/S1526612521007775

2. Sahafnejad-Mohammadi I, Karamimoghadam M, Zolfagharian A, Akrami M, Bodaghi M. 4D printing technology in medical engineering: A narrative review. *J Brazilian Soc Mech Sci Eng*. 2022;44(6). Available from: https://doi.org/10.1007/s40430-022-03514-x

3. Kuhnt T, Camarero-Espinosa S. Additive manufacturing of nanocellulose based scaffolds for tissue engineering: Beyond a reinforcement filler. *Carbohydr Polym*. 2021;252(July 2020):117159. Available from: https://doi.org/10.1016/j.carbpol.2020.117159

4. Arif ZU, Khalid MY, ur Rehman E. Laser-aided additive manufacturing of high entropy alloys: Processes, properties, and emerging applications. *J Manuf Process*. 2022;78:131–71. Available from: https://www.sciencedirect.com/science/article/pii/S1526612522002432

5. Top N, Şahin İ, Gökçe H, Gökçe H. Computer-aided design and additive manufacturing of bone scaffolds for tissue engineering: State of the art. *J Mater Res*. 2021;36(19):3725–45.

6. Zafeiris K, Brasinika D, Karatza A, Koumoulos E, Karoussis IK, Kyriakidou K, et al. Additive manufacturing of hydroxyapatite–chitosan–genipin composite scaffolds for bone tissue engineering applications. *Mater Sci Eng C*. 2021;119:111639. Available from: https://doi.org/10.1016/j.msec.2020.111639

7. Gauss C, Pickering KL, Muthe LP. The use of cellulose in bio-derived formulations for 3D/4D printing: A review. *Compos Part C Open Access*. 2021;4(January):100113. Available from: https://doi.org/10.1016/j.jcomc.2021.100113

8. Durga Prasad Reddy R, Sharma V. Additive manufacturing in drug delivery applications: A review. *Int J Pharm*. 2020;589(June):119820. Available from: https://doi.org/10.1016/j.ijpharm.2020.119820

9. Hann SY, Cui H, Esworthy T, Miao S, Zhou X, Lee S, et al. Recent advances in 3D printing: Vascular network for tissue and organ regeneration. *Transl Res*. 2019;211(April 2019):46–63. Available from: https://doi.org/10.1016/j.trsl.2019.04.002

10. Bayart M, Charlon S, Soulestin J. Fused filament fabrication of scaffolds for tissue engineering; how realistic is shape-memory? A review. *Polymer (Guildf)*. 2021;217(January):1–16.

11. Aldana AA, Houben S, Moroni L, Baker MB, Pitet LM. Trends in double networks as bioprintable and injectable hydrogel scaffolds for tissue regeneration. *ACS Biomater Sci Eng*. 2021;7(9):4077–101.

12. Santoni S, Gugliandolo SG, Sponchioni M, Moscatelli D, Colosimo BM. 3D bioprinting: Current status and trends—A guide to the literature and industrial practice. *Bio-Design Manuf*. 2022;5(1):14–42.

13. Gupta S, Bissoyi A, Bit A. A review on 3D printable techniques for tissue engineering. *Bionanoscience*. 2018;8(3):868–83.

14. Nesic D, Durual S, Marger L, Mekki M, Sailer I, Scherrer SS. Could 3D printing be the future for oral soft tissue regeneration? *Bioprinting*. 2020;20(January):1–11.

15. Mohammadi Zerankeshi M, Bakhshi R, Alizadeh R. Polymer/metal composite 3D porous bone tissue engineering scaffolds fabricated by additive manufacturing techniques: A review. *Bioprinting*. 2022;25:e00191. Available from: https://www.sciencedirect.com/science/article/pii/S240588662200001X

16. Tibbits S, McKnelly C, Olguin C, Dikovsky DHS. 4D printing and universal transformation. In: *Proceedings of the 34th Annual Conference of the Association for Computer Aided Design in Architecture*. 2014. p. 539–548.

17. Zhou W, Qiao Z, Nazarzadeh Zare E, Huang J, Zheng X, Sun X, et al. 4D-printed dynamic materials in biomedical applications: Chemistry, challenges, and their future perspectives in the clinical sector. *J Med Chem*. 2020;63(15):8003–24.

18. Momeni FM, Mehdi Hassani N S, Liu X, Ni J. A review of 4D printing. *Mater Des*. 2017;122:42–79. Available from: http://dx.doi.org/10.1016/j.matdes.2017.02.068

19. Sydney Gladman A, Matsumoto EA, Nuzzo RG, Mahadevan L, Lewis JA. Biomimetic 4D printing. *Nat Mater*. 2016;15(4):413–8.

20. Zhou Y, Huang WM, Kang SF, Wu XL, Lu HB, Fu J, et al. From 3D to 4D printing: Approaches and typical applications. *J Mech Sci Technol*. 2015;29(10):4281–8. Available from: https://doi.org/10.1007/s12206-015-0925-0

21. Tong A, Pham QL, Abatemarco P, Mathew A, Gupta D, Iyer S, et al. Review of low-cost 3D bioprinters: State of the market and observed future trends. *SLAS Technol*. 2021;26(4):333–66.

22. Choi J, Kwon OC, Jo W, Lee HJ, Moon MW. 4D printing technology: A review. *3D Print Addit Manuf*. 2015;2(4):159–67.

23. Khalid MY, Arif ZU, Noroozi R, Zolfagharian A, Bodaghi M. 4D printing of shape memory polymer composites: A review on fabrication techniques, applications, and future perspectives. *J Manuf Process*. 2022;81:759–97. Available from: https://www.sciencedirect.com/science/article/pii/S1526612522005035

24. Eswaramoorthy SD, Ramakrishna S, Rath SN. Recent advances in three-dimensional bioprinting of stem cells. *J Tissue Eng Regen Med*. 2019;13(6):908–24.

25. Noroozi R, Zolfagharian A, Fotouhi M, Bodaghi M. 4D-printed shape memory polymer: Modeling and fabrication. In: *Smart Materials in Additive Manufacturing, Volume 2: 4D Printing Mechanics, Modeling, and Advanced Engineering Applications*. Elsevier; 2022. p. 195–228.

26. Noroozi R, Bodaghi M, Jafari H, Zolfagharian A, Fotouhi M. Shape-adaptive metastructures with variable bandgap regions by 4D printing. *Polymers (Basel)*. 2020;12(3).

27. Tie D, Liu H, Guan R, Holt-Torres P, Liu Y, Wang Y, et al. In vivo assessment of biodegradable magnesium alloy ureteral stents in a pig model. *Acta Biomater*. 2020;116:415–25. Available from: https://doi.org/10.1016/j.actbio.2020.09.023

28. Bardot M, Schulz MD. Biodegradable poly(Lactic acid) nanocomposites for fused deposition modeling 3d printing. *Nanomaterials*. 2020;10(12):1–20.

29. Kabir H, Munir K, Wen C, Li Y. Recent research and progress of biodegradable zinc alloys and composites for biomedical applications: Biomechanical and biocorrosion perspectives. *Bioact Mater*. 2021;6(3):836–79. Available from: https://doi.org/10.1016/j.bioactmat.2020.09.013

30. Melocchi A, Uboldi M, Cerea M, Foppoli A, Maroni A, Moutaharrik S, et al. Shape memory materials and 4D printing in pharmaceutics. *Adv Drug Deliv Rev*. 2021;173:216–37. Available from: https://doi.org/10.1016/j.addr.2021.03.013

31. Evans SE, Harrington T, Rodriguez Rivero MC, Rognin E, Tuladhar T, Daly R. 2D and 3D inkjet printing of biopharmaceuticals – A review of trends and future perspectives in research and manufacturing. *Int J Pharm*. 2021;599(February). https://doi.org/10.1016/j.ijpharm.2021.120443

32. Javaid M, Haleem A. Exploring smart material applications for covid-19 pandemic using 4d printing technology. *J Ind Integr Manag*. 2020;5(4):481–94.

33. Ma SQ, Zhang YP, Wang M, Liang YH, Ren L, Ren LQ. Recent progress in 4D printing of stimuli-responsive polymeric materials. *Sci China Technol Sci*. 2020;63(4):532–44.

34. Zhakeyev A, Zhang L, Xuan J. Photoactive resin formulations and composites for optical 3D and 4D printing of functional materials and devices. In: *3D and 4D Printing of Polymer Nanocomposite Materials*. 2020. p. 387–425.

35. Huang J, Xia S, Li Z, Wu X, Ren J. Applications of four-dimensional printing in emerging directions: Review and prospects. *J Mater Sci Technol.* 2021;91:105–20. Available from: https://doi.org/10.1016/j.jmst.2021.02.040

36. Elkhoury K, Morsink M, Sanchez-Gonzalez L, Kahn C, Tamayol A, Arab-Tehrany E. Biofabrication of natural hydrogels for cardiac, neural, and bone Tissue engineering Applications. *Bioact Mater.* 2021;6(11):3904–23. Available from: https://doi.org/10.1016/j.bioactmat.2021.03.040

37. Askari M, Afzali Naniz M, Kouhi M, Saberi A, Zolfagharian A, Bodaghi M. Recent progress in extrusion 3D bioprinting of hydrogel biomaterials for tissue regeneration: A comprehensive review with focus on advanced fabrication techniques. *Biomater Sci.* 2021;9(3):535–73.

38. Zhu X, Wang Z, Teng F. A review of regulated self-organizing approaches for tissue regeneration. *Prog Biophys Mol Biol.* 2021;167(xxxx):63–78. Available from: https://doi.org/10.1016/j.pbiomolbio.2021.07.006

39. Ramezani M, Mohd Ripin Z. 4D printing in biomedical engineering: Advancements, challenges, and future directions. *J Funct Biomater.* 2023;14(7):347.

40. Ghilan A, Chiriac AP, Nita LE, Rusu AG, Neamtu I, Chiriac VM. Trends in 3D printing processes for biomedical field: Opportunities and challenges. *J Polym Environ.* 2020;28(5):1345–67. Available from: https://doi.org/10.1007/s10924-020-01722-x

41. Javaid M, Haleem A. Additive manufacturing applications in orthopaedics: A review. *J Clin Orthop Trauma.* 2018;9(3):202–6. Available from: https://doi.org/10.1016/j.jcot.2018.04.008

42. Robles-Martinez P, Xu X, Trenfield SJ, Awad A, Goyanes A, Telford R, et al. 3D printing of a multi-layered polypill containing six drugs using a novel stereolithographic method. *Pharmaceutics.* 2019;11(6).

43. Vasiliadis AV, Koukoulias N, Katakalos K. From three-dimensional (3D)- to 6D-printing technology in orthopedics: Science fiction or scientific reality? *J Funct Biomater.* 2022;13(3):2–7.

44. Haleem A, Javaid M, Vaishya R. 5D printing and its expected applications in Orthopaedics. *J Clin Orthop Trauma.* 2019;10(4):809–10. Available from: https://doi.org/10.1016/j.jcot.2018.11.014

45. Mohd Javaid AH. 4D printing applications in medical field: A brief review. In: *Clinical Epidemiology and Global Health.* 2019.

46. Sharma KS. Artificial intelligence assisted fabrication of 3D, 4D and 5D printed formulations or devices for drug delivery. *Curr Drug Deliv.* 2023;20(6):752–69.

47. Naidu N, Trivedi S, Wadher K, Umekar M. 3D and 4D printing: A review on current developments and pharmaceuticals applications. *J Chem Pharm Res.* 2021;13(3).

48. Willemen NGA, Morsink MAJ, Veerman D, da Silva CF, Cardoso JC, Souto EB, et al. From oral formulations to drug-eluting implants: Using 3D and 4D printing to develop drug delivery systems and personalized medicine. *Bio-Design Manuf.* 2022;5(1):85–106. Available from: https://doi.org/10.1007/s42242-021-00157-0

49. Miao S, Castro N, Nowicki M, Xia L, Cui H, Zhou X, et al. 4D printing of polymeric materials for tissue and organ regeneration. *Mater Today.* 2017;20(10):577–91. Available from: https://doi.org/10.1016/j.mattod.2017.06.005

50. Hann SY, Cui H, Nowicki M, Zhang LG. 4D printing soft robotics for biomedical applications. *Addit Manuf.* 2020;36(December 2019):101567. Available from: https://doi.org/10.1016/j.addma.2020.101567

51. Ashammakhi N, Tamimi F, Caterson EJ. Three-dimensional bioprinting, oxygenated tissue constructs, and intravital tissue regeneration. *J Craniofac Surg.* 2021;32(7):2257–8.

52. Costa PDC, Costa DCS, Correia TR, Gaspar VM, Mano JF. Natural origin biomaterials for 4D bioprinting tissue-like constructs. *Adv Mater Technol.* 2021;6(10):1–21.

53. Kuang X, Roach DJ, Wu J, Hamel CM, Ding Z, Wang T, et al. Advances in 4D printing: Materials and applications. *Adv Funct Mater*. 2019;29(2):1–23.

54. Bodaghi M, Damanpack AR, Liao WH. Adaptive metamaterials by functionally graded 4D printing. *Mater Des*. 2017;135:26–36. Available from: https://doi.org/10.1016/j.matdes.2017.08.069

55. Bodaghi M, Damanpack AR, Liao WH. Self-expanding/shrinking structures by 4D printing. *Smart Mater Struct*. 2016;25(10):1–15. Available from: http://doi.org/10.1088/0964-1726/25/10/105034

56. Ge Q, Sakhaei AH, Lee H, Dunn CK, Fang NX, Dunn ML. Multimaterial 4D printing with tailorable shape memory polymers. *Sci Rep*. 2016;6(July):1–11.

57. Jin B, Song H, Jiang R, Song J, Zhao Q, Xie T. Programming a crystalline shape memory polymer network with thermo- and photo-reversible bonds toward a single-component soft robot. *Sci Adv*. 2018;4(1):1–6.

58. Zarek M, Layani M, Cooperstein I, Sachyani E, Cohn D, Magdassi S. 3D printing of shape memory polymers for flexible electronic devices. *Adv Mater*. 2016;28(22):4449–54.

59. Miyazaki S, Otsuka K. Development of shape memory alloys. *ISIJ Int*. 1989;29(5):353–77.

60. Huang WM, Ding Z, Wang CC, Wei J, Zhao Y, Purnawali H. Shape memory materials. *Mater Today*. 2010;13(7–8):54–61. Available from: http://doi.org/10.1016/S1369-7021(10)70128-0

61. Lee AY, An J, Chua CK. Two-way 4D printing: A review on the reversibility of 3D-printed shape memory materials. *Engineering*. 2017;3(5):663–74. Available from: http://doi.org/10.1016/J.ENG.2017.05.014

62. Yao T, Wang Y, Zhu B, Wei D, Yang Y, Han X. 4D printing and collaborative design of highly flexible shape memory alloy structures: A case study for a metallic robot prototype. *Smart Mater Struct*. 2020;30(1):1–14.

63. Korde JM, Kandasubramanian B. Naturally biomimicked smart shape memory hydrogels for biomedical functions. *Chem Eng J*. 2020;379(April 2019):122430. Available from: https://doi.org/10.1016/j.cej.2019.122430

64. Champeau M, Heinze DA, Viana TN, de Souza ER, Chinellato AC, Titotto S. 4D printing of hydrogels: A review. *Adv Funct Mater*. 2020;30(31):1–22.

65. Wu JJ, Huang LM, Zhao Q, Xie T. 4D printing: History and recent progress. *Chinese J Polym Sci* (English Ed. 2018;36(5):563–75.

66. Ding H, Zhang X, Liu Y, Ramakrishna S. Review of mechanisms and deformation behaviors in 4D printing. *Int J Adv Manuf Technol*. 2019;105(11):4633–49.

67. Madbouly SA, Lendlein A. Shape-memory polymer composites. In: *Advances in Polymer Science*. 2010. p. 41–95.

68. Santo L, Quadrini F, Accettura A, Villadei W. Shape memory composites for self-deployable structures in aerospace applications. *Procedia Eng*. 2014;88:42–7. Available from: http://dx.doi.org/10.1016/j.proeng.2014.11.124

69. Zhang W, Wang H, Wang H, Chan JYE, Liu H, Zhang B, et al. Structural multi-colour invisible inks with submicron 4D printing of shape memory polymers. *Nat Commun*. 2021;12(1):1–8.

70. Lin C, Liu L, Liu Y, Leng J. 4D printing of bioinspired absorbable left atrial appendage occluders: A proof-of-concept study. *ACS Appl Mater Interfaces*. 2021;13(11):12668–78.

71. Su JW, Gao W, Trinh K, Kenderes SM, Tekin Pulatsu E, Zhang C, et al. 4D printing of polyurethane paint-based composites. *Int J Smart Nano Mater*. 2019;10(3):237–48.

72. Wagner M, Terentjev E. *Liquid Crystal Elastomers*. 2007. p. Clarendon Press, London.

73. Wen Z, Yang K, Raquez JM. A review on liquid crystal polymers in free-standing reversible shape memory materials. *Molecules*. 2020;25:1–13.

74. Chen Y, Chen C, Rehman HU, Zheng X, Li H, Liu H, et al. Shape-memory polymeric artificial muscles: Mechanisms, applications and challenges. *Molecules*. 2020;25(4246):1–27.

75. White TJ, Broer DJ. Programmable and adaptive mechanics with liquid crystal polymer networks and elastomers. *Nat Mater*. 2015;14(11):1087–98. Available from: http://dx.doi.org/10.1038/nmat4433

76. Thomsen DL, Keller P, Naciri J, Pink R, Jeon H, Shenoy D, et al. Liquid crystal elastomers with mechanical properties of a muscle. *Macromolecules*. 2001;34(17):5868–75.

77. Feng W, Broer DJ, Liu D. Combined light and electric response of topographic liquid crystal network surfaces. *Adv Funct Mater*. 2020;30(2):1–7.

78. Zhang C, Lu X, Fei G, Wang Z, Xia H, Zhao Y. 4D printing of a liquid crystal elastomer with a controllable orientation gradient. *ACS Appl Mater Interfaces*. 2019;11(47):44774–82.

79. He Q, Wang Z, Song Z, Cai S. Bioinspired design of vascular artificial muscle. *Adv Mater Technol*, 2019;4(1):1–7.

80. Zeng H, Wani OM, Wasylczyk P, Priimagi A. Light-driven, caterpillar-inspired miniature inching robot. *Macromol Rapid Commun*. 2018;39(1):1–6.

81. Palagi S, Mark AG, Reigh SY, Melde K, Qiu T, Zeng H, et al. Structured light enables biomimetic swimming and versatile locomotion of photoresponsive soft microrobots. *Nat Mater*. 2016;15(6):647–53.

82. López-Valdeolivas M, Liu D, Broer DJ, Sánchez-Somolinos C. 4D printed actuators with soft-robotic functions. *Macromol Rapid Commun*. 2018;39(5):3–9.

83. Lu X, Ambulo CP, Wang S, Rivera-Tarazona LK, Kim H, Searles K, et al. 4D-printing of photoswitchable actuators. *Angew Chemie - Int Ed*. 2021;60(10):5536–43.

84. Kaiser A, Winkler M, Krause S, Finkelmann H, Schmidt AM. Magnetoactive liquid crystal elastomer nanocomposites. *J Mater Chem*. 2009;19(4):538–43.

85. Momeni F, Ni J. Laws of 4D printing. *Engineering*. 2020;6(9):1035–55. Available from: https://doi.org/10.1016/j.eng.2020.01.015

86. Ahmed A, Arya S, Gupta V, Furukawa H, Khosla A. 4D printing: Fundamentals, materials, applications and challenges. *Polymer* (Guildf). 2021;228(June):123926. Available from: https://doi.org/10.1016/j.polymer.2021.123926

87. Miao S, Zhu W, Castro NJ, Nowicki M, Zhou X, Cui H, et al. 4D printing smart biomedical scaffolds with novel soybean oil epoxidized acrylate. *Sci Rep*. 2016;6(June):1–10.

88. Hendrikson WJ, Rouwkema J, Clementi F, Van Blitterswijk CA, Farè S, et al. Towards 4D printed scaffolds for tissue engineering: Exploiting 3D shape memory polymers to deliver time-controlled stimulus on cultured cells. *Mater Today Proc*. 2019;27:31. Available from: https://doi.org/10.1016/j.jare.2020.01.010%0A

89. Ge Q, Chen Z, Cheng J, Zhang B, Zhang YF, Li H, et al. 3D printing of highly stretchable hydrogel with diverse UV curable polymers. *Sci Adv*. 2021;7(2):1–10.

90. Lai J, Ye X, Liu J, Wang C, Li J, Wang X, et al. 4D printing of highly printable and shape morphing hydrogels composed of alginate and methylcellulose. *Mater Des*. 2021;205(April):109699. Available from: https://doi.org/10.1016/j.matdes.2021.109699

91. Yang Q, Gao B, Xu F. Recent Advances in 4D Bioprinting. *Biotechnol J*. 2020;15(1):1–10.

92. Mehrpouya M, Vahabi H, Janbaz S, Darafsheh A, Mazur TR, Ramakrishna S. 4D printing of shape memory polylactic acid (PLA). *Polymer (Guildf)*. 2021;230(August):1–17. Available from: https://doi.org/10.1016/j.polymer.2021.124080

93. Fu YQ, Huang WM, Luo JK, Lu H. Polyurethane shape-memory polymers for biomedical applications. In: *Shape Memory Polymer Biomedical Applications*. 2015. p. 167–95. Available from: https://doi.org/10.1016/B978-0-85709-698-2.00009-X

94. Zhang L, Lin Z, Zhou Q, Ma S, Liang Y, Zhang Z. PEEK modified PLA shape memory blends: Towards enhanced mechanical and deformation properties. *Front Mater Sci.* 2020;14(2):177–87.

95. Caputo AMP, Berkowitz AE, Peter M, Solomon CV. 4D printing of net shape parts made from Ni-Mn-Ga magnetic shape memory alloys matthew. *Addit Manuf.* 2018;21(2010):579–88.

96. Wan Z, Zhang P, Liu Y, Lv L, Zhou Y. Four-dimensional bioprinting: Current developments and applications in bone tissue engineering. *Acta Biomater.* 2020;101:26–42.

97. Aronsson C, Jury M, Naeimipour S, Boroojeni FR, Christoffersson J, Lifwergren P, et al. Dynamic peptide-folding mediated biofunctionalization and modulation of hydrogels for 4D bioprinting. *Biofabrication.* 2020;12(3).

98. Zhu P, Yang W, Wang R, Gao S, Li B, Li Q. 4D printing of complex structures with a fast response time to magnetic stimulus. *ACS Appl Mater Interfaces.* 2018;10(42):36435–42.

99. Zhang K, Geissler A, Standhardt M, Mehlhase S, Gallei M, Chen L, et al. Moisture-responsive films of cellulose stearoyl esters showing reversible shape transitions. *Sci Rep.* 2015;5:1–13.

100. Yang B, Huang WM, Li C, Lee CM, Li L. On the effects of moisture in a polyurethane shape memory polymer. *Smart Mater Struct.* 2004;13(1):191–5.

101. Chen MC, Tsai HW, Chang Y, Lai WY, Mi FL, Liu CT, et al. Rapidly self-expandable polymeric stents with a shape-memory property. *Biomacromolecules.* 2007;8(9):2774–80.

102. Sidorenko A, Krupenkin T, Taylor A, Fratzl P, Aizenberg J. Reversible switching of hydrogel-actuated nanostructures into complex micropatterns. *Science.* 2007;315(5811):487–90.

103. Zhang Z, Demir KG, Gu GX. Developments in 4D-printing: A review on current smart materials, technologies, and applications. *Int J Smart Nano Mater.* 2019;10(3):205–24. Available from: https://doi.org/10.1080/19475411.2019.1591541

104. Mao Y, Ding Z, Yuan C, Ai S, Isakov M, Wu J, et al. 3D printed reversible shape changing components with stimuli responsive materials. *Sci Rep.* 2016;6(April):1–13. Available from: http://dx.doi.org/10.1038/srep24761

105. du Toit L C, Marimuthu T, Kumar P CYE. Customized shape memory biopolymers, in: V. Pillay, Y.E. Choonara (Eds.). In: *Unfolding the Biopolymer Landscape.* Bentham Science Publishers; 2016. p. 92–123.

106. Zhu Y, Hu J, Luo H, Young RJ, Deng L, Zhang S, et al. Rapidly switchable water-sensitive shape-memory cellulose/elastomer nano-composites. *Soft Matter.* 2012;8(8):2509–17.

107. Georgantzinos SK, Giannopoulos GI, Bakalis PA. Additive manufacturing for effective smart structures: The idea of 6d printing. *J Compos Sci.* 2021;5(5):1–11.

108. TWI Ltd. 2023. What is 5D printing? (A comprehensive guide). Available from: https://www.twi-global.com/technical-knowledge/faqs/what-is-5d-printing#:~:text=The principal difference lies in,layers on a fixed plateau

109. 4D Printing: All you need to know in 2023. 2023.

110. Chu H, Yang W, Sun L, Cai S, Yang R, Liang W, et al. 4D printing: A review on recent progresses. *Micromachines.* 2020;11(9):1–30.

111. Quanjin M, Rejab MRM, Idris MS, Kumar NM, Abdullah MH, Reddy GR. Recent 3D and 4D intelligent printing technologies: A comparative review and future perspective. *Procedia Comput Sci.* 2020;167:1210–9. Available from: https://doi.org/10.1016/j.procs.2020.03.434

112. Bedell ML, Navara AM, Du Y, Zhang S, Mikos AG. Polymeric systems for bioprinting. *Chem Rev.* 2020;120(19):10744–92.

113. Nida S, Moses JA, Anandharamakrishnan C. Emerging applications of 5D and 6D printing in the food industry. *J Agric Food Res.* 2022;10(June):100392. Available from: https://doi.org/10.1016/j.jafr.2022.100392

114. Heinrich MA, Liu W, Jimenez A, Yang J, Akpek A, Liu X, et al. 3D bioprinting: From benches to translational applications. *Small*. 2019;15(23):1–88.

115. Nureddin A, Samad A, Fan Z, Kasinan S, Farnaz L, Gorka O, et al. Advances and future perspectives in 4D bioprinting. *Biotechnol J*. 2018;13(12):1–21.

116. Anas S, Khan MY, Rafey M, Faheem K. Concept of 5D printing technology and its applicability in the healthcare industry. *Mater Today Proc*. 2022;56:1726–32. Available from: https://doi.org/10.1016/j.matpr.2021.10.391

117. Mahmoud DB, Schulz-Siegmund M. Utilizing 4D printing to design smart gastro-retentive, esophageal, and intravesical drug delivery systems. *Adv Healthc Mater*. 2023;12(10).

118. Smith KT. What is 4D printing and how does it differ from 3D printing?. 2020. Available from: https://www.azom.com/article.aspx?ArticleID=19378

119. Mahmood A, Akram T, Chen H, Chen S. On the evolution of additive manufacturing (3D/4D printing) technologies: Materials, applications, and challenges. *Polymers (Basel)*. 2022;14(21):1–31.

120. Van Zeijderveld J. 5D printing: A new branch of additive manufacturing. 2018. Available from: https://www.sculpteo.com/blog/2018/05/07/5d-printing-a-new-branch-of-additive-manufacturing

121. Sossou G, Demoly F, Montavon G, Gomes S. Design for 4D printing: Rapidly exploring the design space around smart materials. *Procedia CIRP*. 2018;70:120–5.

122. Wang W, Caetano G, Ambler WS, Blaker JJ, Frade MA, Mandal P, et al. Enhancing the hydrophilicity and cell attachment of 3D printed PCL/graphene scaffolds for bone tissue engineering. *Materials (Basel)*. 2016;9(12).

123. Cai J. *4D Printing Dielectric Elastomer Actuator Based Soft Robots*. University of Arkansas: Fayetteville, AR; 2016.

124. Raghavendra, K.; Manjaiah, M.; Balashanmugam N. Materials Forming, Machining and Post Processing. Cham, Switzerland: Springer International Publishing; 2020. p. 93–107.

125. Shores JT, Gabriel A, Gupta S. Skin substitutes and alternatives: A review. *Adv Skin Wound Care*. 2007;20(9 Pt 1):493–508.

126. Norouzi M, Boroujeni SM, Omidvarkordshouli N, Soleimani M. Advances in skin regeneration: Application of electrospun scaffolds. *Adv Healthc Mater*. 2015;4(8): 1114–33.

127. Ginsburg GS, Willard HF. Genomic and personalized medicine: Foundations and applications. *Transl Res*. 2009;154(6):277–87. Available from: http://dx.doi.org/10.1016/j.trsl.2009.09.005

128. Moroni S, Bingham R, Buckley N, Casettari L, Lamprou DA. 4D printed multipurpose smart implants for breast cancer management. *Int J Pharm*. 2023;642(June):123154. Available from: https://doi.org/10.1016/j.ijpharm.2023.123154

129. Zhang Y, Wang Q, Yi S, Lin Z, Wang C, Chen Z, et al. 4D printing of magnetoactive soft materials for on-demand magnetic actuation transformation. *ACS Appl Mater Interfaces*. 2021;13(3):4174–84.

130. Liu J, Erol O, Pantula A, Liu W, Jiang Z, Kobayashi K, et al. Dual-gel 4D printing of bioinspired tubes. *ACS Appl Mater Interfaces*. 2019;11(8):8492–8.

131. Cui H, Liu C, Esworthy T, Huang Y, Yu ZX, Zhou X, et al. 4D physiologically adaptable cardiac patch: A 4-month in vivo study for the treatment of myocardial infarction. *Sci Adv*. 2020;6(26):1–12.

132. Kim SH, Seo YB, Yeon YK, Lee YJ, Park HS, Sultan MT, et al. 4D-bioprinted silk hydrogels for tissue engineering. *Biomaterials*. 2020;260(July).

133. Miao S, Cui H, Esworthy T, Mahadik B, Lee S jun, Zhou X, et al. 4D self-morphing culture substrate for modulating cell differentiation. *Adv Sci*. 2020;7(6):1–12.

134. Gioumouxouzis CI, Tzimtzimis E, Katsamenis OL, Dourou A, Markopoulou C, Bouropoulos N, et al. Fabrication of an osmotic 3D printed solid dosage form for controlled release of active pharmaceutical ingredients. *Eur J Pharm Sci.* 2020;143(February 2020):105176. Available from: https://doi.org/10.1016/j.ejps.2019.105176

135. Melocchi A, Uboldi M, Inverardi N, Briatico-Vangosa F, Baldi F, Pandini S, et al. Expandable drug delivery system for gastric retention based on shape memory polymers: Development via 4D printing and extrusion. *Int J Pharm.* 2019;571:118700. Available from: https://doi.org/10.1016/j.ijpharm.2019.118700

136. Villar G, Heron AJ, Bayley H. Formation of droplet networks that function in aqueous environments. *Nat Nanotechnol.* 2011;6(12):803–8.

137. Booth MJ, Bayley H. 3D-printed synthetic tissues. *Biochem (Lond).* 2016;38(4):16–9.

138. Zarek M, Mansour N, Shapira S, Cohn D. 4D printing of shape memory-based personalized endoluminal medical devices. *Macromol Rapid Commun.* 2017;38(2):1–6.

139. Chadwick M, Yang C, Liu L, Gamboa CM, Jara K, Lee H, et al. Rapid processing and drug evaluation in glioblastoma patient-derived organoid models with 4D bioprinted arrays. *iScience.* 2020;23(8):101365. Available from: https://doi.org/10.1016/j.isci.2020.101365

140. Monal Mehta, Khan A, Danish S, Haffty BG, Sabaawy HE. Radiosensitization of primary human glioblastoma stem-like cells with low-dose AKT inhibition. *Mol Cancer Ther.* 2015;14(5):1171–1180.

141. He X, Sun J, Zhuang J, Xu H, Liu Y, Wu D. Microneedle system for transdermal drug and vaccine delivery: Devices, safety, and prospects. *Dose-Response.* 2019;17(4):1–18.

142. Al-Japairai KA, Mahmood S, Almurisi SH, Venugopal JR, Hilles AR, Azmana M, et al. Current trends in polymer microneedle for transdermal drug delivery. *Psychiatry Res.* 2020;14(4):293. Available from: https://pubmed.ncbi.nlm.nih.gov/33276180/

143. Liu G shi, Kong Y, Wang Y, Luo Y, Fan X, Xie X, et al. Microneedles for transdermal diagnostics: Recent advances and new horizons. *Biomaterials.* 2020;232(119740):1–37.

144. Dixon RV, Skaria E, Lau WM, Manning P, Birch-Machin MA, Moghimi SM, et al. Microneedle-based devices for point-of-care infectious disease diagnostics. *Acta Pharm Sin B.* 2021;11(8):2344–61. Available from: https://doi.org/10.1016/j.apsb.2021.02.010

145. García-Guzmán JJ, Pérez-Ràfols C, Cuartero M, Crespo GA. Microneedle based electrochemical (Bio)Sensing: Towards decentralized and continuous health status monitoring. *TrAC - Trends Anal Chem.* 2021;135(February 2021):116148. Available from: https://doi.org/10.1016/j.trac.2020.116148

146. Sabri AH, Ogilvie J, Abdulhamid K, Shpadaruk V, McKenna J, Segal J, et al. Expanding the applications of microneedles in dermatology. *Eur J Pharm Biopharm.* 2019;140(April):121–40. Available from: https://doi.org/10.1016/j.ejpb.2019.05.001

147. Chen X, Wang L, Yu H, Li C, Feng J, Haq F, et al. Preparation, properties and challenges of the microneedles-based insulin delivery system. *J Control Release.* 2018;288:173–88. Available from: https://doi.org/10.1016/j.jconrel.2018.08.042

148. Ingrole RSJ, Azizoglu E, Dul M, Birchall JC, Gill HS, Prausnitz MR. Trends of microneedle technology in the scientific literature, patents, clinical trials and internet activity Rohan. *Physiol Behav.* 2018;176(5):139–48.

149. Dabbagh SR, Sarabi MR, Rahbarghazi R, Sokullu E, Yetisen AK, Tasoglu S. 3D-printed microneedles in biomedical applications. *iScience.* 2021;24(1):102012. Available from: https://doi.org/10.1016/j.isci.2020.102012

150. Olowe M, Parupelli SK, Desai S. A review of 3D-printing of microneedles. *Pharmaceutics.* 2022;14(12):9–12.

151. Rajesh NU, Coates I, Driskill MM, Dulay MT, Hsiao K, Ilyin D, et al. 3D-printed microarray patches for transdermal applications. *JACS Au.* 2022;2(11):2426–45.

152. Caudill C, Perry JL, Iliadis K, Tessema AT, Lee BJ, Mecham BS, et al. Transdermal vaccination via 3D-printed microneedles induces potent humoral and cellular immunity. *Proc Natl Acad Sci U S A*. 2021;118(39):1–8.

153. Han D, Morde RS, Mariani S, La Mattina AA, Vignali E, Yang C, et al. 4D printing of a bioinspired microneedle array with backward-facing barbs for enhanced tissue adhesion. *Adv Funct Mater*. 2020;30(11).

154. Moussi K, Kosel J. 3-D printed biocompatible micro-bellows membranes. *J Microelectromechanical Syst*. 2018;27(3):472–8.

155. Moussi K, Bukhamsin A, Hidalgo T, Kosel J. Biocompatible 3D printed microneedles for transdermal, intradermal, and percutaneous applications. *Adv Eng Mater*. 2020;22(2):1–10.

156. Ross S, Scoutaris N, Lamprou D, Mallinson D, Douroumis D. Inkjet printing of insulin microneedles for transdermal delivery. *Drug Deliv Transl Res*. 2015;5(4):451–61.

157. Uddin MJ, Scoutaris N, Klepetsanis P, Chowdhry B, Prausnitz MR, Douroumis D. Inkjet printing of transdermal microneedles for the delivery of anticancer agents. *Int J Pharm*. 2015;494(2):593–602. Available from: http://dx.doi.org/10.1016/j.ijpharm.2015.01.038

158. Pere CPP, Economidou SN, Lall G, Ziraud C, Boateng JS, Alexander BD, et al. 3D printed microneedles for insulin skin delivery. *Int J Pharm*. 2018;544(2):425–32. Available from: https://doi.org/10.1016/j.ijpharm.2018.03.031

159. Luzuriaga MA, Berry DR, Reagan JC, Smaldone RA, Gassensmith JJ. Biodegradable 3D printed polymer microneedles for transdermal drug delivery. *Lab Chip*. 2018;18(8):1223–30.

160. Tamay DG, Usal TD, Alagoz AS, Yucel D, Hasirci N, Hasirci V. 3D and 4D printing of polymers for tissue engineering applications. *Front Bioeng Biotechnol*. 2019;7(Jul).

161. Lei L, Wang X, Zhu Y, Su W, Lv Q, Li D. Antimicrobial hydrogel microspheres for protein capture and wound healing. *Mater Des*[Internet]. 2022;215:110478. Available from: https://doi.org/10.1016/j.matdes.2022.110478

162. Fernando IPS, Kim D, Nah JW, Jeon YJ. Advances in functionalizing fucoidans and alginates (bio)polymers by structural modifications: A review. *Chem Eng J*. 2019;355:33–48. Available from: https://www.sciencedirect.com/science/article/pii/S1385894718315894

163. Zheng Y, Yang J, Liang J, Xu X, Cui W, Deng L, et al. Bioinspired hyaluronic acid/phosphorylcholine polymer with enhanced lubrication and anti-inflammation. *Biomacromolecules*. 2019;20(11):4135–42.

164. Gao B, Yang Q, Zhao X, Jin G, Ma Y, Xu F. 4D bioprinting for biomedical applications. *Trends Biotechnol*. 2016;34(9):746–56. Available from: http://dx.doi.org/10.1016/j.tibtech.2016.03.004

165. Hong S, Song SJ, Lee JY, Jang H, Choi J, Sun K, et al. Cellular behavior in micropatterned hydrogels by bioprinting system depended on the cell types and cellular interaction. *J Biosci Bioeng*. 2013;116(2):224–30. Available from: http://dx.doi.org/10.1016/j.jbiosc.2013.02.011

166. Caspi O, Lesman A, Basevitch Y, Gepstein A, Arbel G, Huber I, et al. Tissue engineering of vascularized cardiac muscle from human embryonic stem cells. *Circ Res*. 2007;100(2):263–72.

167. Dai W, Guo H, Gao B, Ruan M, Xu L, Wu J, et al. Double network shape memory hydrogels activated by near-infrared with high mechanical toughness, nontoxicity, and 3D printability. *Chem Eng J*. 2019;356:934–49. Available from: https://www.sciencedirect.com/science/article/pii/S1385894718317947

168. Budharaju H, Zennifer A, Sethuraman S, Paul A, Sundaramurthi D. Designer DNA biomolecules as a defined biomaterial for 3D bioprinting applications. *Mater Horiz*. 2022;9(4):1141–66. Available from: http://dx.doi.org/10.1039/D1MH01632F

169. Yang GH, Yeo M, Koo YW, Kim GH. 4D bioprinting: Technological advances in biofabrication. *Macromol Biosci.* 2019;19(5):1–10.

170. Gugulothu SB, Chatterjee K. Visible light-based 4D-bioprinted tissue scaffold. *ACS Macro Lett.* 2023 Apr;12(4):494–502.

171. Foresti R, Rossi S, Pinelli S, Alinovi R, Sciancalepore C, Delmonte N, et al. In-vivo vascular application via ultra-fast bioprinting for future 5D personalised nanomedicine. *Sci Rep.* 2020;10(1):1–13.

172. Anas S, Khan MY, Rafey MA, Faheem K. Concept of 5D printing technology and its applicability in the healthcare industry. *Mater Today Proc.* 2021; Available from: https://api.semanticscholar.org/CorpusID:244015546

173. Foresti R, Rossi S, Magnani M, Guarino Lo Bianco C, Delmonte N. Smart society and artificial intelligence: Big data scheduling and the global standard method applied to smart maintenance. *Engineering.* 2020;6(7):835–46. Available from: https://doi.org/10.1016/j.eng.2019.11.014

174. Gillaspie EA, Matsumoto JS, Morris NE, Downey RJ, Shen KR, Allen MS, et al. From 3D printing to 5D printing: Enhancing thoracic surgical planning and resection of complex tumors. *Ann Thorac Surg.* 2017;176(1):139–48.

175. Rocha-García D, Guerra-Contreras A, Rosales-Mendoza S, Palestino G. Role of porous silicon/hydrogel composites on drug delivery. *Open Mater Sci.* 2016;3(1):93–101.

176. Campisi M, Shin Y, Osaki T, Hajal C, Chiono V, Kamm RD. 3D self-organized microvascular model of the human blood-brain barrier with endothelial cells, pericytes and astrocytes. *Biomaterials.* 2018;176(5):139–48.

177. Haleem A, Javaid M. Expected applications of five-dimensional (5D) printing in the medical field. *Curr Med Res Pract.* 2019;9(5):208–9.

178. Vancauwenberghe V, Baiye Mfortaw Mbong V, Vanstreels E, Verboven P, Lammertyn J, Nicolai B. 3D printing of plant tissue for innovative food manufacturing: Encapsulation of alive plant cells into pectin based bio-ink. *J Food Eng.* 2019;263:454–64. Available from: https://doi.org/10.1016/j.jfoodeng.2017.12.003

179. Ghazal AF, Zhang M, Mujumdar AS, Ghamry M. Progress in 4D/5D/6D printing of foods: Applications and R&D opportunities. *Crit Rev Food Sci Nutr.* 2022:1–24. Available from: https://doi.org/10.1080/10408398.2022.2045896

180. Chiu DT, deMello AJ, Di Carlo D, Doyle PS, Hansen C, Maceiczyk RM, et al. Small but perfectly formed? Successes, challenges, and opportunities for microfluidics in the chemical and biological sciences. *Chem.* 2017;2(2):201–23.

181. What is 5D printing?. 2023. Available from: https://www.twi-global.com/technical-knowledge/faqs/what-is-5d-printing

182. Sheikh A, Abourehab MAS, Kesharwani P. The clinical significance of 4D printing. *Drug Discov Today.* 2023;28(1):1–15.

8 Regulatory Perspective on 3D-Printing in Dermaceuticals

Kantrol Kumar Sahu and Ravi Verma
GLA University, Mathura, India

Ramakant Joshi
Amity Institute of Pharmacy, Madhya Pradesh, India

Ritesh Jain
Chouksey Engineering College, Bilaspur, India

8.1 INTRODUCTION

In August 2015, the U.S. Food and Drug Administration (FDA) authorized the first three-dimensional (3D)-printed medicinal prescription product, setting the stage for an industrial revolution in the pharmaceutical sector (1). The idea of customization has been actively researched in the pharmaceutical industry ever since the human genome project was completed in the middle of the 1990s (2–4). Traditional medication delivery methods, such as the use of tablets, capsules, and other dosage forms, are progressively dwindling. Active components like macromolecules and deoxyribonucleic acid are evolving quickly to become the next wave of pharmaceuticals. Therapeutic approaches may be modified and improved to meet the unique requirements, preferences, and features of each patient. The present bulk production techniques for standardized dose forms, however, are being challenged by the quickly changing medical paradigms. Traditionally, hundreds of thousands of tablets are produced using high-speed, "one size fits all" pharmaceutical-grade machinery. Using these bulk manufacturing procedures, the medicinal product must be chemically and thermally stable for the full two years of its shelf life. Regulatory requirements also call for each product to be equal across all batches in terms of purity, impurities, and defined quality features. A large amount of formulation research has been done to increase the shelf-life of products, yet every year, promising compounds with low physicochemical stability are eliminated from the development pipeline. Nevertheless, these possible candidates may be prepared using a suitable platform for on-demand manufacture with minimal to nonexistent long-term stability for the immediate administration of patients following preparation. The product design

DOI: 10.1201/9781032690926-8

process may become difficult despite the technique's apparent simplicity. While 3D printing has already shown the financial viability of creating pharmaceutical products in bulk, it also amply demonstrates the potential of on-demand production. Over the past 10 years, 3D-printed medical equipment has been certified and controlled by the Center for Equipment and Radiological Health (CDRH), even though 3D printing has only recently entered the pharmaceutical manufacturing of medications (5).

8.2 THINGS TO KEEP IN MIND FOR 3D-PRINTING DEVELOPMENT

8.2.1 PROCESS AND DESIGN OF THE PRODUCT

By using this technique, porous tablets are produced, which dissolve virtually instantly in the mouth (1). Three-dimensional printing is described in previous chapters as a layer-by-layer process that turns computer blueprints into 3D things. Contrary to conventional pharmaceutical processes, also referred to as subtractive processes, the process of 3D printing is bottom-up, in which thin 2D layers are sequentially built and joined to the layer below through the base plate's or the print head's precise movement (2–4). The dosage form and manufacturing technique have a significant impact on the physical product design when employing a conventional pharmaceutical procedure. Additionally, formulation development has a significant impact on how functionally designed a product is (such as modified-release goods). A number of well-known pharmaceutical dosage forms that have been shown to be suitable for 3D printing include tabs, caps, powders, lozenges, MN transdermal patches, films (2D printing), and more. However, creating complex geometries can be facilitated by employing 3D printing in product design. Examples of 3D-printed dosage forms that are spherical, multilayered, pyramidal, cylindrical, and cubic are shown in Figure 8.1 and were created to test the viability of pharmaceuticals (2–4). Three-dimensional printing's flexibility and other technologies enable the fabrication of final dose forms, giving patients the opportunity to receive personalized regimens like polypharmacy (3, 4). There are several 3D-printing platforms, each with a particular technology that makes use of a different kind of input material or working model. As a result, the kind of 3D printer used and vice versa have a significant impact on the platform's product and process design. Specific product designs for the 3D printer exist. For example, Spritam is the first product to be approved by the FDA for 3D printing and a specific production technique called ZipDose technology. It is made using inkjet 3D printing (6–8).

Similar to how complicated functional designs made with 3D-printing technology might impact oral dosage forms' medication release. It would be challenging to formulate a bimodal drug release mechanism using traditional bulk manufacturing techniques. Regulating the rate and volume of medication release from every subsection during the deposition of pharmacological material across a dosage form may require the employment of a progressive concentration gradient and other spatial patterns. More recent studies have shown that by carefully regulating the medication and excipient mixture, 3D-printing technology may be able to produce solid

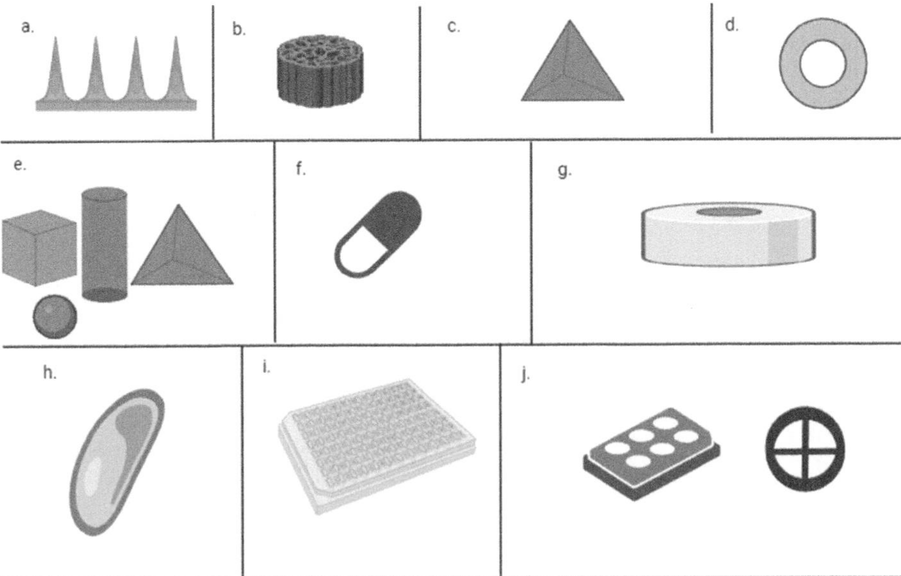

FIGURE 8.1   The following are examples of complex and un-mouldable product designs made with 3D printing: (a) Microneedles miconazole (9); (b) Acetaminophen tabs with various gradient constructions (10); (c) Hot-melt extrusion (HME) filament felodipine (11); (d) Donut shaped tablet with acetaminophen, paracetamol, and regulated release polymers (12); (e) Printed sphere, cube, pyramid, and cylinder in three dimensions (13); (f) Shell-core fused deposition modeling (FDM)-based delayed-release tablet (14); (g) Tablet that is printed in three dimensions and has a bound zone in the center of the device (15); (h) A caplet contained within another caplet (16); (i) Printed patches for medication administration in three dimensions (17); (j) A tablet with several compartments (18).

oral dosage forms. To generate a multimodal drug release profile, adjust densities and diffusivities. A complicated formulation that is based on several research articles is shown in Figure 8.2 (19, 20).

These sophisticated formulations are the only ones that allow for precise regulation of in vivo biodistribution and medication release that is disease-specific and site-specific. These intricately built tablets are believed to be extremely thin slabs or one micro tablet contained within a larger tablet that may release medication either pulsatile or by a mix of several drug release mechanisms (21). The use of an osmotic pump in combination with erosion- and/or diffusion-controlled medication release may be necessary for this (22). They are also reserved for drug candidates that need to be extremely precise, such as those with patient-specific nanotechnology, high potency, restricted therapeutic index, and insoluble (23). These complicated formulation design examples may all be designed and produced using technologies for 3D printing. It is anticipated that the answers to these queries will have a big impact on design and process considerations. First off, all conventional Chemistry, Manufacturing, and Controls (CMC)-related regulations will be used if a commercially produced, 3D-printed object

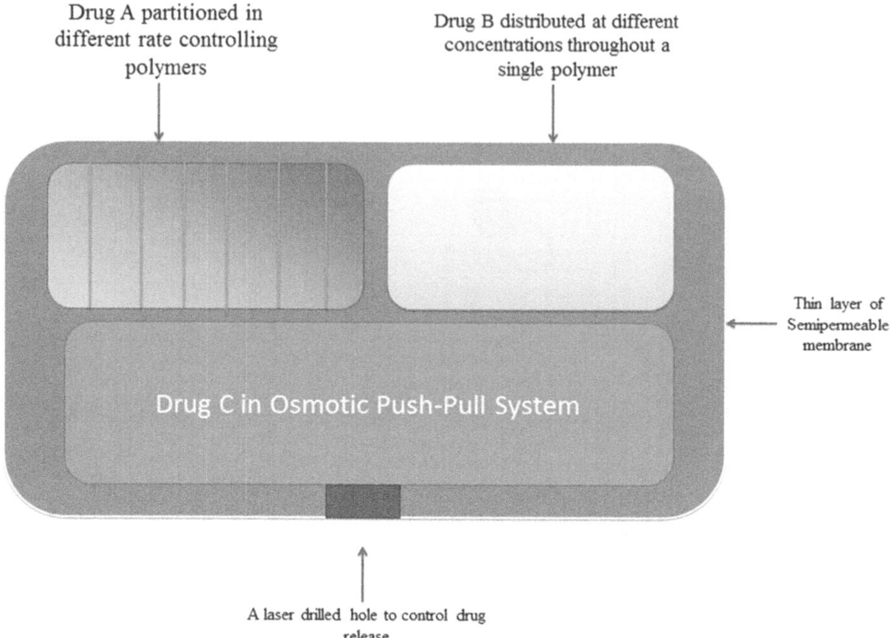

FIGURE 8.2   A multicompartmental tablet with three separate medications included in one fixed dosage combination. Drug A is divided vertically into several polymer types, allowing for regulated drug release through mechanisms such as dissolution and diffusion. Using an erosion-controlled polymer, the print head applies scattered droplets throughout the tablet to distribute Drug B at different concentrations. Consequently, the erosion mechanism is followed to produce drug release. Medication C is an osmotic push–pull device in which osmosis controls the release of the medication.

is designed for a patient population. The final formulation components must be the same for each dosage form unit in order to meet the targeted shelf life and standard. When creating a 3D-printed item, the following aspects are often taken into account in both individual and mass-production 3D-printing scenarios: (1) medicinal product manifestation that takes into account the target patient as opposed to the target patient group; (2) individual or group-specific patient demands, such as localized medicine administration using 3D-printed microneedle transdermal patches; (3) the kind of molecule to be given and its intended use; for example, biologics may need a particular formulation and process design in addition to a particular regulatory framework; (i4) desired dosage and its precision level; (5) degree of customization; (6) the intended distribution path; (7) achieving the desired pharmacokinetic characteristic and in vitro drug release aim; (8) desired qualitative characteristics; (9) target package arrangement; and (10) A desired shelf life.

Depending on how the computer-aided design (CAD) product is designed internally, externally, and functionally, a pharmaceutical business could make use of many 3D-printing systems. Although 3D printers operate according to different philosophies, the majority of 3D-printing procedures adhere to the framework shown in

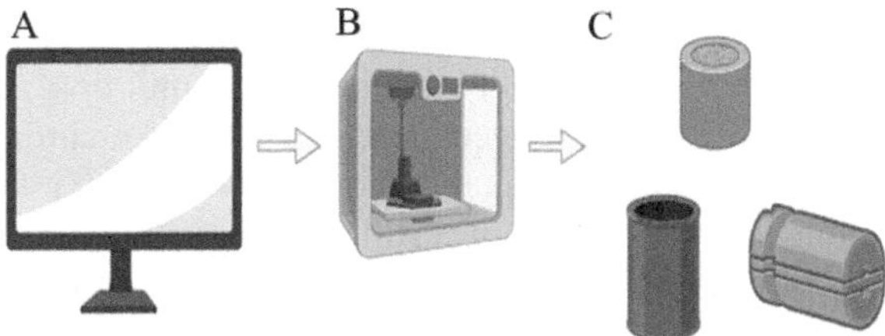

FIGURE 8.3 The 3D-printing methods for pharmaceutical production. A. Using computer-aided design, a pharmaceutical tablet is initially developed in three dimensions. B. The 3D printer receives the product design file. The design is subsequently divided into several 2D layers by the printing software. Layers of the material are deposited onto the build plate under the direction of the software, which also controls the print head. C. Throughout the process, 2D layers are combined to generate a single 3D product, such as a multilayered tablet that contains one or more medications, a simple matrix tablet, or a tablet inside a tablet.

Figure 8.3 and the subsequent step-by-step instructions for producing pharmaceutical products (24–46).

S-1: First, computer-aided design software is used to produce a 3D digital design of the desired object.

S-2: The machine's outside may be read. The surface of a 3D model is then defined using the design's .stl file format. After that, the printing software "slices" these surfaces into distinct 2D-printable layers and electronically transmits layer-by-layer instructions to the printer. Both the overall number of layers and the individual layer thickness can change. The software determines where the scaffolding material for the current print should be produced in addition to controlling the movement of the print head.

S-3: Taking care of the raw resources is stage one. Depending on the type of printing technology being used, the raw components may be processed into granules, dry mixed powder, filaments, or binder solutions. Granules, powder, or print fluid may both include the active medicinal ingredient. A combination of two or more medications may occasionally be used.

S-4: The buildup cycle refers to the subsequent automated layer-by-layer addition and solidification of raw components to create the desired result.

S-5: It is now possible to gather and recycle any unprinted materials so they may be utilized once more throughout the printing process. To characterize the unprinted harvested material further for potential drug breakdown, segregation, and other standard physical characteristics that are looked for while looking at powders, it may be necessary if it includes any active components.

Following the decision on a particular printer type, the following are common process considerations: (1) Is mass production with 3D printing a viable option? (2) When technology is moved from small-scale research and development 3D printers to large-scale production 3D printers, scaling up is challenging; (3) Is production moving quickly enough to meet demand from customers? (4) Does the procedure have the flexibility and ability to reliably duplicate each unit dose? Does the procedure have the capacity to support, if necessary, a structure for cutting-edge pharmaceutical research, production, and quality control (PAT)? (5) Is the procedure user-friendly and able to pass any type of certification or validation in a current Good Manufacturing Practice (cGMP)setting? (6) Is the program effective in controlling the process? and (7) Can you validate the software?

8.2.2 CONTROL OF INTERMEDIATE AND RAW MATERIALS

It takes more control over the raw materials for 3D printing. With 3D printing, the original material may change significantly on a physical and/or chemical level, layer by layer, because each layer may be sparsely spread (as thin as 10 microns or less). Therefore, the characteristics of the finished medicinal product can be significantly influenced by the starting material and any inactive molecules added throughout the production cycle. For example, in powder-bed inkjet 3D printing, changes in layer thickness and inappropriate adhesion between layers may occur if the product's micromeritics and flow properties are not well defined. As a result, the final product that is manufactured may not even closely resemble the desired product design. Typically, the selection of excipients and active pharmaceutical ingredients (APIs)is heavily influenced by their physicochemical stability, printability, and the kind of 3D printer that will be utilized. For instance, powder-based 3D-printing processes will have different material requirements than stereolithography (47, 48).

8.2.3 U.S. FDA CONTRIBUTION TO PHARMACEUTICAL 3D-PRINTING IMPROVEMENTS

Owing to growing interest in and understanding of bioprinting, 3D-printed medical equipment, and, more recently, pharmaceutical medication goods, the FDA has launched a number of internal regulatory science and research initiatives throughout its centers such as Center for Drug Evaluation and Research (CDER), Center for Devices and Radiological Health (CDRH), Center for Biologics Evaluation and Research (CBER). This was put into practice to improve our understanding of how material characteristics and process variables relate to the final product quality of biologics, medical devices, and 3D-printed pharmaceuticals (5). FDA quality experts may support the adoption of novel techniques for pharmaceutical manufacture while offering significant and pertinent regulatory supervision if they are fully versed in the science and how to apply it. Thus far, the FDA has inspected and regulated 3D-printed products in compliance with existing legislation. Within the agency, there has been a great deal of cross-center cooperation, with separate centers developing specialized work groups. Recently, the CDER formed an Emerging Technology Team to engage closely with stakeholders in order to uncover particular scientific challenges related to 3D printing that may impede advancement or adoption. In order to gather feedback from the additive manufacturing (AM) community, the CDRH previously hosted public workshops in 2014 and issued guidelines, both of which were described earlier in this chapter. It is highly challenging to create regulatory advice about the use of 3D printing to manufacture customized medicine that can offer precise prescriptions for each fabrication and patient. Instead, the agency's current focus is on creating a standard framework that will enable this technology to produce 3D-printed goods in compliance with current laws. These are some examples of drugs that are made through stereolithographic (SLA) 3D printing, which are compiled in Table 8.1 (49).

8.2.4 SPECIFYING DRUG PRODUCTS MADE WITH 3D PRINTING

The International Conference on Harmonization (ICH) Q6 guidelines should be followed when creating specifications for drug products that are printed using 3D printing. It is important to keep in mind that this advice only applies to conventional bulk pharmaceutical product manufacturing. A clinically relevant specification that takes into account all important quality attributes associated with these dosage forms—such as capsules, tablets, parenteral, transdermal patches, ointments, and suspensions—should be established in accordance with the guideline if the creation of any common, typical dosage forms using 3D printing is intended. These include United States Pharmacopoeia (USP), the British Pharmacopoeia (BP), and the Japanese Pharmacopoeia (JP). Assay, impurity, content homogeneity, and dissolution are examples of conventional quality qualities in specifications that may not apply to the product created by 3D printing. The tablet's porosity may be an added quality feature and have an extremely porous interior structure, which may influence the tablet's quick disintegration. This feature might also affect the product's tensile strength, which is essential for preventing the product's physical structure from breaking during handling and transportation. These kinds of 3D-printed dosage forms might have their transportation and storage integrity guaranteed by a simulation of the shipping process. Certain characteristics in the specification, however, could differ from patient to patient and/or scenario to scenario. For instance, it is necessary to set up a tailored dosage for a particular patient or group of patients, such as 10 distinct medicine combinations or doses for 10 distinct patients. Similarly, under extreme circumstances such as combat, when a pharmaceutical product is immediately required to save lives, some qualities might not be required (50).

8.3 REGULATORY OMISSIONS AND DIFFICULTIES

Under the present paradigm, the AM community—which includes academics and businesses—now faces the following regulatory shortcomings for pharmaceutical medical goods: (a) In the event that this technology is used to produce customized goods that are ordered on demand, what kind of regulations should be in place? In U.S. hospitals, certain patient demands are met by using certain accepted amounts of compounding, among others. Therefore, institutional review boards, hospital policies, or the practice of medicine may have jurisdiction over the use of 3D printing for this purpose. Compounders that are not registered as outsourcing facilities must comply with state-level regulations under Sections 503B (b) (5)

TABLE 8.1
Examples of Drug Delivery Systems Fabricated Using (SLA)

Drug	Dosage Form	Excipient		Dimensions
		Monomer	Photoinitiator	
Paracetamol & 4-aminosalicylic acid	Oral modified-release dosage form	Polyethylene glycoldiacrylate (PEGDA)	Diphenyl(2,4,6-trimethylbenzoyl) phosphine oxide	Torus shape tablets, 11-mm diameter × 4-mm height, and the central hole of 3-mm diameter
Paracetamol, caffeine, naproxen, chloramphenicol, prednisolone, and aspirin,	Polypills	Polyethylene glycoldiacrylate (PEGDA)	Diphenyl(2,4,6-trimethylbenzoyl) phosphine oxide	Cylinder—10-mm diameter and 3-mm height ring—10-mm diameter and 6-mm height
Berberine chloride	Nano-composite pills	Polyethylene glycoldiacrylate (PEGDA)	Diphenyl(2,4,6-trimethylbenzoyl) phosphine oxide	Height—5 mm Diameter—7.5 mm
Rifampicin	Hollow microneedles (HMNs) array	Dental SG resin	–	MNs per array—49 (7 * 7) Each cubical reservoir with dimensions 13.0 mm × 13.0 mm × 3.5 mm
Dacarbazine	Drug-loaded microneedle arrays	Poly(propylene fumarate): diethyl fumarate (50:50)	Diphenyl(2,4,6-trimethylbenzoyl) phosphine oxide	The length of the microneedle is 700 μm, and the conical tip of 300 μm. While apex diameter is 20 μm.
Lidocaine hydrochloride monohydrate	Urinary bladder insert	Elastic resin	–	Solid Device—130-mm length and 3-mm diameter Hallow device—130-mm length, 3-mm outer diameter, 0.5-mm shell thickness

Implants	Antimicrobial dental implants	Quaternary ammonium methacrylate prepared by incorporating quaternary ammonium groups into diurethanedimethacrylate/ glycerol dimethacrylate	Bisacrylphosphine oxide	Different models with various dimensions
	Prosthetic vascular grafts	α,w-polytetrahydrofuranether-diacrylate	Irgacure 184 (1-Hydroxycyclohexyl phenyl ketone)	Inner diameter—20 µm to 2 m
Ciprofloxacin Fluocinolone acetonide	Drug-eluting hearing aids	Kudo 3DSR Flexible resin & Kudo 3DSR ENG hard resin	–	Circular discs—10-mm diameter * 1-mm height Rectangular slabs—10 mm * 20 mm * 1 mm

Note: Adopted with permission from (49) copyright 2023, Elsevier.

and 503B (a) (10) for medications manufactured in the United States, except for hospitals. Nevertheless, the use of 3D printing for compounding in any circumstance is not expressly covered by these compounding standards. Any compounding business that uses 3D-printing technology should, at the very least, comply with all current compounding rules. (b) Printing in pharmacies, hospitals, and clinical research facilities: All current regulations are applicable if printing is used to produce goods at a clinical location connected to clinical trials and industrial-scale product development (such as the first human safety study). Printing at the pharmacy or hospital raises issues with (a), as previously mentioned. The main issues in both situations are the potential production of unknown harmful degradation products, the usage of organic solvents, and the health and safety risks resulting from these processes. Because 3D-printing technology is portable and has the potential to be used to generate a range of medical products, other factors, such as transportation, climate variability, and resistance to cross-contamination, could be necessary for the regulation procedure (c). Doctor's office or at-home printing: As of right now, there is no legal framework allowing physicians or patients to use 3D printing to produce customized medications either in the doctor's office or at home. Apart from the previously mentioned regulatory apprehensions, the underlying deficiencies are as discussed here: (1) Production of ink toner in bulk that includes excipients and API, as well as their distribution, by whom, and how will this be governed? (2) Who is going to give those cartridges out? Pharmacists or doctors? (3) Who is going to produce the 3D printers? Will they be subject to medical device regulations? (4) Who will keep an eye on how prescription drugs are made at home? (5) Which product specifications should be measured, how should they be used, and how should they be measured? (6) How long would the product last on the shelf? and (7) Is it necessary to verify the shelf life of print cartridges containing drugs? (50).

8.4 EMERGING 3D-PRINTING TECHNOLOGIES FOR DRUG DELIVERY DEVICES

Because traditional drug delivery platforms cannot be tailored to each patient's unique pharmacokinetic characteristics, its "one-size-fits-all" approach frequently limits its applicability in the pharmaceutical sector. Three-dimensional-printed drug-delivery medical devices are becoming more and more common due to the advancements in AM technology. These devices have several benefits over conventional drug administration methods. The capacity to create 3D buildings with complex architecture and adjustable designs is one of the main advantages; maybe more significantly, however, is the simplicity of creating customized pharmaceuticals. Additionally, the development of 4D printing and multi-material printing combines the advantages of several functional materials, opening up a wide range of possibilities for the evolution of customized drug delivery systems. Even with AM methods' amazing advancements, challenges with cost-effectiveness, scalability, and regulatory compliance still loom large (51).

8.5　MEDICAL DEVICES THAT DISPENSE DRUGS

Notwithstanding its unique ability to create complex, multifunctional structures, regulatory approval is still a hurdle that might prevent 3D printing from being used in the biomedical field. Before being released onto the commercial market, drug delivery devices made using AM methods must meet all FDA regulations. Nonetheless, there are a few key issues that need to be addressed and merged correctly, including medication degradation, the device's biocompatibility and biodegradability, and hazardous responses. A major turning point for 3D-printed pharmaceutical dosage forms was the FDA's approval of Spritam, the first 3D-printed medication (52).

8.6　REGULATORY RESTRICTION

The FDA released *Technical Considerations for Additive Manufactured Devices Guidelines* in 2017. The design, materials, software processing, printing process parameters, post-processing parameters, and process validation of 3D-printed medical goods are the main topics covered by these standards. It also lists the printed product's quality concerns, including material chemistry, mechanical attributes, dimensions, and biocompatibility (53). Nevertheless, no guidelines pertaining to medical items manufactured using 3D printing were released. In the future, guidelines could be released with perhaps stricter rules than those governing medical devices. In contrast to traditional goods, where the FDA gave the approval of the drug product without giving much thought to the manufacturing process, 3D-printed pharmaceutical regulations are anticipated to incorporate process controls. Pharmaceutical businesses would continue to be interested in using 3D printer technology on hard turf if these difficulties were resolved. Furthermore, producers have an increased burden to comply with the many sets of requirements linked with various regulatory authorities due to the lack of concordance across regulatory organizations (53, 54).

8.7　CONCLUSION

Since its debut in the last 10 years, interest in and knowledge of the age of customized medicine and the genetic revolution have expanded significantly. In this kind of environment, 3D printing has already proven to be a cutting-edge manufacturing method for producing medical equipment. However, in the adaptability of generating final dosage forms that facilitate the administration of patient-specific regimens, 3D printing has shown a lot of promise. It would have looked like science fiction to use 3D printing to design and manufacture our medications, but this is quickly becoming a reality, and the technology will only advance.

ACKNOWLEDGMENTS

The authors express their sincere gratitude to the host institutions for generously providing all the necessary facilities throughout the course of this study.

FUNDING

None.

CONFLICT OF INTEREST

None.

REFERENCES

1. United States Food and Drug Administration. Highlights of prescribing information – Spritam. 2015. Available from: http://www.accessdata.fda.gov/drugsatfda_docs/label/2015/207958s000lbl.pdf
2. Norman J, Madurawe RD, Moore CMV, Khan MA, Khairuzzaman A. A new chapter in pharmaceutical manufacturing: 3D printed drug products. *Adv Drug Deliv Rev* 2017;108:39–50.
3. Trenfield SJ, Awad A, Goyanes A, Gaisford S, Basit AW. 3D printing pharmaceuticals: Drug development to frontline care. *Trends Pharmacol Sci* 2018;39(5):440–445.
4. Awad A, Trenfield SJ, Goyanes A, Gaisford S, Basit AW. Reshaping drug development using 3D printing. *Drug Discov Today* 2018; https://doi.org/10.1016/j.drudis.2018.05.025
5. Prima MD, Coburn J, Hwang D, Kelly J, Khairuzzaman A, Ricles L. Additively manufactured medical products – the FDA perspective. *3D Print Med* 2016;2:1.
6. United States Government Accountability Office. 3D printing: Opportunities, challenges, and policy implications of additive manufacturing. 2015. Available from: http://www.gao.gov/assets/680/670960.pdf
7. Chhaya MP, Poh PS, Balmayor ER, van Griensven M, Schantz JT, Hutmacher DW. Additive manufacturing in biomedical sciences and the need for definitions and norms. *Expert Rev Med Devices* 2015;12(5):537–543.
8. International Standards Organization. ISO/ASTM 52900 Additive manufacturing – General principles – Terminology. [under development] Available from: http://www.iso.org/iso/catalogue_detail.htm?csnumber=69669
9. Prasad LM, Smyth H. 3D printing technologies for drug delivery: A review. *Drug Dev Ind Pharm* 2016;42(7):1019–1031.
10. Yu DG, Yang XL, Huang WD, Liu J, Wang YG, Xu H. Tablets with material gradients fabricated by three-dimensional printing. *J Pharm Sci* 2007;96(9):2446–2456.
11. Alhijjaj M, Belton P, Qi S. An investigation into the use of polymer blends to improve the printability of and regulate drug release from pharmaceutical solid dispersion prepared via fused deposition modeling (FDM) 3D printing. *Eu J Pharm Biopharm* 2016;108:111–125.
12. Wang J, Goyanes A, Gaisford S, Basit AW. Stereolithographic (SLA) 3D printing of oral modified-release dosage forms. *Int J Pharm* 2016; 503:207–212.
13. Goyanes A, Martinez PR, Buanz A, Basit A, Gaisford S. Effect of geometry on drug release from 3D printed tablets. *Int J Pharm* 2015;494:657–663.
14. Okwuosa TC, Pereira BC, Arafat B, Cieszynska M, Isreb A, Alhnan MA. Fabricating a ShellCore delayed release tablet using dual FDM 3D printing for patient-centred therapy. *Pharm Res* 2017;34:427–437.
15. Acosta-Vélez GF, Wu BM. 3D pharming: Direct printing of personalized pharmaceutical tablets. *Pol Sci* 2016;1:2.
16. Goyanes A, Wang J, Buanz A, Martinez-Pacheco R, Telford R, Gaisford S, et al. 3D printing of medicines: Engineering novel oral devices with unique design and drug release characteristics. *Mol Pharm* 2015;12(11):4077–4084.

17. Yi HG, Cho YJ, Kang KS, Hong JM, Pati RG, Park MN, et al. A 3D printed local drug delivery patch for pancreatic cancer growth suppression. *J Control Release* 2016;238:231–241.
18. Khaled SA, Burley JC, Alexander MR, Yang J, Roberts CJ. 3D printing of tablets containing multiple drugs with defined release profiles. *Int J Pharm* 2015;494(2):643–650.
19. Katstra WE, Palazzolo RD, Rowe CW, Giritlioglu B, Teung P, Cima MJ. Oral dosage forms fabricated by three dimensional printing. *J Control Release* 2000;66(1):1–9.
20. Sun Y, Soh S. Printing tablets with fully customizable release profiles for personalized medicine. *Adv Mater* 2015;27(47):7847–7853.
21. Wu BM, Borland SW, Giordano RA, Cima LG, Sachs EM, Cima MJ. Solid free-form fabrication of drug delivery devices. *J Control Release* 1996;40(1–2):77–87.
22. Vogel BJ. Intellectual property and additive manufacturing/3D printing: Strategies and challenges of applying traditional IP Laws to a transformative technology. *Minn J L Sci Tech* 2016;17(2):880–906.
23. Beck RCR, Chaves PS, Goyanes A, Vukosavljevic B, Buanz A, Windbergs A, et al. 3D printed tablets loaded with polymeric nanocapsules: An innovative approach to produce customized drug delivery systems. *Int J Pharm* 2017;528(1–2):268–279.
24. Alhnan MA, Okwuosa TC, Sadia M, Wan KW, Ahmed W, Arafat B. Emergence of 3D printed dosage forms: Opportunities and challenges. *Pharm Res* 2016;33(8):1817–1832.
25. Fina F, Goyanes A, Gaisford S, Basit AW. Selective laser sintering (SLS) 3D printing of medicines. *Int J Pharm* 2017;529(1–2):285–293.
26. Fina F, Madla CM, Goyanes A, Zhang J, Gaisford S, Basit AW. Fabricating 3D printed orally disintegrating printlets using selective laser sintering. *Int J Pharm* 2018;541(1–2):101–107.
27. Fina F, Goyanes A, Madla CM, Awad A, Trenfield SJ, Kuek JM, et al. 3D printing of drug loaded gyroid lattices using selective laser sintering. *Int J Pharm* 2018;547:44–52.
28. Genina N, Boetker JP, Colombo S, Harmankaya N, Rantanen J, Bohr A. Anti-tuberculosis drug combination for controlled oral delivery using 3D printed compartmental dosage forms: From drug product design to in vivo testing. *J Control Release* 2017;268:40–48.
29. Gioumouxouzis CI, Katsamenis OL, Bouropoulos N, Fatouros DG. 3D printed oral solid dosage forms containing hydrochlorothiazide for controlled drug delivery. *J Drug Deliv Sci Technol* 2017;40:164–171.
30. Goyanes A, Chang H, Sedough D, Hatton GB, Wang J, Buanz A, et al. Fabrication of controlled-release budesonide tablets via desktop (FDM) 3D printing. *Int J Pharm* 2015;496(2):414–420.
31. Goyanes A, Det-Amornrat U, Wang J, Basit AW, Gaisford S. 3D scanning and 3D printing as innovative technologies for fabricating personalized topical drug delivery systems. *J Control Release* 2016;234:41–48.
32. Goyanes A, Kobayashi M, Martínez-Pacheco R, Gaisford S, Basit AW. Fused-filament 3D printing of drug products: Microstructure analysis and drug release characteristics of PVAbased caplets. *Int J Pharm* 2016;514(1):290–295.
33. Goyanes A, Fina F, Martorana A, Sedough D, Gaisford S, Basit AW. Development of modified release 3D printed tablets (printlets) with pharmaceutical excipients using additive manufacturing. *Int J Pharm* 2017;527(1–2):21–30.
34. Goyanes A, Scarpa M, Kamlow M, Gaisford S, Basit AW, Orlu M. Patient acceptability of 3D printed medicines. *Int J Pharm* 2017;530(1–2):71–78.
35. Goyanes A, Fernández-Ferreiro A, Majeed A, Gomez-Lado N, Awad A, Luaces-Rodríguez A, et al. PET/CT imaging of 3D printed devices in the gastrointestinal tract of rodents. *Int J Pharm* 2018;536(1):158–164.
36. Awad A, Trenfield SJ, Gaisford S, Basit AW. 3D printed medicines: A new branch of digital healthcare. *Int J Pharm* 2018;548(1):586–596.

37. Goyanes A, Buanz AB, Hatton GB, Gaisford S, Basit AW. 3D printing of modified-release aminosalicylate (4-ASA and 5-ASA) tablets. *Eur J Pharm Biopharm* 2015;89:157–162.

38. Melocchi A, Parietti F, Maroni A, Foppoli A, Gazzaniga A, Zema L. Hot-melt extruded filaments based on pharmaceutical grade polymers for 3D printing by fused deposition modeling. *Int J Pharm* 2016;509(1–2):255–263.

39. Okwuosa TC, Stefaniak S, Arafat B, Isreb A, Wan KW, Alhnan MA. A lower temperature FDM 3D printing for the manufacture of patient-specific immediate release tablets. *Pharm Res* 2016;33(11):2704–2712.

40. Muwaffak Z, Goyanes A, Clark V, Basit AW, Hilton ST, Gaisford S. Patient-specific 3D scanned and 3D printed antimicrobial polycaprolactone wound dressings. *Int J Pharm* 2017;527(1–2):161–170.

41. Sadia M, Sośnicka A, Arafat B, Isreb A, Ahmed W, Kelarakis A, et al. Adaptation of pharmaceutical excipients to FDM 3D printing for the fabrication of patient-tailored immediate release tablets. *Int J Pharm* 2016;513(1–2):659–668.

42. Skowyra J, Pietrzak K, Alhnan MA. Fabrication of extended-release patient-tailored prednisolone tablets via fused deposition modelling (FDM) 3D printing. *Eur J Pharm Sci* 2015;68:11–17.

43. Solanki NG, Tahsin M, Shah AV, Serajuddin ATM. Formulation of 3D printed tablet for rapid drug release by fused deposition modeling: Screening polymers for drug release, drug polymer miscibility and printability. *J Pharm Sci* 2018;107(1):390–401.

44. Goyanes A, Buanz AB, Basit AW, Gaisford S. Fused-filament 3D printing (3DP) for fabrication of tablets. *Int J Pharm* 2014;476(1–2):88–92.

45. Kollamaram G, Croker DM, Walker GM, Goyanes A, Basit AW, Gaisford S. Low temperature fused deposition modeling (FDM) 3D printing of thermolabile drugs. *Int J Pharm* 2018;545(1–2):144–152.

46. Zhang J, Yang W, Vo AW, Feng X, Ye X, Kim DW, Repka MA. Hydroxypropyl methylcellulose based controlled release dosage by melt extrusion and 3D printing: Structure and drug release correlation. *Carbohydr Polym* 2017;177:49–57.

47. Martinez PR, Goyanes A, Basit AW, Gaisford S. Fabrication of drug-loaded hydrogels with stereolithographic 3D printing. *Int J Pharm* 2017;532:313–317.

48. Martinez PR, Goyanes A, Basit AW, Gaisford S. Influence of geometry on the drug release profiles of stereolithographic (SLA) 3D printed tablets. *AAPS PharmSciTech* 2018; https://doi.org/10.1208/s12249-018-1075-3

49. Lakkala P, Munnangi SR, Bandari S, Repka M. Additive manufacturing technologies with emphasis on stereolithography 3D printing in pharmaceutical and medical applications: A review. *Int J Pharm: X* 2023 Dec;5:100159.

50. Khairuzzaman A. Regulatory perspectives on 3D printing in pharmaceuticals. *AAPS Adv Pharm Sci Ser* 2018;31:215–236.

51. Wang J, Zhang Y, Aghda NH, Pillai AR, Thakkar R, Ali N, Maniruzzaman M. Emerging 3D printing technologies for drug delivery devices; Current status and future perspective. *Adv Drug Deliv Rev* 2021;174:294–316.

52. Rowe CW, Katstra WE, Palazzolo RD, Giritlioglu B, Teung P, Cima MJ. Multimechanism oral dosage forms fabricated by three dimensional printing. *J Control Release* 2000;66:11–17.

53. Rahman Z, Barakh Ali SF, Ozkan T, Charoo NA, Reddy IK, Khan MA. Additive manufacturing with 3D printing: progress from bench to bedside. *AAPS J* 2018;206(20):1–14.

54. Xu X, Awad A, Robles-Martinez P, Gaisford S, Goyanes A, Basit AW. Vat photopolymerization 3D printing for advanced drug delivery and medical device applications. *J Control Release* 2021 Jan; 329:743–757.

9 Basic Concept of Microfluidics and Its Application in Dermatological Conditions

Kiran Sharma
Charles Sturt University, Orange, Australia

Pankaj Kumar Bhatt
Lloyd Institute of Management and Technology,
Greater Noida, India

Monika Kaurav
KIET School of Pharmacy, Ghaziabad, India

9.1 INTRODUCTION

Microfluidics is a phrase that is increasingly appearing in articles and scientific periodicals; nevertheless, what precisely is microfluidics is still debatable. In reality, the term *microfluidics* refers to both a science and a technology. In fact, microfluidics is basically the regulation of fluids at the micron-scale (1×10^{-6}), which demands the design of devices with incredibly small footprints and microchannels as well as a deep understanding of fluid physics at this scale (1). Microfluidics has its roots in three separate fields: microanalysis, biodefense, and microelectronics. Microfluidics was originally used in microbiology as an analytical technique because it allows for the use of exceptionally small amounts of material and chemicals, which is a particularly appealing aspect of microanalysis (2). Furthermore, the ability to perform several functionalities in a compact and inexpensive device has significantly enhanced the attractiveness of microfluidics-based applications in this field.

The primary idea underlying microfluidics is to do activities that would previously need a full laboratory in just one micro-sized device. This idea is not new in science; in fact, it was the same necessity that motivated scientists to take on the task of microelectronics. Microfluidics is simply a topic dedicated to "miniaturized

DOI: 10.1201/9781032690926-9

"

plumbing and fluidic manipulation" since microelectronics is the study and technology of electronic components under the micron (10^{-6} m) scale (3). However, there's a significant distinction between the two: in microfluidics, the underlying physics of the system alters more quickly with size. Despite the fact that current microelectronic devices are reaching the nanoscale, electrons within them behave similarly to the macroscopic environment. The contents within microchannels of microfluidic systems, on the contrary, develop novel properties at this size (4).

Microfluidic systems now have a variety of options in the area of tissue engineering because of recent advancements in microscale technological developments. The benefits of microfluidics have been successfully incorporated into the area of tissue engineering using organ-on-chip systems. These systems provide live organs with dynamic biomechanical conditions and spatiotemporal biochemical gradients, enabling the creation of biomimetic tissues and organs that may stand alone as prototypes for drug discovery purposes. An organ-on-a-chip is a microfluidic system made up of diverse cell types that may interact with one another in a carefully regulated microenvironment, simulating the complicated cell–cell, and cell–matrix interactions (5, 6).

In this chapter, we briefly examine the biology of skin and some of the most significant skin illnesses before talking about the current skin models and the improvements being made through tissue engineering and microfluidics in skin simulations. We go on to discuss how forthcoming skin-on-chip platforms made by combining microfluidics, cells, biomaterials, and biosensors would be able to accurately reproduce the structure and function of skin in the research and treatment of in vitro skin disorders. Skin-on-chip models of diseases have the possibility to be used in pharmaceutical research, medication discovery, and environmental safety evaluation.

9.2   DERMATOLOGICAL STUDIES AND CONCERN PROBLEMS

To protect dangerous substances and germs from the body, the major organ in the human body—the skin—forms a biological barrier. There are still many things that can impact and influence human skin, even if it is covered by a cornified layer. Consequently, it is critical to identify and evaluate allergies, drug/pathogen penetration, chemicals' aging effects, and a wide range of skin problems (7). Preclinical investigations pertaining to novel pharmaceutical compounds and the enhancement of cosmetics formulations presently depend on the implementation of diverse in vitro models that are reproducible. Nevertheless, animal models possess certain constraints, including but not limited to ethical dilemmas and substantial investments of time and labor. Moreover, variations in thickness, hair density, and morphology across different models may introduce unpredictability and lack of repeatability in the experimental outcomes that are obtained (8, 9). Animal experimentation in the European Union for the purpose of assessing the toxicology of cosmetics has been outlawed since 2009 due to the aforementioned factors [(76/768/EEC, February 2003)]. The reduction, refinement, and replacement of animals in studies (3R principles) and (10, 11) have been emphasized. Skin models based on cells and Transwell have gained popularity, and their complexity has been growing. Nevertheless, despite these advancements, neither the models nor their culture procedures can completely replicate the skin microenvironment, a critical prerequisite for the proliferation of original human cells (12, 13).

Dermatological studies, integral to understanding skin health and addressing various skin conditions, delve into the complex interplay of cells, tissues, and external factors. While animal models have traditionally been employed for dermatological research, they pose significant challenges. Species differences often limit the translatability of findings to human skin, impacting the accuracy of drug responses and disease mechanisms (14). Additionally, ethical concerns surrounding animal testing have prompted a search for alternative approaches. Animal models may not fully capture the complexity of human skin responses, hindering translatability to clinical outcomes. As dermatology seeks more accurate and ethically sound methodologies, advancements like microfluidics offer innovative in vitro solutions to replicate human skin environments, providing researchers with tools that bridge the gap between traditional animal models and the complexities of human dermatology (15).

Microfluidic technology has emerged as a transformative solution in dermatological research, offering advanced in vitro models to overcome these challenges. Skin-on-a-chip (SoC) platforms on microfluidic devices precisely replicate the microenvironment of human skin, incorporating multiple cell types and enabling dynamic fluid flow to mimic blood circulation. These systems allow for realistic drug testing, disease modeling, and barrier function assessments, offering more accurate predictions of human responses. Importantly, microfluidics reduces the need for animal testing, aligning with ethical considerations, while providing a more human-relevant, cost-effective, and high-throughput alternative for studying skin biology. The integration of microfluidic technology into dermatological research signifies a paradigm shift, offering researchers unprecedented tools to explore skin-related conditions and therapies with greater precision, efficiency, and ethical consciousness (16).

9.3 FUNDAMENTALS OF MICROFLUIDICS

Microfluidics is a field that manipulates small amounts of fluids, typically in channels with dimensions on the micrometer scale. The basic principle involves precise control and manipulation of fluids to perform various tasks, such as mixing, separating, and analyzing samples. Utilizing the unique properties of fluids at the microscale, microfluidic devices enable efficient and rapid processes, often enhancing sensitivity and reducing sample volume. Applications include medical diagnostics, chemical synthesis, and biotechnological research. The key elements include miniaturization, precise fluid handling, and the ability to exploit laminar flow for controlled reactions, making microfluidics valuable in diverse scientific and technological domains (17).

Microscale fluid behavior differs from macroscale behavior due to increased surface-to-volume ratios and dominance of surface tension and viscous forces. At the microscale, flow patterns are influenced by molecular interactions, exhibiting unique phenomena like capillary action and dominant laminar flow. Surface effects become prominent, impacting wetting and contact angles. Fluid inertia diminishes, making diffusion and viscous effects more pronounced. These distinctions lead to enhanced mixing efficiency, reduced sample volumes, and distinctive transport phenomena (18).

At the microscale, the skin's intricate topography influences fluid flow, impacting drug delivery and skin care formulations. Microfluidic principles enable precise control over small volumes, enhancing the efficacy of transdermal drug delivery systems and skin care products. Unique phenomena, such as capillary-driven transport, play a pivotal role, offering tailored solutions for dermatological challenges. Recognizing microscale fluid behavior in this context facilitates the development of innovative, efficient, and patient-friendly solutions in dermatology, optimizing the benefits of microfluidic technologies for skin health (19).

9.4 KEY ELEMENTS OF THE MICROFLUIDIC SYSTEM

Microfluidic systems are intricate devices designed for the precise manipulation of minute volumes of fluids, typically on the scale of microliters or nanoliters. The key components of a microfluidic system collectively enable controlled fluid handling, mixing, and analysis in a miniaturized format (Figure 9.1). First, microchannels are small pathways etched or fabricated into materials like glass, silicon, or polymers, defining the flow paths within the system. Microchannels play a fundamental role in guiding fluids through the device.

After that, microfluidic pumps generate controlled flow rates, facilitating the movement of fluids within the microchannels. Various types of pumps, such as syringe

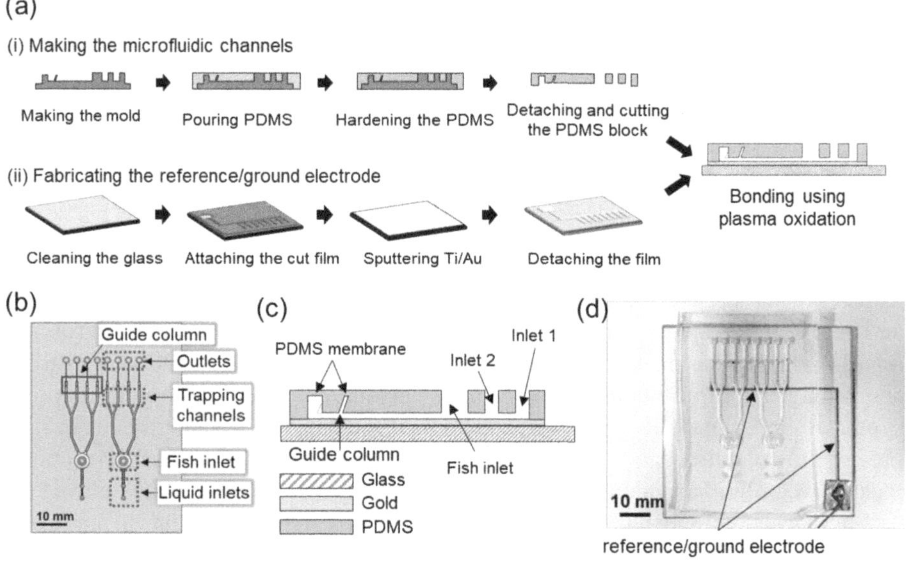

FIGURE 9.1 Design and fabrication of the microfluidic chip. (a) Manufacture a microfluidic block that features (i) PDMS microchannels and (ii) ground/reference electrodes made of glass. PDMS microchannels block and ground electrode joined by a plasma method. This figure provides the microfluidic channel schematics (b: top view, c: side view). (d) A picture of a fabricated microfluidic chip showing gold patterns of reference/ground electrode at the bottom of channels. (Adapted from reference (22).

pumps or pneumatic pumps, are employed to achieve precise fluid control. Another component is valves, which regulate fluid flow and direction within the microchannels. They enable precise control over when and where fluids move, allowing for automation and programmability in microfluidic operations. Most importantly, sensors and detectors are integrated into microfluidic systems for real-time monitoring and analysis. These components may include optical sensors, electrochemical sensors, or other specialized detectors, depending on the application. Mixing devices is also crucial for homogenizing fluids in microscale environments. Passive or active mixing elements, such as chaotic mixers or micro stirrers, ensure efficient blending of reagents or samples within the microchannels. Reservoir containers for holding and introducing samples or reagents into the microfluidic system. Reservoirs may connect to the microchannels through inlet ports, allowing controlled loading of liquids. In microfluidic devices temperature controlling panels, also installed to maintain stable temperature conditions, are vital for many applications. Integrated heaters and coolers, along with thermal sensors, enable precise temperature control within the microfluidic system. Except for the arrangements, surface modifications are employed to control wetting and interactions with biological materials, enhancing compatibility and performance in applications like cell culture or biosensing (20, 21).

Microfluidic systems find applications in various fields, including chemistry, biology, medicine, and environmental monitoring, offering advantages such as reduced sample volumes, rapid analyses, and automation. The synergy of these components allows for the development of innovative solutions in areas like point-of-care diagnostics, lab-on-a-chip technologies, and drug discovery. In dermatological applications, microfluidic systems revolutionize skin care by precisely delivering therapeutic agents through microchannels, optimizing drug penetration. These devices enable the controlled release of skin care formulations tailored to individual needs, enhancing treatment efficacy. Microfluidics also facilitates on-chip analysis of skin samples, offering rapid diagnostics for conditions like melanoma. The miniaturized scale allows for reduced sample volumes, minimizing discomfort during testing. With applications ranging from personalized skin care to point-of-care dermatology, microfluidic systems contribute to advanced, patient-centric solutions for skin health, showcasing their potential to transform diagnostics and treatments in the field of dermatology (23).

Microfluidic devices offer precise drug delivery, reducing side effects in dermatological treatments. Their miniaturized scale allows efficient use of limited samples and facilitates personalized skin care formulations. SoC models mimic realistic microenvironments for studying drug responses and disease mechanisms. Microfluidics enables rapid point-of-care diagnostics, while high-resolution imaging aids in detailed skin analysis. These devices streamline cosmetic formulation development, providing cost-effective and automated solutions. Overall, microfluidic devices enhance accuracy, efficiency, and innovation in dermatology research and treatment (24).

9.5 TYPES OF MICROFLUIDIC MATERIALS

A number of substances, including glass, silicon, and polymers, were used to make microfluidic devices over the course of time. Undoubtedly, there is nothing known as a "perfect" material, since each one has benefits as well as drawbacks when used in microfluidics (25). It is the application that directs the researcher's choice. The materials that are most frequently used in microfluidics are explored briefly in this chapter.

9.5.1 POLYMERS FOR MICROFLUIDIC APPLICATIONS

The high biochemical functionality and inexpensive cost of polymer materials make them a popular choice for creating microfluidic devices. Among these, polydimethylsiloxane (PDMS) is one of the most popular. The siloxane family's mineral-organic polymer Polydimethylsiloxane is denoted by the abbreviation PDMS (26). There are many variables that make PDMS an excellent choice for chip production, but the key ones are (a) transparency: clear viewing of microchannels and their material; (b) elasticity: PDMS is highly elastic, and this characteristic can be applied in a number of ways, such as channel distortion for valve integration. Additionally, its flexibility of it may be "tuned" by crosslinking agents; (c) price: PDMS is significantly less costly than the other substances used in the manufacturing of microfluidic chips; (d) gas-permeable PDMS can be utilized for gas sensors, cell culture, and other applications (27). Of course, employing PDMS to make microfluidic chips has its drawbacks as well. Examples include material aging, which reduces chip efficiency over time, and PDMS's low chemical suitability with several organic solvents, which renders it best suited for water-based applications. Additionally, hydrophobic compounds and water vapor that may unintentionally be released during the experiment are absorbed by PDMS. Even while this may be overcome by placing the electrical components in the glass cover slide rather than the chip itself, the inability to integrate electrodes inside the chip is still a disadvantage of PDMS microfluidic systems (28).

Polystyrene (PS), a polymer often used in drug development for cell-culture plates, is one example of a different polymer utilized for microfluidic chips. PS is biocompatible, inert, stiff, and optically clear, and its exterior may be easily functionalized. Its hydrophobic surface may also be easily converted to a hydrophilic state using a variety of physical and chemical processes, such as corona release, gas plasma, and radiation (29). Polycarbonate (PC) and polymethylmethacrylate (PMMA) are two other polymers that are frequently utilized for microfluidic devices. PMMA is less thermally resistant than PC, allowing PC to be utilized across a broader temperature range. PMMA is an elastomer that deforms less than PDMS; therefore, it is used when stiffness is needed, such as when building canalization for microvalves (30).

9.5.2 THERMOSETS FOR MICROFLUIDIC CHIP

Thermosets are polymers that are connected by chemical interactions, as indicated by their name. These substances are given a strongly crosslinked polymeric framework as a result of this process, which accounts for their great mechanical and physical durability but low elasticity when compared to thermoplastics and elastomers. The major characteristics of thermosets are their insolubility, lack of melting, lack of swelling when exposed to specific solvents, and strong creep resistance (31).

Thermoset polyester (TPE) is one of the most commonly used thermoplastics for microfluidic purposes. The benefits of utilizing thermosets are inexpensiveness, quick and simple chip creation, and great visibility. Additionally, thermosets frequently work with solvents that are not polar, which makes PDMS-based microfluidic chips expand. However, because thermosets are not elastomeric like PDMS chips, there are significant drawbacks to employing thermoset devices in microfluidic systems. They need fluidic interconnectors that are distinct from those utilized by PDMS because when they cure, they turn into materials that are hard (32).

9.5.3 Silicon and Glass Microfluidic Chips

Silicon was one of the earliest substances utilized in microfluidics. This is due to the close relationship between the initial microfluidics chips and the microelectronics sector, where silicon has been and continues to be one of the most frequently utilized materials. Silicon has benefits in microfluidic usage because of its solvent compatibility, surface strength, and thermal conductivity (33). Since optical detection is difficult in the visual electromagnetic spectrum, silicon microfluidic chips' fundamental flaw is their optical opacity. Glass has been a pioneering substance in the creation of microfluidic chips. The benefits of silicon are also present in this substance. It is the finest option for numerous purposes in particular because of its renowned surface chemistries, outstanding optical clarity, and good high-pressure durability (34). Additionally, glass is hydrophilic in nature, inert to chemicals, biocompatible, and enables effective coatings. Glass microfluidic chips' primary drawback is the relatively expensive cost of the basic component.

9.5.4 Paper-Based Microfluidic Chips

Paper has also been considered as a possible component for microfluidic chip manufacturing. The primary cause of this is the low cost of paper as a starting point. The benefits of employing paper for projects using microfluidic devices, however, go beyond only due to their extremely low costs. Paper is thin, light, and simple to handle, store, and move. Additionally, it may be altered chemically to interact with chemicals or proteins and is biocompatible with biological material. Last but not least, paper is a very environmentally friendly medium for microfluidic chips since it is simple to discard after usage (35). The fundamental drawback of microfluidic devices made from paper is the challenge of channel patterning on the chip. There simply is not one "perfect" patterned technique because each one involves trade-offs among expenses, simplicity, and resolution that must be considered individually.

9.5.5 Hydrogel for Microfluidic Devices

A colloid called a hydrogel is composed of polymeric chains of monomers dispersed in liquid. Sodium polyacrylate is one popular polymer utilized in the production of hydrogel. Their appropriateness for physiological investigations determines how they might be used in microfluidic systems. They work well as diffusion matrices since most cell nutrition and growth agents are soluble in hydrogel. Indeed, it has been demonstrated that the diffusivity of the majority of solutes in agarose gels—a popular hydrogel utilized in microfluidic chips is remarkably similar to that of water. Due to its extreme malleability, hydrogel can accommodate features of all shapes and sizes (36). Additionally, hydrogel is readily accessible, safe for cells, and inexpensive.

9.6 SoC MODELS

An SoC bioengineered model on a microfluidic platform is an in vitro system that mimics human skin's microenvironment (37). Microchannels re-create vascular and tissue structures, allowing dynamic fluid flow. Cell layers, including keratinocytes and fibroblasts, replicate the epidermis and dermis. This model facilitates realistic drug testing, disease modeling, and barrier function assessment. It supports real-time imaging, reduces reliance on animal testing, and enables personalized medicine by incorporating patient-specific cells (38, 39). The platform accelerates research through high-throughput screening, providing a sophisticated, ethically sound tool for studying skin biology, diseases, and therapeutic responses in a controlled setting.

Conversely, the 3D interactions among cells and then cells with matrix in the body cannot be reproduced by conventional 2D models. However, such types of studies can be performed using a 3D SoC model instead. Several researchers constructed a 3D human skin tissue model via bioprinting consisting of keratinocytes and fibroblasts to represent the epidermal and dermal layers (40, 41). Primarily, it has three layers: a top one, an intermediate layer, and a bottom layer. The bottom layer is where the microvascular channel is located. In contrast, there is a porous membrane separating the top and bottom layers that resides in the middle/intermediate layer, while the culture chamber as well as side pneumatic channels are included in the upper layer. By comparison, in Lee et al. (40) a basic SoC design utilized 3D-bioprinted epidermal cells (keratinocytes and fibroblasts) to create this area of skin called epidermis or dermis. Three levels usually make up the system: a top layer, a middle layer, and a bottom layer. The microvascular channel is located in the bottom layer. The top layer contains the culture chamber and the laterally pneumatic passages, while the porous membrane that divides the upper and lower layers is located in the middle/intermediate layer. The establishment of the endothelium monolayer is mechanically supported by a microvascular channel. Hemostasis, inflammation, and transport are all regulated by the endothelium layer–formed capillary walls. Mechanical stimulation is the main purpose of pneumatic channels (42).

9.6.1 EVOLUTIONARY HISTORY OF SoC MODELS

Since the development of the first SoC model in 2013, still the challenges lie in replicating the intricate structure of the skin, requiring advancements in technology, industry maturity, and continuous research efforts to propel organ-on-a-chip (OoC) platforms for skin cultivation beyond their current infancy (43). After that, several SoC platforms have been developed via the implementation of a variety of techniques. In this book chapter, we reported the classification of present SoC models into three categories, 2D SoC models, 3D SoC with perfusable lumens, and 3D SoC with microfluidic channels, which was previously published by Zoio et al. (44; Figure 9.2). Here mentioned SoC models were much more advanced in design and working as compared to the earliest developed OoC.

The main purpose of the development of the SoC models is to maintain good skin tissue integrity and durability throughout the experiment with continuous blood supply channels to establish a co-culture tissue model for different organs. The transferred SoC is developed by integration of skin tissues removed via biopsies on the chips (45–47) or biomimetic fibroblasts derived full-thickness skin models (FTSms) developed off-chip (43, 48–50; Figure 9.2a). This research offers important insights into the application of SoC devices and their intended therapeutic uses for cosmetics

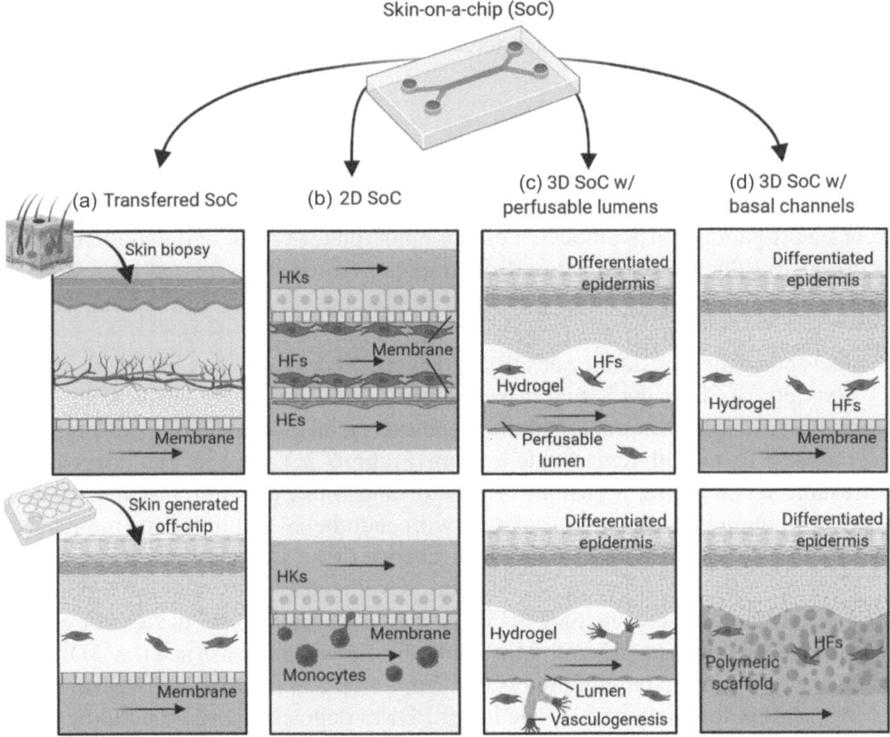

FIGURE 9.2 Schematic diagram showing strategies to create models of SoC. (a) Transferred SoC devices in which skin biopsies (top) or skin models generated off-chip (bottom) are transferred on-chip. (b) 2D SoC devices (i) 2D SoC with 3 compartments/2 membrane (top) and (ii) 2D SoC with 2 compartments/1membrane (bottom). (c) 3D SoC with perfusable lumens constructed via 3D patterning techniques with vasculature establishment (bottom). (d) 3D SoC with microfluidic channels constructed via layer arrangement of membrane-based SoC device microfluidic layers and a porous membrane and skin tissue constructed on it or a porous scaffold integrated inside it, without employment of porous membrane and hydrogel. Abbreviations: HKs, human keratinocytes; HFs, human fibroblasts, HEs, human endothelial cells. (Adopted from (44).)

and novel drug technologies evaluation including medication efficacy, sensitivity safety, and toxicity as well as multi-organ interaction.

9.6.2 2D SoC Models

In these types of models, 2D cell culture systems are developed using keratinocytes and fibroblasts that form monolayers on porous membranes as models for human skin structure and functional responses. SoC 2D models are now very useful drug testing tools, safety assessment platforms, and aids to biomedical research which better reflects human skin physiology (Figure 9.2b). In their approach, Wufuer et al. (37) constructed an SoC device with three layers; epidermal, dermal, and vascular layers were co-cultured in this device. Interlayer communication is enabled through porous membranes separating each layer. These 2D SoC models consist of cultures of skin cells on microfluidic chips to create an in situ natural skin mimic microenvironment. However, they do not have complex features or exhibit 3D architecture.

9.6.3 3D SoC Models

In vitro, 3D SoC models use microfluidic technologies and 3D skin tissue. These skin models simulate skin physiology for pharmacological and cosmetic testing. For complete investigations, these models contain epidermal, dermal, and endothelial cells to create full-thickness skin. Based on studies performed by researchers, 3D skin models are categorized into two types: The first model consists of skin compartments with ample vascular networks (Figure 9.2c), and the second is based on microfluidic channels consisting of skin tissues tissue (Figure 9.2d).

A variety of 3D manufacturing techniques such as multicellular techniques, 3D bioprinting, vascularization, templating, and sacrificial molding have been employed to produce FTSms with replaceable lumens (Figure 9.2c). Groeber et al. developed a perfusable FTSm using a custom bioreactor and a pig jejunum vascular scaffold. While achieving in-vivo-like vasculature with endothelial cell lining, its impracticality for large-scale production arises from reliance on an animal organ (51).

More recently, a number of SoC devices developed FTSms with basal perfusion using microfluidic-based methods (Figure 9.2d). Recently, SoC devices developed perfusable FTSms with microfluidic methods. Lee et al. constructed a 3D FTSm using a unique gravity-based flow system with a chip composed of two PDMS deposits over a glass foundation (52). The lower PDMS deposits housed the fluidic chamber, while the upper PDMS deposits hosted the skin model creation. The model included a collagen layer along with primary human dermal fibroblasts, epidermal keratinocytes, and human umbilical vein endothelial cells (HUVECs) to replicate the vascular structure. Their findings showed similar expressions of key markers such as filaggrin, keratin5, and involucrin compared to traditional transwell-based skin models, presenting a promising microfluidic-based approach. Few studies based on all types of models discussed in a table such as 2D SoC (37, 53, 54), 3D SoC with perfusable lumens (51, 55–58), 3D SoC with basal perfusion (44, 51–52, 59–68), and transferred SoC (43, 45–47, 69–70) (Table 9.1).

TABLE 9.1

Types of SoC Models: A Summary of Different Types of SoC Models

Cell Types	Dermal Matrix	Flow Pattern Type and Features	Construction Material Membrane/Device	Fabrication Technique	Type of Platform	Applications	References
2D SoC models							
HaCaT + HS27 + HUVECS	–	Gravity flow/Not stated	PDMS/PET membrane	Photolithography;	In situ SoC	For inflammation and edema studies	(37)
HaCaT + U937 dendritic cells	–	Syringe pump flow	PMMA and PDMS/ PET membrane	Rapid prototyping;	In situ SoC	Immune competent model; TEER measurement, cell tight junction	(53)
HaCaT	–	Syringe pump flow	PMMA and PDMS/ PET membrane	Laser cutter	In situ SoC	Irritation testing with potassium dichromate	(54)
3D SoC models with perfusable lumens							
Primary HEKs + primary HDFs + hDMECC	Decellularizedporcine jejunum	PeristalticPump flowNot stated	PEEK/PC	Rapid prototyping	Vascularized HSE	TEER measurement	(51)
Primary HEKs + primary HDFs+ HUVECs	Collagen	PeristalticPump flow	Not stated	3D printing and templating	Vascularized HSE	Permeation studies of drugs	(55)
Normal human fibroblasts + Keratinocytes + HUVECs	Collagen	Perfusion, simulated vasculature	Flexible silicone rubber (PDMS and EcoflexVR)	3D printing	Vascularized HSE	Improved skin equivalents for biological investigations	(56)

(Continued)

TABLE 9.1
(Continued)

Cell Types	Dermal Matrix	Flow Pattern Type and Features	Construction Material Membrane/Device	Fabrication Technique	Type of Platform	Applications	References
Primary HEKs + primary HDFs + HUVECs + primary HPAs	Fibrinogen, ECM porcine skin	PeristalticPump flow	PCL	3D printing;	Vascularized HSE	Bioprinting and Integration of hypodermis	(57)
Primary HEKs + primary HDFs + HUVECs	Collagen	PeristalticPump flow	PCL	3D printing and templating	Vascularized HSE	Topical and systemic drug permeability of drugs and pollutants	(58)
3D SoC Model with basal perfusion							
Primary fibroblasts + keratinocytes	Collagen	Pumpless, gravity flow	PDMS	Not stated	In situ SoC	Drug efficacy and side effects evaluation	(59)
Primary fibroblasts + keratinocytes	Collagen	Pumpless, gravity flow	PDMS	Soft lithography	In situ SoC	Cosmetics and pharmaceuticals testing	(60)
Primary fibroblasts + Keratinocytes + HUVECs	collagen	Pumpless, gravity flow	PDMS	Lithography	In situ SoC	Studies of drugs and cosmetics transport	(52)
Primary fibroblasts + keratinocytes	collagen	perfusion	PDMS and glass	Soft lithography	In situ SoC	Antiwrinkle drugs and cosmetics testing	(61)
Primary human fibroblasts + HaCaT keratinocytes	fibrin	perfusion	Adhesive PVCPDMS and glass/PC	Micro-machining	In situ SoC	Complex skin disease model	(62)

Primary fibroblasts + keratinocytes	Different type collagens	Pumpless, gravity flow	PDMS	Lithography	In situ SoC	Effect of scaffold material on model working	(63)
Primary fibroblasts + keratinocytes	collagen	Pumpless, gravity flow	PDMS	lithography	In situ SoC	Human skin equivalent model	(64)
Primary fibroblasts + Immortalized N/TERT keratinocytes	Fibrin-PEG complex	perfusion	PMMA/PC	Micro milling	In situ SoC	Better model with advanced skin dermis properties along with Higher differentiation and barrier function	(65)
Primary HEKs + primary HDFs	Collagen	PeristalticPump flow	PTFE/PET membrane	Not stated	In situ SoC	Skin barrier function and drug permeability studies	(66)
HaCaT + primary HDFs	Fibrin	Syringe pump flow	PMMA, PDMS/ PVC and PC membrane	Edge plotter	In situ SoC	Controlled Parallel flowBased bilayer skin model	(67)
Primary HEKs + primary HDFs	FDM + PS scaffold	Syringe pump flow	PMMA	Rapid prototyping	In situ SoC	Improved barrier properties, irritation studies, TEER measurements on-chip	(44)
Primary HEKs + primary HDFs + HUVECS	ECM-coating of single cells (FN and G)	PeristaticPump flow		3D printing	In situ SoC	High-thickness skin model suitable for 3D-wound healing assay	(68)

(Continued)

TABLE 9.1
(Continued)

Cell Types	Dermal Matrix	Flow Pattern Type and Features	Construction Material Membrane/Device	Fabrication Technique	Type of Platform	Applications	References
			Transferred SoC models				
L929 murine fibroblasts + EpiDerm ™	Commercial platform transwell insert	Perfusion	Commercial platform/transwell insert	Bioprinting	Transferred SoC	TEER and EAR measurement	(69)
EpiDermFT™ + ex vivo subcutaneous tissue	EpiDermFT TM (commercial)	Perfusion, on-chip micropump	PDMS	Not stated	Transferred SoC	Improved culture conditions for in-vitro skin models	(43)
Primary fibroblasts+ keratinocytes	Collagen	Pumpless, gravity-driven	PDMS, PCL	lithography techniques	Transferred SoC	Skin disease treatment drugs testings on human skins	(70)
Blood cells + human biopsy	Biopsy	Static	PDMS	photolithography	Transferred SoC	Study of neutrophil migration into skin during microbial infections	(45)
Human biopsy	Biopsy	Perfusion, on-chip micropump	PDMS, PET membrane	low-pressure plasma oxidation	Transferred SoC	Pharmacokinetics and pharmacodynamics studies of drugs	(47)
Human biopsy	Biopsy	Perfusion, on-chip micropump	PDMS	low-pressure plasma oxidation	Transferred SoC	Systemic drug testing	(46)

Abbreviations: HUVECS, human umbilical vein endothelial cells; HEKs, human epidermal keratinocytes; HDFns, human dermal fibroblasts; hDMECs, human dermal microvascular endothelial cells; HUVECS, human umbilical vein endothelial cells; HPAs, human preadipocytes subcutaneous; dECM, decellularized extracellular matrix; dECM, decellularized extracellular matrix HSE, human skin equivalent HUVEC, human umbilical vein endothelial cells PS, polystyrene PVC, polyvinyl chloride FDM,fibroblast-derived matrix PS, polystyrene ECM, extracellular matrix FN, fibronectin G, gelatin PTFE, polytetrafluoroethylene; PDMS, polydimethylsiloxane; PEG, polyethylene glycol; PET, polyethylene terephthalate; PMMA, poly(methylmethacrylate); PEEK, polyether ether ketone; PC, polycarbonate; PET, polyethylene terephthalate; PCL, polycaprolactone; TEER, transepithelial electrical resistance.

9.7 APPLICATIONS

Applications of microfluidics for skin disease modeling and skin tissue regeneration are still in their infancy. However, several studies on cell migration and wound healing suggested that this technique could be able to repair skin damage.

9.7.1 PERSPIRATION MODELING

By creating a bilayer artificial skin in a microfluidic system, Hou et al. produced the first perspiration simulator. Comparable to human sweating, they were able to maintain a steady sweat rate in all pores at minimal flow rates. Since the smaller holes remained dry due to the Laplace pressure differential between the exterior and interior of a curved surface, evaluating single-layered systems revealed that membranes were unable to function correctly at low flow rates. Consequently, a novel solution was put out to solve this important issue by creating a bilayer artificial perspiration simulation (71). The skin-replica substance, dry film photoresist layer, and polyester film were used to create the upper membrane of this simulation that was intended to imitate the right pore density and roughness of the surface. The layer of the membrane at the bottom resembled eccrine glands. Continuous sweat flow depends on certain bottom-layer pore characteristics, including small size, appropriate density, and significant hydrophilicity. Available polycarbonate membranes with track etching fulfilled these requirements (72).

9.7.2 DIFFUSION CHARACTERIZATION

In terms of safety, effectiveness, and toxicities, percutaneous penetration of novel ingredients employed in medicinal or cosmetic formulations is crucial. Therefore, at the very beginning of the development process, sufficient knowledge about the permeability coefficient of new elements is required. Provin et al. created a microfluidic system to measure the percutaneous absorption of seven distinct drugs by creating a repeatable artificial stratum corneum using a lipid layer. The instrument's donor chamber was within the top layer, which had been filled with saturated solution, and the bottom chamber, which was loaded with media via inlets and outlets, was empty. A membrane made of lipids made up of a combination of fatty acids, cholesterol, and other substances was present in the middle layer. Soft lithography was used to include an optical fiber channel into the bottom channel, allowing for sophisticated ultraviolet (UV)- visible absorption spectroscopy to track the penetration in real time. Three states of the permeation processes were shown by the outcomes: the first transient state; steady-state diffusion, whose accuracy is greatly dependent on high sampling rates since it uses an online detecting approach; and the last transient state (73).

9.7.3 BACTERIAL INFECTION AND BIOFILM REMOVAL

In order to study the impact of Dispersin B combined with Gentamycin on methicillin-resistant *Staphylococcus pseudintermedius* (MRSP) biofilms, Terry et al. created an in vitro microfluidic-based wound prototype. In this work, the topmost channels of a Y-shaped microfluidic system with three inlets and one exit were filled with either water or a solution of Dispersin B and Gentamycin. The channels held a bacterial mix that had been incubated and coated with collagen, and 25–50% of the device's interior was covered in biofilm, which had parabolic shapes in various channel sections. Even though Dispersin B-Gentamycin had been used, an image examination of the sample taken from the outlet revealed a higher light intensity. However, the efficacy of Dispersin B–Gentamycin was not noticeably greater than water on average. Additionally, a model modeling an animal with wound infections was created, and the outcomes with the microfluidic model were contrasted. Another way to achieve antimicrobial resistance in biofilms is by using microfluidic devices to create dynamic gradients of concentration (74).

9.7.4　Wound Healing

One of the immune system's defense strategies is inflammation, which consists of physiological and behavioral actions regulated by cytokines that promote the attraction of efficient cells. It causes the stimulation of phagocytosis and leukocytes, T-cell migration, and the development of new cells. The epithelial tissues that serve as barriers in the skin and define relationships between the human surface and the outside world depend on inflammation and immunological homeostasis. Serious disorders like psoriasis are brought on by improper control of immunological epithelial responses (75). Electric fields and chemical gradients of concentration are replicated using microfluidic devices to characterize cell movement. For the purpose of researching neutrophil cell movement, a microfluidic device had already been created that enabled a variety of dynamic temporal and spatial concentration gradients. Lin et al. investigated the reaction of human peripheral blood T lymphocytes to chemotaxis in an individual and superimposed gradient of concentration of two chemokines (CCL19 and CXCL12) using a "Y"-type microfluidic system constructed of a series of microchannels. The findings demonstrated that T cells migrated more quickly in the direction of the CCL19 gradient than they did toward the CXCL12 gradient. Due to constant flow in the region being studied area, which accurately imitated an in vivo environment, the gradient profile remained steady (76).

9.7.5　Skin Cancer

In skin cancer, the microenvironment significantly influences the initiation, proliferation, metastasis, invasion, drug resistance, and cell–cell and complicated cell–matrix interactions, as well as tumor invasions and metastasis. These all point to the concept that tumor growth is influenced by both the tumor microenvironment and malignant cells. Microfluidic systems have the capability of precisely modeling the interactions between tissues as well as the biochemical and biophysical variables that control the tumor microenvironment, including mechanical forces, endothelial and inflammatory cells, as well as the physical characteristics of biomaterials and the extracellular matrix (ECM) (77). With various microchannel networks that are parallelizable and have variable fluid flow, such devices may be compared to the size of blood arteries.

This approach can provide an accurate high-throughput well-plate design and is now being utilized to characterize the relationship of endothelial cells, fibroblasts, and leukocytes with cancer cells utilizing hanging-drop spheroid models. Mattei et al. have recently utilized knocked-out (KO) mice in interferon regulatory factor (IRF)-8 and a microfluidic system independently to study the interaction between skin cancer and immune cells. The rodents used in the in vivo study were injected subcutaneously with B16.F10 cells, which are mouse skin melanoma. B16.F10 has the ability to suppress the immune system of KO mice. B16.F10 cells and immune system cells were co-cultured in three culturing compartments that were linked by microchannels on the microfluidic device (78).

9.7.6 INNERVATED SKIN MODELS

Touch, pain, and temperature perception are all senses that are processed by sensory neurons that are innervated into the skin. This process is known as somatosensation. Blais et al. looked at the integration of Schwann cells in RS both in vitro and in vivo to optimize the process of nerve migration and regeneration. They investigated the impact of Schwann cells on axonal migration in vitro using a tissue-engineered innervated reconstructed dermis (IRD) model, and they found that nerve migration in the IRD increased 2.15 times in just 14 days. They also used RS samples to graft on thymic mice for 90 days in order to study the potential of Schwann cells in vivo (79). In comparison to RS without these cells, the RS with implanted Schwann cells had 1.8 and 1.7 times more nerve fibers. By grafting rebuilt human SE on dorsal wounds in highly immunosuppressed pigs, Ferretti et al. were able to characterize the relationships between vascularization and re-innervation. They investigated the healing mechanism employing fluorescent microscopy and discovered that angiogenesis happens prior to nerve growth, corroborating the idea that the vascular system's provision of nutrients is essential for the development of neural cells with high metabolic requirements. Given the significant advancements in vascularized and innervated microfluidic chips, it is expected that microfluidics will soon be able to provide an autonomous nerve layer supplied by a vasculature layer to be inserted into the existing skin tissues (80).

9.7.7 SWEAT ANALYSIS

Sweat is very characteristic in nature and noninvasive and contains several disease markers, making it valuable for monitoring physiological health and detecting disorders (81–86). Quantitative sweat rate measurements can avoid overheating and stroke in hot weather (87). Since sweat pH is related to alkalosis, it can be measured noninvasively from sweat (87, 88). Sweat electrolytes and metabolites can also indicate blood glucose, electrolyte balance, hydration, and health (such as lactate, sodium, potassium, chloride, and glucose; 89, 90). Early sweat collection methods use cotton swabs and gauze, filter paper, or absorbent pads. Sweat analysis is done on benchtop equipment after centrifuging sweat from absorbent pads. This technique requires costly materials equipment and skilled workers for sample collection and result analysis (90).

Optional wearable microfluidic devices provide real-time sweat collection and analysis for military readiness, sports performance, and customized therapy. Zhang and colleagues introduced a sweat analysis SoC device with hydrophobic valves at the chamber-microfluidic channel contact to reduce the evaporation of sweat from the device. Due to the presence of blockage of liquids front flow coming from the hydrophilic microchannel into the other chambers, generates the initial curved upper surface, and occupies them throughout (91).

9.8   CONCLUSION

A SoC microfluidics model is a milestone in biomedical research, with very complex and physiologically relevant environments for studying skin biology and drug testing. The complexity of cellular interactions, the presence of blood vessels, and the response to external stimuli are some of the key aspects of the human skin that have been replicated by these microscale systems. Microfluidic technology has also increased the accuracy and reproducibility of these models through better control over fluid flow, nutrient delivery, and waste management.

Onward, there is a wide range of opportunities presented by SoC microfluidics models. Such platforms could be used for personalized medicine where patient-specific responses to drugs and treatments can be assessed in a more realistic in vitro setting. This approach could also revolutionize toxicity testing as it would minimize the use of animals, hence being more ethical and cost-effective. Additionally, future advances may include the incorporation of sensors or monitoring devices that can capture real-time data about cellular responses, thereby making our understanding of skin physiology more dynamic and comprehensive.

Refinement and optimization of SoC microfluidics models to address issues like scalability and long-term stability will rely on the cooperation of researchers, engineers, and pharmaceutical companies. The possibility of revolutionizing drug discovery and our comprehension of skin disorders lies in these new approaches due to ongoing advances in materials science, microfabrication techniques, and our knowledge of skin biology. Making such a transition from laboratory-based models to actual applications in the medical and pharmaceutical domains offers great potential for enhancing human health and welfare.

ACKNOWLEDGMENT

None.

CONFLICT OF INTEREST

None.

REFERENCES

1. Naderi A, Bhattacharjee N, Folch A. Digital manufacturing for microfluidics. *Annu Rev Biomed Eng* 2019 Jun 4;21:325–64.
2. Venkatesan S, Jerald J, Asokan P, Prabakaran R. A Comprehensive Review on Microfluidics Technology and its Applications. In: Kumar H, Jain P, editors. *Recent Advances in Mechanical Engineering*. Lecture Notes in Mechanical Engineering. Springer, Singapore. 2019:235–45.
3. Nunes JK, Stone HA. Introduction: Microfluidics. *Chem Rev* 2022;122(7):6919–20.
4. Yeo LY, Chang HC, Chan PP, Friend JR. Microfluidic devices for bioapplications. *Small* 2011;7(1):12–48.
5. Gharib G, Bütün I, Muganlı Z, Kozalak G, Namlı I, Sarraf SS, Ahmadi VE, Toyran E, van Wijnen AJ, Koşar A. Biomedical applications of microfluidic devices: A review. *Biosensors (Basel)* 2022 Nov 16;12(11):1023.
6. Karimi M, Bahrami S, Mirshekari H, Basri SM, Nik AB, Aref AR et al. Microfluidic systems for stem cell-based neural tissue engineering. *Lab Chip* 2016;16(14):2551–71.
7. Li Q, Wang C, Li X, Zhang J, Zhang Z, Yang K et al. Epidermis-on-a-chip system to develop skin barrier and melanin mimicking model. *J Tissue Eng* 2023;14:20417314231168529.
8. Moniz T, Costa Lima SA, Reis S. Human skin models: From healthy to disease-mimetic systems; characteristics and applications. *Br J Pharmacol* 2020;177(19):4314–29.
9. Van Gele M, Geusens B, Brochez L, Speeckaert R, Lambert J. Three-dimensional skin models as tools for transdermal drug delivery: Challenges and limitations. *Expert Opin Drug Deliv* 2011;8(6):705–20.
10. van den Broek LJ, Bergers LIJC, Reijnders CMA, Gibbs S, et al. Progress and future prospectives in skin-on-chip development with emphasis on the use of different cell types and technical challenges. *Stem Cell Rev Rep* 2017;13(3):418–29.
11. Zhang Q, Sito L, Mao M, He J, Zhang YS, Zhao X. Current advances in skin-on-a-chip models for drug testing. *Microphysiol Syst* 2018;2:4.
12. Pires de Mello CP, Carmona-Moran C, McAleer CW, Perez J, Coln EA, Long CJ, et al. Microphysiological heart-liver body-on-a-chip system with a skin mimic for evaluating topical drug delivery. *Lab Chip* 2020;20(4):749–59.
13. Lee JH, Kim HW. Emerging properties of hydrogels in tissue engineering. *J Tissue Eng* 2018;9:2041731418768285.
14. Zhang J, Zhong F, He K, Ji M, Li S, Li C. Recent advancements and perspectives in the diagnosis of skin diseases using machine learning and deep learning: A review. *Diagnostics (Basel)* 2023;13(23):3506.
15. Kiani AK, Pheby D, Henehan G, Brown R, Sieving P, Sykora P, et al. Ethical considerations regarding animal experimentation. *J Prev Med Hyg* 2022;63(2);Suppl 3:E255–66.
16. Fernandez-Carro E, Angenent M, Gracia-Cazaña T, Gilaberte Y, Alcaine C, Ciriza J. Modeling an optimal 3D skin-on-chip within microfluidic devices for pharmacological studies. *Pharmaceutics* 2022;14(7):1417.
17. Niculescu AG, Chircov C, Bîrcă AC, Grumezescu AM. Fabrication and applications of microfluidic devices: A review. *Int J Mol Sci* 2021;22(4):2011.
18. Sackmann EK, Fulton AL, Beebe DJ. The present and future role of microfluidics in biomedical research. *Nature* 2014;507(7491):181–9.
19. Nguyen NT, Shaegh SA, Kashaninejad N, Phan DT. Design, fabrication and characterization of drug delivery systems based on lab-on-a-chip technology. *Adv Drug Deliv Rev* 2013;65(11–12):1403–19.

20. Song Y, Cheng D, Zhao L, Lei KF. Introduction: The origin, current status, and future of microfluidics. In: Song Y, Cheng D, Zhao L, editors. *Microfluidics: Fundamental, Devices and Applications*; 2018. © 2018 Wiley-VCH Verlag GmbH & Co. KGaA. Published 2018 by Wiley-VCH Verlag GmbH & Co. KGaA.

21. Kashaninejad N, Moradi E, Moghadas H. Micro/nanofluidic devices for drug delivery. *Prog Mol Biol Transl Sci* 2022;187(1):9–39.

22. Lee Y, Seo HW, Lee KJ, Jang JW, Kim S. A microfluidic system for stable and continuous EEG monitoring from multiple larval zebrafish. *Sensors (Basel)* 2020;20(20):5903.

23. Hu N, Cheng K, Zhang S, Liu S, Wang L, Du X et al. Advancements in microfluidics for skin cosmetic screening. *Analyst* 2023;148(8):1653–71.

24. Damiati S, Kompella UB, Damiati SA, Kodzius R. Microfluidic devices for drug delivery systems and drug screening. *Genes (Basel)* 2018;9(2):103.

25. Alrifaiy A, Lindahl OA, Ramser K. Polymer-based microfluidic devices for pharmacy, biology and tissue engineering. *Polymers* 2012;4(3):1349–98.

26. Borók A, Laboda K, Bonyár A. PDMS bonding technologies for microfluidic applications: A review. *Biosensors* 2021;11(8):292.

27. Fornells E, Murray E, Waheed S, Morrin A, Diamond D, Paull B et al. Integrated 3D printed heaters for microfluidic applications: Ammonium analysis within environmental water. *Anal Chim Acta* 2020;1098:94–101.

28. Raj M K, Chakraborty S. PDMS microfluidics: A mini review. *J Appl Polym Sci* 2020;137(27):48958.

29. Agostini M, Greco G, Cecchini M. Polydimethylsiloxane (PDMS) irreversible bonding to untreated plastics and metals for microfluidics applications. *APL Mater* 2019;7(8).

30. Faghih MM, Sharp MK. Solvent-based bonding of PMMA–PMMA for microfluidic applications. *Microsyst Technol* 2019;25(9):3547–58.

31. Liao S, He Y, Chu Y, Liao H, Wang Y. Solvent-resistant and fully recyclable perfluoropolyether-based elastomer for microfluidic chip fabrication. *J Mater Chem A* 2019;7(27):16249–56.

32. Fan Y, Huang L, Cui R, Zhou X, Zhang Y. Thermoplastic polyurethane-based flexible multilayer microfluidic devices. *J Micro Nanolithogr MEMS MOEMS* 2020;19(2):024501.

33. Lebedev D, Malyshev G, Ryzhkov I, Mozharov A, Shugurov K, Sharov V et al. Focused ion beam milling based formation of nanochannels in silicon-glass microfluidic chips for the study of ion transport. *Microfluid Nanofluid* 2021;25(6):51.

34. Pattanayak P, Singh SK, Gulati M, Vishwas S, Kapoor B, Chellappan DK et al. Microfluidic chips: Recent advances, critical strategies in design, applications and future perspectives. *Microfluid Nanofluid* 2021;25(12):99.

35. Jin Y, Aziz AUR, Wu B, Lv Y, Zhang H, Li N et al. The road to unconventional detections: Paper-based microfluidic chips. *Micromachines* 2022;13(11):1835.

36. Akther F, Little P, Li Z, Nguyen NT, Ta HT. Hydrogels as artificial matrices for cell seeding in microfluidic devices. *RSC Adv* 2020;10(71):43682–703.

37. Wufuer M, Lee G, Hur W, Jeon B, Kim BJ, Choi TH et al. Skin-on-a-chip model simulating inflammation, edema and drug-based treatment. *Sci Rep* 2016;6:37471.

38. Zhang B, Korolj A, Lai BFL, Radisic M. Advances in organ-on-a-chip engineering. *Nat Rev Mater* 2018;3(8):257–78.

39. Zhang Q, Sito L, Mao M, He J, Zhang YS, Zhao X. Current advances in skin-on-a-chip models for drug testing. *Microphysiol Syst* 2018;2:4.

40. Lee J, Soper SA, Murray KK. Microfluidic chips for mass spectrometry-based proteomics. *J Mass Spectrom* 2009;44(5):579–93.

41. Lee W, Debasitis JC, Lee VK, Lee JH, Fischer K, Edminster K et al. Multi-layered culture of human skin fibroblasts and keratinocytes through three-dimensional freeform fabrication. *Biomaterials* 2009;30(8):1587–95.

42. Lee V, Singh G, Trasatti JP, Bjornsson C, Xu X, Tran TN et al. Design and fabrication of human skin by three-dimensional bioprinting. *Tissue Eng Part C Methods* 2014;20(6):473–84.

43. Ataç B, Wagner I, Horland R, Lauster R, Marx U, Tonevitsky AG et al. Skin and hair on-a-chip: In vitro skin models versus ex vivo tissue maintenance with dynamic perfusion. *Lab Chip* 2013;13(18):3555–61.

44. Zoio P, Oliva A. Skin-on-a-chip technology: Microengineering physiologically relevant in vitro skin models. *Pharmaceutics* 2022;14(3):682.

45. Kim JJ, Ellett F, Thomas CN, Jalali F, Anderson RR, Irimia D et al. A microscale, full-thickness, human skin on a chip assay simulating neutrophil responses to skin infection and antibiotic treatments. *Lab Chip* 2019;19(18):3094–103.

46. Wagner I, Materne EM, Brincker S, Süssbier U, Frädrich C, Busek M; et al. A dynamic multi-organ-chip for long-term cultivation and substance testing proven by 3D human liver and skin tissue co-culture. *Lab Chip* 2013;13(18):3538–47.

47. Maschmeyer I, Lorenz AK, Schimek K, Hasenberg T, Ramme AP, Hübner J; et al. A four-organ-chip for interconnected long-term co-culture of human intestine, liver, skin and kidney equivalents. *Lab Chip* 2015;15(12):2688–99.

48. Abaci HE, Gledhill K, Guo Z, Christiano AM, Shuler ML. Pumpless microfluidic platform for drug testing on human skin equivalents. *Lab Chip* 2015;15(3):882–8.

49. Kühnl J, Tao TP, Brandmair K, Gerlach S, Rings T, Müller-Vieira U; et al. Characterization of application scenario-dependent pharmacokinetics and pharmacodynamic properties of permethrin and hyperforin in a dynamic skin and liver multi-organ-chip model. *Toxicology* 2021;448:152637.

50. Tavares RSN, Tao TP, Maschmeyer I, Maria-Engler SS, Schäfer-Korting M, Winter A et al. Toxicity of topically applied drugs beyond skin irritation: Static skin model vs. two organs-on-a-chip. *Int J Pharm* 2020;589:119788.

51. Groeber F, Engelhardt L, Lange J, Kurdyn S, Schmid FF, Rücker C et al. A first vascularized skin equivalent as an alternative to animal experimentation. *ALTEX Altern Anim Exp* 2016;33(4):415–22.

52. Lee S, Jin SP, Kim YK, Sung GY, Chung JH, Sung JH. Construction of 3D multicellular microfluidic chip for an in vitro skin model. *Biomed Microdevices* 2017;19(2):22.

53. Ramadan Q, Ting FCW. In vitro micro-physiological immune-competent model of the human skin. *Lab Chip* 2016;16(10):1899–908.

54. Sasaki N, Tsuchiya K, Kobayashi H. Photolithography-free skin-on-a-chip for parallel permeation assays. *Sens Mater* 2019;31(1):107–15.

55. Mori N, Morimoto Y, Takeuchi S. Skin integrated with perfusable vascular channels on a chip. *Biomaterials* 2017;116:48–56.

56. Mori N, Morimoto Y, Takeuchi S. Perfusable and stretchable 3D culture system for skin-equivalent. *Biofabrication* 2018;11(1):011001.

57. Kim BS, Gao G, Kim JY, Cho DW. 3D cell printing of perfusable vascularized human skin equivalent composed of epidermis, dermis, and hypodermis for better structural recapitulation of native skin. *Adv Healthc Mater* 2019;8(7):e1801019.

58. Salameh S, Tissot N, Cache K, Lima J, Suzuki I, Marinho PA, Rielland M, Soeur J, Takeuchi S, Germain S, Breton L. A perfusable vascularized full-thickness skin model for potential topical and systemic applications. *Biofabrication* 2021;13(3).

59. Jeon HM, Kim K, Choi KC, Sung GY. Side-effect test of sorafenib using 3-D skin equivalent based on microfluidic skin-on-a-chip. *J Ind Eng Chem* 2020;82:71–80.

60. Kim K, Jeon HM, Choi KC, Sung GY. Testing the effectiveness of Curcuma longa leaf extract on a skin equivalent using a pumpless skin-on-a-chip model. *Int J Mol Sci* 2020;21(11):1–15.

61. Lim HY, Kim J, Song HJ, Kim K, Choi KC, Park S et al. Development of wrinkled skin-on-a-chip (WSOC) by cyclic uniaxial stretching. *J Ind Eng Chem* 2018;68:238–45.

62. Risueño I, Valencia L, Holgado M, Jorcano JL, Velasco D. Generation of a simplified three-dimensional skin-on-a-chip model in a micromachined microfluidic platform. *J Vis Exp* 2021;171(171):e62353.

63. Song HJ, Lim HY, Chun W, Choi KC, Sung JH, Sung GY. Fabrication of a pumpless, microfluidic skin chip from different collagen sources. *J Ind Eng Chem* 2017;56:375–81.

64. Song HJ, Lim HY, Chun W, Choi KC, Lee T, Sung JH et al. Development of 3D skin-equivalent in a pump-less microfluidic chip. *J Ind Eng Chem* 2018;60:355–9.

65. Sriram G, Alberti M, Dancik Y, Wu B, Wu R, Feng Z et al. Full-thickness human skin-on-chip with enhanced epidermal morphogenesis and barrier function. *Mater Today* 2018;21(4):326–40.

66. Strüver K, Friess W, Hedtrich S. Development of a perfusion platform for dynamic cultivation of in vitro skin models. *Skin Pharmacol Physiol* 2017;30(4):180–9.

67. Valencia L, Canalejas-Tejero V, Clemente M, Fernaud I, Holgado M, Jorcano JL et al.. A new microfluidic method enabling the generation of multi-layered tissues-on-chips using skin cells as a proof of concept. *Sci Rep* 2021;11(1):13160.

68. Rimal R, Marquardt Y, Nevolianis T, Djeljadini S, Marquez AB, Huth S; et al. Dynamic flow enables long-term maintenance of 3-D vascularized human skin models. *Appl Mater Today* 2021;25:101213.

69. Alexander FA, Eggert S, Wiest J. Skin-on-a-chip: Transepithelial electrical resistance and extracellular acidification measurements through an automated air-liquid interface. *Genes (Basel)* 2018;9(2):114.

70. Abaci HE, Guo Z, Coffman A, Gillette B, Lee WH, Sia SK et al. Human skin constructs with spatially controlled vasculature using primary and iPSC-derived endothelial cells. *Adv Healthc Mater* 2016;5(14):1800–7.

71. Rabost-Garcia G, Farré-Lladós J, Casals-Terré J. Recent impact of microfluidics on skin models for perspiration simulation. *Membranes* 2021;11(2):150.

72. Naik AR, Zhou Y, Dey AA, Arellano DLG, Okoroanyanwu U, Secor EB et al. Printed microfluidic sweat sensing platform for cortisol and glucose detection. *Lab Chip* 2021;22(1):156–69.

73. Ho TM, Razzaghi A, Ramachandran A, Mikkonen KS. Emulsion characterization via microfluidic devices: A review on interfacial tension and stability to coalescence. *Adv Colloid Interf Sci* 2022;299:102541.

74. Tang PC, Eriksson O, Sjögren J, Fatsis-Kavalopoulos N, Kreuger J, Andersson DI. A microfluidic chip for studies of the dynamics of antibiotic resistance selection in bacterial biofilms. *Front Cell Infect Microbiol* 2022;12:896149.

75. Zhao W, Zhang Y, Liu L, Gao Y, Sun W, Sun Y et al. Microfluidic-based functional materials: New prospects for wound healing and beyond. *J Mater Chem B* 2022;10(41):8357–74.

76. Shabestani Monfared G, Ertl P, Rothbauer M. Microfluidic and lab-on-a-chip systems for cutaneous wound healing studies. *Pharmaceutics* 2021;13(6):793.

77. Coughlin MF, Kamm RD. The use of microfluidic platforms to probe the mechanism of cancer cell extravasation. *Adv Healthc Mater* 2020;9(8):e1901410.

78. Mohamadali M, Ghiaseddin A, Irani S, Amirkhani MA, Dahmardehei M. Design and evaluation of a skin-on-a-chip pumpless microfluidic device. *Sci Rep* 2023;13(1):8861.

79. Ahn J, Ohk K, Won J, Choi DH, Jung YH, Yang JH et al. Modeling of three-dimensional innervated epidermal like-layer in a microfluidic chip-based coculture system. *Nat Commun* 2023;14(1):1488.

80. Guichard A, Remoué N, Honegger T. In vitro sensitive skin models: Review of the standard methods and introduction to a new disruptive technology. *Cosmetics* 2022;9(4):67.

81. Sonner Z, Wilder E, Heikenfeld J, Kasting G, Beyette F, Swaile D et al. The microfluidics of the eccrine sweat gland, including biomarker partitioning, transport, and biosensing implications. *Biomicrofluidics* 2015;9(3):031301.
82. Koh A, Kang D, Xue Y, Lee S, Pielak RM, Kim J et al.A soft, wearable microfluidic device for the capture, storage, and colorimetric sensing of sweat. *Sci Transl Med* 2016;8(366):366ra165.
83. Kim SB, Lee K, Raj MS, Lee B, Reeder JT, Koo J et al. Soft, skin-interfaced microfluidic systems with wireless, battery-free electronics for digital, real-time tracking of sweat loss and electrolyte composition. *Small* 2018;14(45):e1802876.
84. Curto VF, Coyle S, Byrne R, Angelov N, Diamond D, Benito-Lopez F. Concept and development of an autonomous wearable micro-fluidic platform for real time pH sweat analysis. *Sensors Actuators B Chem* 2012;175:263–70.
85. Wang Z, Gui M, Asif M, Yu Y, Dong S, Wang H et al. A facile modular approach to the 2D oriented assembly MOF electrode for non-enzymatic sweat biosensors. *Nanoscale* 2018;10(14):6629–38.
86. Epstein Y, Roberts WO. The pathopysiology of heat stroke: An integrative view of the final common pathway. *Scand J Med Sci Sports* 2011;21(6):742–8.
87. Zhang Y, Guo H, Kim SB, Wu Y, Ostojich D, Park SH et al. Passive sweat collection and colorimetric analysis of biomarkers relevant to kidney disorders using a soft microfluidic system. *Lab Chip* 2019;19(9):1545–55.
88. Zhu C, Chortos A, Wang Y, Pfattner R, Lei T, Hinckley AC et al. Stretchable temperature-sensing circuits with strain suppression based on carbon nanotube transistors. *Nat Electron* 2018;1(3):183–90.
89. Mena-Bravo A, Luque de Castro MD. Sweat: A sample with limited present applications and promising future in metabolomics. *J Pharm Biomed Anal* 2014;90:139–47.
90. Sekine Y, Kim SB, Zhang Y, Bandodkar AJ, Xu S, Choi J et al. A fluorometric skin-interfaced microfluidic device and smartphone imaging module for in situ quantitative analysis of sweat chemistry. *Lab Chip* 2018;18(15):2178–86.
91. Zhang Y, Chen Y, Huang J, Liu Y, Peng J, Chen S et al. XSkin-interfaced microfluidic devices with one-opening chambers and hydrophobic valves for sweat collection and analysis. *Lab Chip* 2020;20(15):2635–45.

10 Materials and Techniques for Microfabrication of Microfluidic Device

Shashikant Chandrakar
Columbia Institute of Pharmacy, Raipur, India

Krishna Yadav
Rungta College of Pharmaceutical Sciences and Research,
Bhilai, India

Madhulika Pradhan
Gracious College of Pharmacy, Abhanpur, India

10.1 INTRODUCTION

Research in dermatology is rapidly expanding into the field of microfluidic systems and materials for microfluidic device production. "The science and technology of devices that process or control tiny volumes of fluids, employing channels with size of tens to hundreds of micrometers," said George Whitesides in his pioneering work on microfluidics. The field of microfluidics, which aims to miniaturize conventional biological studies, is summed up in this brief description (1–3). Miniaturizing biological investigations is made possible by microfluidics, which allows for the integration of a whole laboratory procedure onto a single chip, which shortens reaction times, reduces reagent quantities, and enables numerous operations. One day, these gadgets will be able to do everything from transporting samples to detecting biological molecules—all with a single device (4, 5). A major step forward in dermatological research has been the creation of in vitro skin models of humans. Both as a platform for the development and testing of biochemical and pharmacological compounds and as a tool for improving our knowledge of skin physiology in a controlled setting, these models perform a double duty. Examples of recent inventive achievements include the development of skin-on-a-chip devices that provide dynamic perfusion via microfluidic channels and the creation of in vitro three-dimensional (3D) skin models (6).

DOI: 10.1201/9781032690926-10

The main goal of using microfluidic systems in skin engineering is to make in vitro human skin models that are very accurate representations of the complex structure and functions of real skin. The regulated and reproducible environment allows these skin-on-a-chip devices to function, providing a degree of accuracy and realism that cannot be achieved using conventional means.

Microfluidic systems provide a dynamic and physiologically appropriate platform, in contrast to traditional static cell cultures or basic tissue models. Emulating complex skin physiological processes, including feed and oxygen delivery, waste disposal, and the dynamic interplay between various cell types, is made possible by these devices that use microscale channels to circulate fluids. If we want to show how different skin diseases, treatments, or medication molecules affect real people, we need this dynamic simulation.

This development has the potential to greatly improve the precision and applicability of pharmacological drug preclinical testing, yielding more trustworthy information on the medicines' effectiveness, safety, and adverse effects for researchers and pharmaceutical businesses (7).

In vitro, skin models and skin grafts are often created using tissue engineering and microfluidic platforms. Additionally, these platforms may be used for the detection of new skin disorders and the screening of new bioactive compounds for potential therapeutic applications (8, 9).

This chapter delves into the topic of microfluidic devices and their use in transdermal drug administration, specifically touching on the design and construction of such devices utilizing different materials. Introduction to microfluidic systems, microfabrication techniques, and various materials utilized in dermatological microfluidic devices are all covered. Choosing skin-safe materials is also covered in detail in this chapter, with an emphasis on mechanical characteristics, biodegradability, and biocompatibility.

10.2 MATERIALS UTILIZED IN MICROFLUIDIC DEVICES FOR DERMATOLOGY

Microfluidic devices have been made from a wide variety of materials in the last few years. Paper, polydimethylsiloxane (PDMS), inorganic materials like glass or silicon, polymers, and mixtures of these materials created by 3D printing (3P) are all materials that are used in microfluidics. Extensive research and inexpensive costs have led to thermoplastics and PDMS's widespread adoption (4).

10.2.1 INORGANIC MATERIALS

Prior to its replacement by materials with better optical properties, steady electro-osmotic flow, and resistance to organic solvents, silicon was the material of choice for microfabrication in microfluidics due to its systematically characterized surface qualities (10, 11). Glass is a popular medium for biochemical investigation due to its compatibility with several biological samples and its high optical transparency. Microfluidic manufacturing using silicon and glass may be costly due to the need for cleanrooms and high-tech equipment (12).

10.2.1.1 Silicon

Because of its semiconducting properties, silicon has been used in microfabrication for a long time. Thanks to its chemical resilience, design flexibility, and well-documented surface modification capabilities, silicon is an ideal material for creating microfluidic devices. This is thanks in large part to the silanol group. The high elastic modulus of silicon, however, makes the pumps and valves more complex (150 GPa) (13, 14). Because they are transparent to visible light, silicon devices are also unsuitable for typical fluorescence-based detection or direct fluid imaging. One common solution to this issue is to wrap silicon microchannels in a transparent material, such as glass or polymers (15). Due to the high expense of creating a single microfluidic device wafer, batch production procedures often entail stacking many devices onto a single silicon wafer (12).

A hollow array of silicon microneedles was designed and built, according to Ashraf et al. The interior lumen of a hollow microneedle is designed to facilitate the passage of drugs. Every microneedle is arranged on a substrate with one on top of the other. For the microneedle array, inductively coupled plasma (ICP) etching is used to create the mask pattern. Computerized fluid dynamics allows for the regulation of the stress distribution and fluid flow rate inside the microneedles array. The results of the simulation demonstrate that the volume grows in tandem with the excitation voltages (16) Microneedles with tapered tips were described by Bodhale et al. Skin implantation is made easy with the microneedles packed into an array of hollow cylindrical silicon microneedles. Initial reports focused on the design and manufacturing procedures for mask layouts that made use of deep reactive ion etching on silicon wafers. A series of combined isotropic and anisotropic etching procedures are used to create silicon hollow microneedles using ICP etching technology. To describe the microneedles' functionality, structural and connected multifield analyses are used (17).

10.2.2 Polymer

10.2.2.1 Polydimethylsiloxane

An often used substrate for microfabrication, polydimethylsiloxane (PDMS) is inexpensive and easy to work with. Device molds may be created using conventional machining or photolithography processes, and then PDMS microstructures can be cast onto these molds. To link various layers via holes, multilayer channel constructions may be built using several layers. It is suitable for cell culture because it has a higher gas permeability than other materials. The microchip allowed for a more controlled microenvironment than was possible with macroscale cultivation. However, PDMS might be troublesome for cell culture due to bubble formation when gas is passed through it. Another drawback is that PDMS oligomer chains with low molecular weight might leach out of solutions (18, 19). A microfluidic platform was created by Hasan Erbil Abaci et al., which allows for the long-term preservation of full-thickness human skin equivalents (HSE) using PDMS for drug testing. The platform has both dermal and epidermal compartments. To estimate intrinsic skin transport features including diffusion rate and drug partitioning, these skin-on-chip devices may recirculate the medium at specified flow rates without the need for a pump (20).

Microfluidic channels were created using soft lithography. The blood-loading channel and the column-loading channel were made by cutting the cured PDMS and punching out their respective inlets and outlets. A punched PDMS channel was attached to glass-bottom well plates by plasma treatment, and the combination was then baked. This microchip might promote the growth and differentiation of skin cells. Researchers studying skin diseases and cutaneous medication delivery have used the state-of-the-art microfluidic skin chip as an in vitro platform (21–23).

10.2.2.2 Polycaprolactone

The biological potential of polycaprolactone (PCL), an aliphatic polyester with a low glass transition temperature and low melting point, has been extensively investigated (24). As a biomedical material, PCL has been extensively explored due to its low melting point and glass transition temperature, which make it an aliphatic polyester (25). Another intriguing property of PCL is its capacity to create appropriate mixes with other polymers. The high elongation at breaking and excellent elastic properties of PCL are due to its low tensile strength (~23 MPa). It is now believed that PCL is nontoxic and tissue-compatible, according to the toxicity studies conducted as part of the Capronor evaluation (26).

10.2.2.3 Polymethylmethacrylate

A second popular material for microchips is polymethylmethacrylate or PMMA. An amorphous thermoplastic, PMMA is somewhat more solvent-compatible than PDMS but does not absorb tiny molecules. PMMA has the ability to be optically transparent, has high mechanical properties, and may be used for small-scale production proto-typing and surface modification. Particularly relevant to micro-physiological systems and organ-on-a-chip technologies, these features may help researchers. A thermoplas-tic polymer often used in microfluidics, polymethylmethacrylate has excellent opti-cal transparency, little autofluorescence, and great biocompatibility. Microfluidics makes extensive use of thermoplastic polymethylmethacrylate because of its excel-lent optical clarity, low autofluorescence, and good biocompatibility. Another reason it might be useful in capillary-driven microfluidic devices is its relative hydrophilic-ity. Nevertheless, PMMA is usually structured using industrial-scale polymer struc-turing processes such as hot embossing or injection molding. The bulk of PMMA fast prototyping has been carried out using subtractive processes such as laser structuring or high-precision milling, as well as laboratory-scale imprinting techniques such as solvent replication or room temperature imprinting. From many unique master archi-tectures, such as stainless steel or polydimethylsiloxane, microfluidic PMMA chips have been successfully manufactured using PMMA prepolymers, which consist of the polymer PMMA and the monomer methylmethacrylate (MMA) (27).

10.3 BIOCOMPATIBILITY AND TOXICITY OF THE DIFFERENT MICROFLUIDIC MATERIALS

To promote tissue and cell development, a biomaterial must be compatible with liv-ing organisms. The accuracy of the model and the findings might be impacted by the use of a biocompatible substance, which is nontoxic to cells. Additionally, the presence of a biocompatible material implies that the carbon dioxide, pH, and oxygen levels are optimal for the chosen cell type to undergo tissue formation. The ideal substance also should not have any negative reactions to the cell culture media (28, 29).

One of the best materials to use as a base for microfluidic devices and skin sensors that you may wear, like fitness bands, is PMMA. The poly(dimethylsiloxane) toxicity research, which was reported by R. A. Paret, mainly included skin irritation and sensitization. New Zealand albino rabbits were used in the skin irritation investigation. Researchers used albino guinea pigs to explore skin sensitivity. The albino rabbits that participated in the experiment showed very little reddening on their severely damaged skin. No animal showed any indications of swelling. This silicone oil is considered to be somewhat irritating to albino rabbit skin according to Draize's grading standards (30).

For the purpose of rejuvenating hands, Vitor Manuel Figueiredo investigated the effectiveness and safety of dermal fillers composed of PLC.

The five volunteers had PLC dermal filler applied to the backs of their hands. The participants were scheduled for follow-up appointments. Dermal filler made of PLC was determined to be an effective, safe, and well-tolerated method of regenerating the hands (31).

10.4 SELECTION OF APPROPRIATE MATERIALS FOR USE IN THE SKIN

One of the most crucial first stages in designing skin-on-chip devices is choosing the biomaterial that will be used as the basis for tissue production and chip system operation.

10.4.1 BIOCOMPATIBILITY

For the biomaterial to function as a habitat for cell growth and repair, it must be able to maintain a consistent oxygen supply, promote cell adhesion, and maintain a pH balance. Biocompatibility is an important consideration in skin-on-chip systems in general and in the pursuit of a completely integrated system with the human body in particular (32, 33).

10.4.2 BIODEGRADABILITY

There are some potential benefits to using biodegradable materials as well. In order for the system to be integrated into the body's extracellular matrix in the future, the biomaterial must be biodegradable (34). The rate of degradation should also be inversely proportionate to the formation of biological tissues by the cells in order for the system to be balanced and sustain homeostasis (35). The biomaterial's biodegradable properties are useful for evaluating small molecules as well. By analyzing the material's kinetics and degradation rates, a more accurate model may be built for drug testing and assessing drug response in specific organ models (36).

10.4.3 MECHANICAL PROPERTIES

The selected biomaterial must possess enough mechanical properties that align with the mechanical features of the intended organ. A few critical mechanical properties of microfluidic chips may decide the outcome. The biomaterial's response to fluid shear stress dictates how the cells multiply, develop, and survive inside the chip. Physical pressure activates surface and intracellular signaling molecules, and it alters the polarity axis of microorganisms and cells (37, 38).

Microfluidic chips typically operate in a laminar flow pattern, which controls the mixing rate but causes slow diffusion. This results in a consistent gradient inside the chip, which may influence biological processes like cell migration and motility or even imitate developmental processes like angiogenesis. In the context of tissue simulation or continuous loading and physiological change, the biomaterial's capacity to dynamically react to mechanical stress might be a benefit. Mechanical properties such as ductility, Young's modulus, and Poisson's ratio often also characterize these characteristics. You may utilize them to find a biomaterial that acts more like the target tissue (39, 40).

10.5 METHODS OF MICROFABRICATION

Specialized demands, such as the ability to work with very tiny objects and high levels of detail, limit the mass manufacturing of micro-sized structures. Consequently, novel manufacturing processes have emerged as a result of scientific and technological advancements. We examined the broad manufacturing processes to establish the scope in three parts. The first group includes molding processes; the second, 3DP; and the third, nanoimprinting lithography and etching procedures (41).

10.5.1 MOLDING

One common method for making microfluidic devices for use in medicine is soft lithography, which is a kind of replica molding. Making silicon molds is a procedure that has been fine-tuned. Using photolithography, patterns are created on silicon wafers to form negative photoresist. The silicon substrate is first covered with the photoresist using a spin coater set to the correct speed to get the desired thickness. The next step is to use mask aligner ultraviolet (UV)-lithography equipment to expose the wafer to UV light via the photomask that was previously generated. The next step is to dip the sample into a developer to remove the exposed portion. At this stage, the SU-8 master, also known as the silicon mold, is prepared. After placing the SU-8 master in a glass Petri dish, the mixture is then poured over it. The curing agent and PDMS prepolymer base are mixed in a 10:1 ratio. Before curing in the oven, the PDMS mixture must be degassed. When the PDMS is taken out of the mold, it is fused to microscope glass slides using an oxygen plasma device to make the microchannel. This method is rapidly becoming the norm in the industry due to the use of a biocompatible polymer (PDMS) that is high-resolution, flexible, optically transparent, and used to make microfluidic devices. A cell's physicochemical environment may be controlled via PDMS microfluidic devices by adjusting the flow conditions. One disadvantage of soft lithography is the increased cost caused by the need for a clean room. Another factor that might affect the biological reaction is the molecule that takes in PDMS (4, 42–44).

10.5.2 Injection Molding

Because of its great productivity, injection molding is a very appealing process for producing microfluidics. This method is quite popular since it is simple to implement and compatible with a broad range of thermoplastics. Compressing the mold's two sides after melting the thermoplastic in a compressible chamber creates the mold cavity. Once cooled, the cast item is removed from the mold (4). The techniques and materials used for mold inserts are dictated by the required production time of the mold. In their discussion of the pros and disadvantages of rapid injection molding, Lee et al. provided design guidance for making good use of this method in the fabrication of microscale cell-based assays (45). In their demonstration, Convery et al. showed how to print inlays in three dimensions for use in injection molding. Poor resolution, expensive mold construction, and material constraints with respect to thermoplastics are frequently the main drawbacks of microinjection molding. The use of injection molding microfluidics, a new method for single-cell analysis, was considered (46, 47).

10.5.3 Hot Embossing

This method involves applying high heat and pressure to thermoplastics or polymers in order to transfer their form from the mold. The process involves heating the thermoplastic film in a vacuum while it is sandwiched between two molds. Pressing the molds down into the pliable polymer transfers the mold's form. Removing the treated polymer from the mold is the last step after cooling (4, 48). Research by Al-Aqbi et al. examined the three-minute process of hot embossing PMMA to separate drugs from whole blood (49). Glass and other amorphous materials may be easily made for microfluidic channels utilizing a versatile approach described by Jiang et al., which involves hot embossing. The effect of process factors on the filling behavior of N-BK7 glass in a silicon carbide microhole mold was investigated. Process variables included embossing force, temperature, soaking duration, and annealing rate. The goal was to create a tool for quick hot embossing; therefore, this was done. Because the thermoplastic flows at a closer distance during hot embossing, compared to injection molding, there is less stress on material was occurs.

This approach cannot build complicated structures in less than 3 minutes, and it does not make very good use of the available materials (50).

10.5.4 3D Printing

One innovative approach to making various microfluidic devices is three-dimensional printing, which involves building them up from many layers of material. The utilization of several materials with different physical and mechanical qualities in a single build process is possible with this additive manufacturing method (48). There are several restrictions to consider while using 3DP, even though it is an inexpensive way to produce detailed features. Some of these issues include a lack of accuracy in the fabrication of hollow and empty parts, a limited variety of transparent materials, poor z-resolution, and less-than-perfect surface finishes. Biomedical devices that are difficult to build using conventional methods, such as molding or machining, may now be engineered with the help of smart additive manufacturing techniques, such as 3DP. The many advantages of 3D-printed microfluidics, such as precise design, low production costs, and rapid manufacture of a wide range of products—even devices with intricate geometrical structures—have recently garnered a lot of interest. To fabricate various parts, 3D printers are used in many different systems and applications. The advent of 3DP has revolutionized the microfluidics discipline and allowed for the creation of novel microfluidic devices that would have been previously unimaginable. A game-changer in the realms of science and technology, 3DP enables the production of cheap, tailor-made machinery that relies on specialized tools. A 3D reaction ware matrix may be printed with chemicals directly into it, allowing for digital control over the design, construction, and functioning of the reaction ware. This is a fascinating but untested use case (51, 52).

10.5.5 Fused Deposition Modeling

One method for creating 3D objects via extrusion is fused deposition modeling (FDM). This approach involves melting thermoplastic filament, forcing it through a nozzle, and then allowing it to cool until it solidifies. Despite the method's efficiency, adaptability, and ease of usage, the created structures are more susceptible to compressive stress fractures. The reason for this is that the fusion between neighboring layers is inadequate (27). Obtaining microchannels that are both transparent and of the appropriate size is also challenging. Printing resolution-influencing factors were investigated by Quero et al., including nozzle properties and frame (53).

10.5.6 Vat Polymerization

Microfluidics printed in three dimensions are made possible by vat polymerization, which employs ultraviolet light to cure the resin. Combining digital light processing (DLP) with stereolithography (SLA) is a quick prototyping technology for producing tiny features (48). A printing platform that acts as a container for reactions, precursor materials that are sensitive to light and contain reactants (photoinitiators), and a light source that enables specific reactions make up the three main components of this technology. To harden the photopolymer, an SLA device utilizes a scanning galvano mirror and a focused light-emitting diode (LED) laser that is aimed at a certain set of coordinates. In the DLP process, the liquid polymer is exposed utilizing a build plate that moves in very small increments in response to a fixed UV light.

For transdermal medicine distribution, biocompatible resin was used to build 3D-printed microneedle arrays. Commercially accessible photopolymers for SLA were the subject of a biocompatibility investigation. In a detection trial conducted using a smartphone, the DLP approach was shown to be suitable for developing a paper-based microfluidic analysis device that could simultaneously identify several biomarkers (54).

10.5.7 MULTI-JET PRINTING

This technology of 3DP, which is marketed as PolyJet, allows for the fabrication of diverse materials and microfluidic devices with excellent precision. Light from a light source attached to the inkjet print head solidifies a droplet of photosensitive resin ejected by the print head (55). Utilizing multi-jet printing, some researchers developed finger-powered, electric power-free sub-millifluidic and microfluidic actuators that were completely 3D-printed (56, 57).

Another research produced a microfluidic device that may be worn to collect perspiration from the skin. Microfluidic valves, an essential part of fluid control, were also produced using this method (58).

10.5.8 TWO-PHOTON POLYMERIZATION

Complex nanoscale structures can be made with this method (48). Due to the non-linear nature of photo excitation, when a concentrated laser is used to cure a volume of liquid resin, part of the liquid is evacuated while the remaining liquid is cured. This 3DP method allowed for the design of biomimetic placental barrier structures, microneedle arrays, microstructures composed of transparent fused silica glass, and coaxial lamination mixers (59–61).

10.5.9 OTHER FABRICATION METHODS

10.5.9.1 Nanofabrication

Normal photolithography's low resolution is because the light source utilized to pattern the substrate has a longer wavelength. Three techniques—nanoimprint lithography (NIL), electron beam lithography (EBL), and extreme ultraviolet lithography—allow for the creation of very minute features by decreasing the wavelength (4).

EBL eschews light in favor of a high-energy electron beam, which reveals an electron resist layer. Nevertheless, these methods are underutilized in nanofluidic design due to their exorbitant prices and poor throughput. One kind of replica molding with several applications in microfluidics is NIL. A prefabricated mold is mechanically pushed into a substance that acts as a resist, and then the resist is solidified utilizing heat, chemicals, or light. Research has shown that NIL has the potential to be used in the fabrication of polymer nanostructured biological detection chips (62, 63).

10.5.9.2 Lab-on-chip Technology

Lab-on-chip (LoC) refers to a device that may transfer one or more laboratory processes to a chip format. In terms of size, this chip falls anywhere between a few millimeters to a few square centimeters. Volumes of fluid less than picoliters are no problem with LoC (64). Since the advent of microfluidic systems, there has been tremendous progress in the creation of LoC technologies, which integrate several operations onto a single substrate. These little devices have the potential to become a tool for faster analytical testing due to their high efficiency and accuracy (65, 66). One potential application for LoC devices is doing on-site sample testing. In laboratory settings, they are useful tools for rapid investigation of potential pathogens. Due to their low waste and little reagent and sample requirements, these devices are both safe and cost-effective. In order to create unique flow patterns for controlled mixing and detection, many methods for constructing LOC devices have been explored (67, 68). Most often, fabrication procedures including photolithography, inkjet printing, screen printing, plasma oxidation, and laser treatment are used in the production of LOCs (69). According to the rules of fluid dynamics, there are two types of mixing technologies: passive mixing, which makes use of geometrical properties and capillarity to propel fluid flow, and active mixing, which makes use of an outside force. How effective a microfluidic device is depends on its design characteristics, mixing patterns, fluid flow parameters, and fluid composition. Understanding the mixing performance and developments in device design has come a long way in the last several years. An affordable 3D-printed microfluidic device was created, for instance, by using a solvent-bonding approach with polymethyl methacrylate and acrylonitrile butadiene styrene (70, 71).

10.5.9.3 Digital Microfluidic

Digital microfluidics is an alternate way of thinking about microfluidic systems that focus on making and manipulating individual droplets and bubbles. Digital microfluidics (DMF) is a novel approach to liquid management that manipulates liquids in discrete droplets using integrated microfluidic devices (72). In contrast to systems that control droplets in isolated microchannels, DMF describes integrated systems that manipulate droplets on many electrodes. Two popular configurations of DMF devices are single-plate (or open) and two-plate (or closed). In a two-plate configuration, droplets are placed between two electrode-patterned surfaces. In most cases, the top plate will have a continuous ground electrode made of a transparent, conductive layer of indium tin oxide (ITO) (73). The bottom plate has a multitude of actuation electrodes. The ground and actuation electrodes on a single substrate are used to assemble the droplets in the one-plate configuration. In both cases, a hydrophobic coating covers all surfaces, and an insulating dielectric layer protects the bottom-plate electrodes. Substituting silicone oil or another filler medium for air in two-plate devices helps reduce the voltage needed for droplet movement, but it is not an ideal solution (74, 75).

Digital microfluidics is a branch of microfluidics that borrows concepts from emulsion science. The most common method for producing droplets or bubbles involves manipulating the flow rates of fluids applied at a microfluidic junction. This approach is simple to implement. Emulsion processing in microfluidics is based on controlling flow rates at the junction of micro-channels while injecting a continuous phase and a dispersed phase. The joining of microchannels at their junction defines the drop/bubble maker's shape (76, 77).

10.6 CURRENT AND EMERGING MICROFLUIDIC DEVICES IN DERMATOLOGY

10.6.1 SKIN-ON-A-CHIP

Skin-on-a-chip technology was first used in drug and cosmetic testing. By using microfluidic devices, it is now feasible to cultivate this tissue while manipulating several physical and biological variables, including flows, stressors, and chemical gradients. It is difficult to classify skin-on-a-chip procedures since they vary greatly in the manufacturing process, materials employed, and tissue preservation, among other areas (7, 8, 78).

Based on the chip's skin production mechanism, we have classified the gadgets from this angle. Two primary approaches have been established for the fabrication of microfluidic chips for use in skin modeling. Two methods exist for constructing artificial tissues on microchips; one is known as "transferred skin-on-a-chip," and it entails directly transferring a piece of skin from a biopsy or an HSE into the chip (79–81).

10.6.2 TRANSFERRED SKIN-ON-A-CHIP

The techniques that generate skin-on-a-chip models by directly inserting tissue into the device have seen the greatest use. These transplanted tissue pieces may be derived from two main sources: a donor skin biopsy or an HSE grown in a lab. A variety of HSEs, including both commercially available and laboratory-made versions, have been used to simulate skin microfluidic chips. Skin chip transplantation models with a dermal compartment are more prevalent, while dermo-epidermal models also exist in the literature (21, 80).

It is possible to construct more accurate models using these mature tissue pieces as they include all the skin layers (82). The development of these skin models has allowed researchers to investigate a wide range of topics related to the maintenance and clinical and experimental usage of the equivalents, including drug sensitivity and toxicity, multiorgan interaction, and the diffusion of chemicals (78).

Kim et al. built a skin-on-a-chip device with two channels separated by a red blood cell filter to study neutrophil responses to skin germs. The procedure included loading blood samples into one channel and exposing a segment of human skin biopsy that had been grown with bacteria into the other. In one channel, blood samples were loaded, and a human skin biopsy fragment that had been cultivated with bacteria was injected (21).

A bottom channel enabled culture media to flow on the chip that Abaci et al. constructed, while a well retained the HSE fragment for testing and maintenance. Growing the HSE on a permeable membrane allowed nutrients to diffuse from the channel. Drug testing and transdermal delivery were two of the possible uses identified by the researchers (20).

Despite being used in single-tissue models, the transferred skin chip technique is often used for constructing multi-organ chips. A multi-organ chip including hair and skin was also developed by Atac et al. A commercially available bilayered alternative,

EpiDerm FTTM, and subcutaneous tissue extracted from human skin biopsies were used to create skin models. Using this device, they demonstrated that the dermo-epidermal construct is more viable with the addition of subcutaneous tissue and extended the lifetime of the commercial version (80).

10.6.3 In Situ Skin-on-a-Chip

With this alternative approach, we want to build the skin model right on the chip. Tissue is made by hand in an open structure inside the equipment. The main distinction is the methodology used to provide the culture media or other ingredients to the skin construct. The original perfusion approach included hollow tubes that crossed the dermal compartment; however, with current skin-on-chip systems, fluid circulation takes place via a microfluidic channel below the tissue construct (83, 84).

Building the skin directly onto an internal hole in the device, Lee et al. developed and optimized a gravity-driven skin-on-a-chip utilizing PDMS. The dermal compartment was mimicked by embedding the fibroblasts in collagen gel and placing them on top of a porous membrane. Next, keratinocytes were planted and cultured on top of the gel to generate fully developed skin (85).

In their study, Song et al. looked at how different types of collagen-affected skin cell differentiation and maturation. Comparing collagen derived from pig skin and duck feet, they discovered that rat tail collagen outperformed the others. The same team also utilized this apparatus to evaluate traditional transwell skin cultures in comparison to dynamic and static microfluidic chips. Compared to the dynamic chip, the static circumstances yielded superior results. Different drug tests also made use of this skin-on-a-chip concept. In a similar vein, Lim et al. developed a device to mechanically stimulate the skin equivalent while holding it in place (30, 86). Along with the manual tissue production that occurred within a cell compartment over a microfluidic channel, an electromagnet was also included in the chip construction this time. This magnet was used to stretch the tissue by means of a magnetic field. There are certain drawbacks to employing the channels as compartments for growing the tissue, mainly because it is difficult to precisely reproduce the 3D structure of the skin (87, 88).

10.6.4 Pumpless Devices

To better manage the physical and chemical components of the cell microenvironment, it has been recently employed to transfer several micro-physiological organ models onto microfluidic platforms, such as skin. To improve the accuracy of toxicity, effectiveness, and delivery assessments, in vitro skin models may be transferred into microfluidic systems. This paves the way for the physiologically appropriate delivery of nutrients and foreign chemicals to the skin (20, 89, 90) Collaborating using a commercial full-thickness skin model or human hair or liver microtissues, Wagner et al. and Atac et al. used a multi-organ platform to cultivate the samples. Media perfusion required the use of an integrated micro pump in each study. The effective long-term preservation of HSEs in skin-on-chip devices demonstrates

TABLE 10.1

Some Microfluidic Materials and Technology Used for Device Fabrication

Device Material	Flow Mechanism	Types of Platform	References
PDMS	Perfusion, on-chip micropump	Transferred skin-on-a-chip	(80)
PDMS	Pumpless, gravity-driven	Transferred skin-on-a-chip	(20)
PDMS	Pumpless, gravity-driven	Pumpless, gravity-driven	(86)
PDMS	Static	Transferred skin-on-a-chip	(92)
PCL	Perfusion	Vascularized HSE	(21)
PDMS and glass	Perfusion	In situ skin-on-a-chip	(93)
PDMS	Perfusion	In situ skin-on-a-chip	(84)
PDMS	Pumpless, gravity-driven	In situ skin-on-a-chip	(94)
PMMA	Perfusion	In situ skin-on-a-chip	(95)
PMMA, PS, and PDMS	Perfusion (negative pressure)	In situ skin-on-a-chip	(96)
PDMS	Pumpless, gravity-driven	In situ skin-on-a-chip	(97)
PDMS	Perfusion, on-chip Micropump	Transferred skin on-a-chip	(91)
Adhesive vinyl (PVC), PDMS, and glass	Perfusion	In situ skin-on-a-chip	(98)

Notes: HSE, human skin equivalent; PCL, polycaprolactone; PDMS, polydimethylsiloxane; PMMA, poly(methyl methacrylate); PS, polystyrene.

their potential relevance in drug testing research (91). A user-friendly, pumpless HSE-on-a-chip platform was developed by a group of researchers. Similar to previous organ-on-a-chip systems, the HSE-on-a-chip was positioned on a platform to accomplish recirculating gravity-driven flow (20). Table 10.1 lists some of the microfluidic materials and technologies that were used in the manufacture of the devices.

10.7 CONCLUSION

A new and exciting area of dermatological research is the investigation of microfluidic systems and materials for the construction of microfluidic devices. Microfluidics, the study and practice of controlling tiny fluid flows via microscopic channels, has significantly reduced the size and scope of conventional biological studies. To identify biological molecules and transport, this revolutionary method combines whole laboratory methods onto a single chip, shortens reaction times, and decreases reagent quantities; the end goal is to enable the total analysis of samples.

Microfluidic systems are dynamic and physiologically realistic platforms that accurately mimic complex skin processes, allowing researchers to better understand how the skin reacts to different environments, treatments, and chemical molecules. This development improves the reliability of data on pharmacological medication effectiveness, safety, and possible adverse effects by increasing the precision of preclinical testing. Additional uses in drug screening, skin disease diagnostics, in vitro skin models, and skin transplant production have been expanded by the combination of microfluidic systems and tissue engineering. Material selection for skin-related microfluidic devices is highlighted in this chapter, with a focus on mechanical qualities, biodegradability, and biocompatibility. As a whole, this area of study has a lot of potential for the future of dermatology and pharmaceuticals.

ACKNOWLEDGMENT

The authors would like to acknowledge their affiliated institution.

CONFLICT OF INTEREST

None.

REFERENCES

1. Whitesides GM. The origins and the future of microfluidics. *Nature* 2006;442(7101):368–73.
2. Qin D, Xia Y, Rogers JA, Jackman RJ, Zhao XM, Whitesides GM. Microfabrication, Microstructures and Microsystems. In: Manz A, Becker H, editors. *Microsystem Technology in Chemistry and Life Science*. Berlin, Heidelberg: Springer Berlin Heidelberg; 1998. pp. 1–20.
3. Gharib G, Bütün I, Muganlı Z, Kozalak G, Namlı I, Sarraf SS, et al. Biomedical applications of microfluidic devices: A review. *Biosensors* 2022;12(11):1023.
4. Gale BK, Jafek AR, Lambert CJ, Goenner BL, Moghimifam H, Nze UC, et al. A review of current methods in microfluidic device fabrication and future commercialization prospects. *Inventions* 2018;3(3):60.
5. Wang K, Man K, Liu J, Liu Y, Chen Q, Zhou Y, et al. Microphysiological systems: Design, fabrication, and applications. *ACS Biomaterials Science & Engineering* 2020 Jun 8;6(6):3231–57.
6. Risueño I, Valencia L, Jorcano JL, Velasco D. Skin-on-a-chip models: General overview and future perspectives. *APL Bioengineering* 2021;5(3).
7. Zoio P, Oliva A. Skin-on-a-chip technology: Microengineering physiologically relevant in vitro skin models. *Pharmaceutics* 2022 Mar;14(3):682.
8. Lukács B, Bajza Á, Kocsis D, Csorba A, Antal I, Iván K, et al. Skin-on-a-chip device for ex vivo monitoring of transdermal delivery of drugs—Design, fabrication, and testing. *Pharmaceutics* 2019;11(9):445.
9. Mohammadi MH, Heidary Araghi B, Beydaghi V, Geraili A, Moradi F, Jafari P, et al. Skin diseases modeling using combined tissue engineering and microfluidic technologies. *Advanced Healthcare Materials* 2016;5(19):2459–80.
10. Jensen KF. Silicon-based microchemical systems: Characteristics and applications. *MRS Bulletin* 2006;31(2):101–7.
11. Yadav K, Dubey S, Singh S, Sharma G, Pradhan M, Subbiah N, et al. Theranostics inorganic nano-particles for brain tumor diagnosis and treatment. In 2023. pp. 201–21.
12. Lavoie E, Wangdi T, Kazmierczak B. Advances in microfluidic materials, functions, integration and applications. *Chemical Reviews* 2012;13(9):1133–45.
13. Nielsen JB, Hanson RL, Almughamsi HM, Pang C, Fish TR, Woolley AT. Microfluidics: Innovations in materials and their fabrication and functionalization. *Analytical Chemistry* 2020;92(1):150–68.

14. Grover WH, Skelley AM, Liu CN, Lagally ET, Mathies RA. Monolithic membrane valves and diaphragm pumps for practical large-scale integration into glass microfluidic devices. *Sensors and Actuators B: Chemical* 2003;89(3):315–23.

15. Yadav K, Pradhan M, Singh D, Singh MR. Chapter 16 - Targeting Autoimmune Disorders through Metal Nanoformulation in Overcoming the Fences of Conventional Treatment Approaches. In: Rezaei N, editor. *Translational Autoimmunity*. Academic Press; 2022. pp. 361–93. (Translational Immunology; vol. 2). Available from: https://www.sciencedirect.com/science/article/pii/B9780128243909000177

16. Ashraf MW, Tayyaba S, Nisar A, Afzulpurkar N, Tuantranont A. Coupledfield microfluidic analysis of integrated MEMS based device for transdermal drug delivery applications. *INMIC 2009 - 2009 IEEE 13th International Multitopic Conference*; 2009.

17. Bodhale DW, Nisar A, Afzulpurkar N. Design, fabrication and analysis of silicon microneedles for transdermal drug delivery applications. *IFMBE Proceedings* 2010;27:84–9.

18. Kastrup CJ, Runyon MK, Lucchetta EM, Price JM, Ismagilov RF. Using chemistry and microfluidics to understand the spatial dynamics of complex biological networks. *Accounts of Chemical Research* 2008;41(4):549–58.

19. Agrawal M, Pradhan M, Singhvi G, Patel R, Ajazuddin, Alexander A. Thermoresponsive in situ gel of curcumin loaded solid lipid nanoparticle: Design, optimization and in vitro characterization. *Journal of Drug Delivery Science and Technology*. 2022;71:103376. Available from: https://www.sciencedirect.com/science/article/pii/S1773224722002866

20. Abaci HE, Gledhill K, Guo Z, Christiano AM, Shuler ML. Pumpless microfluidic platform for drug testing on human skin equivalents. *Lab on a Chip* 2015;15(3):882–8.

21. Kim JJ, Ellett F, Thomas CN, Jalali F, Anderson RR, Irimia D, et al. A microscale, full-thickness, human skin on a chip assay simulating neutrophil responses to skin infection and antibiotic treatments. *Lab on a Chip* 2019;19(18):3094–103.

22. O'Neill AT, Monteiro-Riviere NA, Walker GM. Characterization of microfluidic human epidermal keratinocyte culture. *Cytotechnology* 2008;56(3):197–207.

23. Sriram G, Alberti M, Dancik Y, Wu B, Wu R, Feng Z, et al. Full-thickness human skin-on-chip with enhanced epidermal morphogenesis and barrier function. *Materials Today* 2018;21(4):326–40.

24. Miguel SP, Ribeiro MP, Coutinho P. Biomedical Applications of Biodegradable Polymers in Wound Care. *Wound Healing Research: Current Trends and Future Directions*. 2021;49(12):509–97.

25. Engelberg I, Kohn J. Physico-mechanical properties of degradable polymers used in medical applications: A comparative study. *Biomaterials* 1991;12(3):292–304.

26. Koleske JV. Blends Containing Poly(ε-caprolactone) and Related Polymers. In *Polymer Blends*. Vol. 2. Academic Press, Inc.; 1978. pp. 369–89.

27. Mader M, Rein C, Konrat E, Meermeyer SL, Lee-Thedieck C, Kotz-Helmer F, et al. Fused deposition modeling of microfluidic chips in transparent polystyrene. *Micromachines* 2021;12(11):5–8.

28. Hosic S, Murthy SK, Koppes AN. Microfluidic sample preparation for single cell analysis. *Analytical Chemistry* 2016;88(1):354–80.

29. Yadav K, Singh D, Rawat Singh M, Chauhan N, Minz S, Pradhan M. Nanobiomaterials as Novel Modules in the Delivery of Artemisinin and Its Derivatives for Effective Management of Malaria. In *Natural Products in Vector-Borne Disease Management*. Academic Press; 2023. pp. 447–66.

30. Parent RA. Acute toxicity of a mercapto - functional silicone oil. *Drug and Chemical Toxicology* 1979;2(3):295–307.

31. Figueiredo VM. A five-patient prospective pilot study of a polycaprolactone based dermal filler for hand rejuvenation. *Journal of Cosmetic Dermatology* 2013;12(1):73–7.

32. Cao UMN, Zhang Y, Chen J, Sayson D, Pillai S, Tran SD. Microfluidic organ-on-a-chip: A guide to biomaterial choice and fabrication. *International Journal of Molecular Sciences* 2023;24(4).

33. Geraghty RJ, Capes-Davis A, Davis JM, Downward J, Freshney RI, Knezevic I, et al. Guidelines for the use of cell lines in biomedical research. *British Journal of Cancer* 2014;111(6):1021–46.

34. Sahu KK, Kaurav M, Bhatt P, Minz S, Pradhan M, Khan J, et al. 5 - Utility of Nanomaterials in Wound Management. In: Solanki PR, Kumar A, Pratap Singh R, Singh J, Singh RB, editors. *Nanotechnological Aspects for Next-Generation Wound Management*. Academic Press; 2024. pp. 101–30. Available from: https://www.sciencedirect.com/science/article/pii/B978032399165000006X

35. Sung HJ, Meredith C, Johnson C, Galis ZS. The effect of scaffold degradation rate on three-dimensional cell growth and angiogenesis. *Biomaterials* 2004;25(26):5735–42.

36. Taylor MS, Daniels AU, Andriano KP, Heller J. Six bioabsorbable polymers: In vitro acute toxicity of accumulated degradation products. *Journal of Applied Biomaterials* 1994;5(2):151–7.

37. Yadav H, Mahalvar A, Pradhan M, Yadav K, Kumar Sahu K, Yadav R. Exploring the potential of phytochemicals and nanomaterial: A boon to antimicrobial treatment. *Medicine in Drug Discovery*. 2023;17:100151. Available from: https://www.sciencedirect.com/science/article/pii/S2590098623000015

38. Yadav R, Pradhan M, Yadav K, Mahalvar A, Yadav H. Present scenarios and future prospects of herbal nanomedicine for antifungal therapy. *Journal of Drug Delivery Science and Technology* 2022;74:103430.

39. Wu Q, Liu J, Wang X, Feng L, Wu J, Zhu X, et al. Organ-on-a-chip: Recent breakthroughs and future prospects. *Biomedical Engineering*. 2020;19(1):1–19.

40. Ding C, Chen X, Kang Q, Yan X. Biomedical Application of Functional Materials in Organ-on-a-Chip. *Frontiers in Bioengineering and Biotechnology* 2020;8(July):1–9.

41. Niculescu AG, Chircov C, Bîrcă AC, Grumezescu AM. Fabrication and applications of microfluidic devices: A review. *International Journal of Molecular Sciences* 2021;22(4):1–26.

42. Souza A, Sousa P, Castanheira EMS, Lima R. Properties and applications of PDMS for biomedical engineering: A review. *Journal of Functional Biomaterials* 2022;13:2.

43. Faustino V, Catarino SO, Lima R, Minas G. Biomedical microfluidic devices by using low-cost fabrication techniques: A review. *Journal of Biomechanics* 2016;49(11):2280–92.

44. van Meer BJ, de Vries H, Firth KSA, van Weerd J, Tertoolen LGJ, Karperien HBJ, et al. Small molecule absorption by PDMS in the context of drug response bioassays. *Biochemical and Biophysical Research Communications* 2017;482(2):323–8.

45. Lee UN, Su X, Guckenberger DJ, Dostie AM, Zhang T, Berthier E, et al. Fundamentals of rapid injection molding for microfluidic cell-based assays. *Lab on a Chip* 2018;18(3):496–504.

46. Convery N, Samardzhieva I, Stormonth-Darling JM, Harrison S, Sullivan GJ, Gadegaard N. 3D printed tooling for injection molded microfluidics. *Macromolecular Materials and Engineering* 2021;306(11):1–11.

47. Li Y, Motschman JD, Kelly ST, Yellen BB. Injection molded microfluidics for establishing high-density single cell arrays in an open hydrogel format. *Analytical Chemistry* 2020 Feb;92(3):2794–801.

48. Scott SM, Ali Z. Fabrication methods for microfluidic devices: An overview. *Micromachines (Basel)* 2021;12(3):319.

49. Al-Aqbi ZT, Yap YC, Li F, Breadmore MC. Integrated microfluidic devices fabricated in poly (Methyl methacrylate) (PMMA) for on-site therapeutic drug monitoring of amino-glycosides in whole blood. *Biosensors* 2019;9(1).

50. Jiang K, Li K, Xu G, Gong F, Wu X, Diao D, et al. A novel and flexible processing for hot embossing of glass microfluidic channels. *Ceramics International* 2021;47(1):1447–55.

51. Alapan Y, Hasan MN, Shen R, Gurkan UA. Three-dimensional printing based hybrid manufacturing of microfluidic devices. *Journal of Nanotechnology in Engineering and Medicine* 2015 May;6(2):021007.

52. Kassem T, Sarkar T, Nguyen T, Saha D, Ahsan F. 3D printing in solid dosage forms and organ-on-chip applications. *Biosensors* 2022;12(4):186.

53. Quero RF, Domingos da Silveira G, Fracassi da Silva JA, de Jesus DP. Understanding and improving FDM 3D printing to fabricate high-resolution and optically transparent microfluidic devices. *Lab on a Chip* 2021 Sep;21(19):3715–29.

54. Xenikakis I, Tzimtzimis M, Tsongas K, Andreadis D, Demiri E, Tzetzis D, et al. Fabrication and finite element analysis of stereolithographic 3D printed microneedles for transdermal delivery of model dyes across human skin in vitro. *European Journal of Pharmaceutical Sciences* 2019;137:104976.

55. Paydar OH, Paredes CN, Hwang Y, Paz J, Shah NB, Candler RN. Characterization of 3D-printed microfluidic chip interconnects with integrated O-rings. *Sensors and Actuators, A: Physical* 2014;205:199–203.

56. Keating SJ, Gariboldi MI, Patrick WG, Sharma S, Kong DS, Oxman N. 3D printed multimaterial microfluidic valve. *PLoS One* 2016;11(8):1–12.

57. Hwang Y, Paydar OH, Candler RN. 3D printed molds for non-planar PDMS microfluidic channels. *Sensors and Actuators, A: Physical* 2015;226:137–42.

58. Gowers SAN, Curto VF, Seneci CA, Wang C, Anastasova S, Vadgama P, et al. 3D printed microfluidic device with integrated biosensors for online analysis of subcutaneous human microdialysate. *Analytical Chemistry* 2015;87(15):7763–70.

59. Mandt D, Gruber P, Markovic M, Tromayer M, Rothbauer M, Adam Kratz SR, et al. Fabrication of biomimetic placental barrier structures within a microfluidic device utilizing two-photon polymerization. *International Journal of Bioprinting*. 2018;4(2):1–12.

60. Faraji Rad Z, Prewett PD, Davies GJ. High-resolution two-photon polymerization: The most versatile technique for the fabrication of microneedle arrays. *Microsystems & Nanoengineering* 2021;7(1):71.

61. Kotz F, Quick AS, Risch P, Martin T, Hoose T, Thiel M, et al. Two-photon polymerization of nanocomposites for the fabrication of transparent fused silica glass microstructures. *Advanced Materials* 2021;33(9):2006341.

62. Basiri A, Heidari A, Nadi MF, Fallahy MTP, Nezamabadi SS, Sedighi M, et al. Microfluidic devices for detection of RNA viruses. *Reviews in Medical Virology* 2021;31(1):1–11.

63. Li Z, Gu Y, Wangs L, Ge H, Wu W, Xia Q, et al. Hybrid nanoimprint-soft lithography with sub-15 nm resolution. *Nano Letters* 2009;9(6):2306–10.

64. Weigl BH, Bardell RL, Cabrera CR. Lab-on-a-chip for drug development. *Advanced Drug Delivery Reviews* 2003;55(3):349–77.

65. Huh D, Matthews BD, Mammoto A, Montoya-Zavala M, Yuan Hsin H, Ingber DE. Reconstituting organ-level lung functions on a chip. *Science* 2010;328(5986):1662–8.

66. Giannitsis AT. Biomeditsiiniliste kiiplaborite valmistamine. *Estonian Journal of Engineering* 2011;17(2):109–39.

67. Livak-Dahl E, Sinn I, Burns M. Microfluidic chemical analysis systems. *Annual Review of Chemical and Biomolecular Engineering* 2011;2(July 2011):325–53.

68. Waldbaur A, Rapp H, Länge K, Rapp BE. Let there be chip - Towards rapid prototyping of microfluidic devices: One-step manufacturing processes. *Analytical Methods* 2011;3(12):2681–716.

69. Ho CMB, Ng SH, Li KHH, Yoon YJ. 3D printed microfluidics for biological applications. *Lab on a Chip* 2015;15(18):3627–37.

70. Kitson PJ, Rosnes MH, Sans V, Dragone V, Cronin L. Configurable 3D-Printed millifluidic and microfluidic "lab on a chip" reactionware devices. *Lab on a Chip* 2012;12(18):3267–71.

71. Ho CMB, Ng SH, Li KHH, Yoon YJ. 3D printed microfluidics for biological applications. *Lab on a Chip* 2015;15(18):3627–37.

72. Choi K, Ng AHC, Fobel R, Wheeler AR. Digital microfluidics. *Annual Review of Analytical Chemistry* 2012;5(July 2019):413–40.

73. Abdelgawad M, Wheeler AR. Rapid prototyping in copper substrates for digital microfluidics. *Advanced Materials* 2007;19(1):133–7.

74. Jebrail MJ, Bartsch MS, Patel KD. Digital microfluidics: A versatile tool for applications in chemistry, biology and medicine. *Lab on a Chip* 2012;12(14):2452–63.

75. Xu X, Cai L, Liang S, Zhang Q, Lin S, Li M, et al. Digital microfluidics for biological analysis and applications. *Lab on a Chip* 2023;23(5):1169–91.

76. Abdelgawad M, Wheeler AR. Low-cost, rapid-prototyping of digital microfluidics devices. *Microfluidics and Nanofluidics* 2008;4(4):349–55.

77. Brassard D, Malic L, Normandin F, Tabrizian M, Veres T. Water-oil core-shell droplets for electrowetting-based digital microfluidic devices. *Lab on a Chip* 2008;8(8):1342–9.

78. Online VA, Wagner I, Horland R, Lauster R, Marx U, Tonevitsky G, et al. Lab on a chip skin and hair on-a-chip: In vitro skin models versus ex vivo tissue maintenance with dynamic perfusion. *Lab on a Chip* 2013;13:3555–61.

79. Abd E, Yousef SA, Pastore MN, Telaprolu K, Mohammed H, Namjoshi S, et al. Skin models for the testing of transdermal drugs. *Clinical Pharmacology: Advances and Applications* 2016;8:163–76.

80. Wagner I, Atac B, Lindner G, Horland R, Busek M, Sonntag F, et al. Skin and hair-on-a-chip: Hair and skin assembly versus native skin maintenance in a chip-based perfusion system. *BMC Proceedings* 2013;7(Suppl 6):6–7.

81. Varga-Medveczky Z, Kocsis D, Naszlady MB, Fónagy K, Erdő F. Skin-on-a-chip technology for testing transdermal drug delivery—Starting points and recent developments. *Pharmaceutics* 2021;13(11):1852.

82. Yadav K, Sahu KK, Sucheta, GSPE, Sure P, Vijayalakshmi R, et al. Biomedical applications of nanomaterials in the advancement of nucleic acid therapy: Mechanistic challenges, delivery strategies, and therapeutic applications. *International Journal of Biological Macromolecules* 2023;241:124582. Available from: https://www.sciencedirect.com/science/article/pii/S0141813023014769

83. Maschmeyer I, Lorenz AK, Schimek K, Hasenberg T, Ramme AP, Hübner J, Lindner M, Drewell C, Bauer S, Thomas A, Sambo NS. A four-organ-chip for interconnected long-term co-culture of human intestine, liver, skin and kidney equivalents. *Lab on a Chip* 2015;15(12):2688–99.

84. Sasaki N, Tsuchiya K, Kobayashi H. Photolithography-free skin-on-a-chip for parallel permeation assays. *Sensors and Materials* 2019;31(1):107–15.

85. Lee S, Jin SP, Kim YK, Sung GY, Chung JH. Construction of 3D multicellular microfluidic chip for an in vitro skin model. *Biomedical Microdevices* 2017;19:1–14.

86. Mi H, Kim K, Chan K, Yong G. Side-effect test of sorafenib using 3-D skin equivalent based on micro fl uidic skin-on-a-chip. *Journal of Industrial and Engineering Chemistry* 2019;82:71–80.

87. Lim HY, Kim J, Song HJ, Kim K, Choi KC, Park S, et al. Development of wrinkled skin-on-a-chip (WSOC) by cyclic uniaxial stretching. *Journal of Industrial and Engineering Chemistry* 2018;68:238–45.

88. Mori N, Morimoto Y. Perfusable and stretchable 3D culture system for skin-equivalent. *Biofabrication* 2019;11:01101.

89. Paquin F, Rivnay J, Salleo A, Stingelin N, Silva C. Multi-phase semicrystalline micro-structures drive exciton dissociation in neat plastic semiconductors. *Journal of Materials Chemistry C* 2015;3:10715–22.

90. Yang Y, Fathi P, Holland G, Pan D, Wang NS, Esch MB. Pumpless microfluidic devices for generating healthy and diseased endothelia. *Lab on a Chip* 2019;19(19):3212–9.

91. Wagner I, Materne EM, Brincker S, Süßbier U, Frädrich C, Busek M, et al. A dynamic multi-organ-chip for long-term cultivation and substance testing proven by 3D human liver and skin tissue co-culture. *Lab on a Chip* 2013;13(18):3538–47.

92. Kim BS, Gao G, Kim JY, Cho DW. 3D cell printing of perfusable vascularized human skin equivalent composed of epidermis, dermis, and hypodermis for better structural recapitulation of native skin. *Advanced Healthcare Materials* 2019;8(7):1–11.

93. Lee S, Jin SP, Kim YK, Sung GY, Chung JH, Sung JH. Construction of 3D multicellular microfluidic chip for an in vitro skin model. *Biomedical Microdevices* 2017;19(2):1–14.

94. Song HJ, Lim HY, Chun W, Choi KC, Sung JH, Sung GY. Fabrication of a pump-less, micro fluidic skin chip from different collagen sources. *Journal of Industrial and Engineering Chemistry* 2017;56:375–81.

95. Sriram G, Alberti M, Dancik Y, Wu B, Wu R, Feng Z, et al. Full-thickness human skin-on-chip with enhanced epidermal morphogenesis and barrier function. *Materials Today* 2018;21(4):326–40.

96. Ramadan Q, Ting FCW. In vitro micro-physiological immune-competent model of the human skin. *Lab on a Chip* 2016;16(10):1899–908.

97. Wufuer M, Lee GH, Hur W, Jeon B, Kim BJ, Choi TH, et al. Skin-on-a-chip model simulating inflammation, edema and drug-based treatment. *Scientific Reports* 2016;6(August):1–12.

98. Risueño I, Valencia L, Holgado M, Jorcano JL, Velasco D. Generation of a simplified three-dimensional skin-on-a-chip model in a micromachined microfluidic platform. *Journal of Visualized Experiments: JoVE* 2021 May;171:e62353.

11 Biomedical Applications of Microfluidics

Leena Kumari
NSHM Knowledge Campus, Kolkata, India

Barnali Maiti Sinha
Techno India University, Kolkata, India

Madhuri Baghel
Apollo College of Pharmacy, Durg, India

Kalyani Sakure
Rungta College of Pharmaceutical Sciences and Research,
Bhilai, India

Alok Singh Thakur and Hemant Badwaik
Shri Shankaracharya Institute of Pharmaceutical Science
and Research, Bhilai, India

Tapan Kumar Giri
Jadavpur University, Kolkata, India

11.1 INTRODUCTION

The implementation of engineering theories and concepts in medical sciences and biological sciences is referred to as biomedical engineering. It aims to focus on cutting-edge, modern technologies that support the advancement of therapeutic and diagnostic healthcare treatment. Among the significant applications of biomedical engineering are the bioassays development for clinical diagnostics, tissue engineering, and the fabrication of novel biomaterials for the pharmaceutical and clinical sectors. Developing physiologically accurate tissue and organ models of human beings in vitro will be extremely helpful for both basic research and pharmacological advancements. These applications benefit from the approaches enabled by microfluidics (1, 2). Microfluidic devices (MDs) have gained increasing attention over the last

DOI: 10.1201/9781032690926-11

few decades, including not only their principles but also the fabrication of devices and their utilization (3). A microchannel networking system, which has become an effective and affordable tool, and can now be used to miniaturize traditional biochemical laboratory protocols due to recent advancements in the MD. These devices contain integrated structures made up of several micro- and nano-sized integrated devices, where a variety of operations, including particle manipulation and sensing, are carried out in the platform (4). The two types of MDs are commonly known as passive and active devices. In passive/inertial MD, the effects of secondary flows, diffusion, and internal forces operate within geometry-dependent restrictions despite being quite efficient at particle manipulation and fluid mixing. In comparison to passive microfluidic chips, the restriction in active MDs requires the interaction between an external energy source and the target. For instance, only structures with magnetic qualities can be impacted by magnetic fields. Various sources of energy, including pressure fields and acoustic fields, remove manipulation constraints even in the presence of a limit between the target structure and source of energy. Over time, many biological applications have been gained from the introduction of MDs(5, 6).

Organ-on-a-chip (OOAC) systems have recently been developed by employing microfluidic chips in combination with biomimetic principles, microengineering, and cell biology (7–9). A scaffold, appropriate cellular microenvironments, and synthetic organ-level stimuli are frequently used in an OOAC to promote the development of functional tissues and organs. The diagnosis of illnesses, including infectious diseases and cancer, is one of the prospective uses of microfluidics (10, 11). Furthermore, cell manipulation, biosensors, and POCT are a few applications where microfluidics-biosensing technology has gained popularity (12). The exact control of pressures and dynamic fluids at a micrometer scale is an additional feature of microfluidics. As a result, it can offer three-dimensional (3D) scaffolds and carefully controlled microenvironments with appropriate physicochemical and biochemical stimuli when used in conjunction with microengineering methods. The development of single- or multi-organ physiologically realistic, functional models on a single chip using these cutting-edge technologies is increasingly being used for pharmaceutical applications, as well as physiological and pathological research (13). Many top-notch evaluations highlighted their developmental processes and applications by implementing microfluidic chips (1, 2). These evaluations have primarily concentrated on microfluidic technologies and their biomedical uses. The use of MDs in the biomedical field has, however, received scant attention in papers. We give a thorough summary of recent developments in microfluidic applications for biomedical engineering in this book chapter. We conclude by addressing the present difficulties and potential of microfluidics in the biomedical field.

11.2 DETECTION AND ANALYSIS OF VARIOUS DISEASES BY MICROFLUIDICS TECHNOLOGY

11.2.1 Cardiovascular Disease Detection

Cardiovascular diseases (CVDs), encompassing conditions like hypertension, heart disease, and stroke, occur due to the malfunctioning of the heart and its associated blood vessels. CVD stands as the leading global cause of premature mortality. Various factors, including social, environmental, cardiometabolic, and behavioral risks, contribute to CVD (14, 15). However, one significant risk factor for CVD is aging, which induces oxidative stress, disrupting biological processes and generating reactive oxygen species (ROS;16). Effective control of CVD is imperative for reducing mortality. Currently, clinical practice employs numerous research techniques based on biomarkers and molecular imaging (MOI). Nevertheless, there is a need for enhancement in the sensitivity, accuracy, and specificity of existing diagnostic tests for the early identification of CVD (17).

Microfluidic diagnostic devices offer mobility and swift analysis advantages. Some studies have employed specific antigens to modify microchannels for CVD biomarker detection (18–23). Several serum biomarkers, such as fibrinogen, C-reactive protein (CRP), and cardiac troponin I (cTnI), have been associated with CVD. However, current diagnostic tests are costly, time-consuming, and subject to batch-to-batch variability. Sinha and colleagues have introduced a portable MD that utilizes aptamer probes and sensor arrays comprising field-effect transistors (FETs) (24). This device swiftly and accurately detects four CVD-related biomarkers, including N-terminal pro-B-type natriuretic peptide (NT-proBNP), fibrinogen, cTnI, and CRP, using small laboratory samples. It holds promise as a POCT solution for CVD. One prevalent CVD, heart failure (HF), correlates with changes in serum NT-proBNP levels. Although an elevated heart rate pattern can indicate heart failure, current CVD screening tools are inadequate in measuring the progression of heart disease. The threshold value of the NT-proBNP biomarker remains underutilized. For example, Baker et al. have developed a microfluidic biosensor chip to monitor changes in NT-proBNP levels by labeling them with silver nanoparticles (AgNPs;25). This involves the use of flow analysis (FIA) in combination with electrochemical and laminar flow analysis (LFA) to simultaneously investigate drug-modified AgNPs. The biosensor's design facilitates accurate and user-friendly NT-proBNP testing at home with a fingerstick sample. Acute myocardial infarction (AMI) is a potentially fatal CVD event that can be challenging to identify due to symptoms that can be mistaken for other conditions. Yin et al. have presented a snail-shaped MD capable of detecting creatine kinase MB (CKMB), cTnI, and myoglobin (Myo) biomarkers for AMI diagnosis (26). They achieve this by employing microfluidic sheets with a central chemiluminescence (CL) detector and a reactive layer based on specific antibodies. As a result, they have developed a potential POCT solution for rapidly and accurately measuring three biomarkers associated with AMI.

11.2.2 Cancer Detection

Cancer, a globally prevalent and highly lethal disease, can originate in various tissues (27). The significance of early cancer detection cannot be overstated. Presently, cancer masses are diagnosed and staged through a range of techniques, such as positron emission tomography, magnetic resonance imaging, and computed tomography (10).

Given that current cancer diagnostic and treatment methods often entail exposing patients to substantial doses of chemotherapy or radiation, there is an undeniable need for innovative approaches (28).

Microfluidics presents promise in diverse biomedical applications, including POCT, DNA amplification, cell culture, and precise drug administration, which involve miniature devices and meticulous analytical methods. Chemotherapy drugs used in cancer treatment frequently result in numerous side effects. Combining imaging or localized agents with nanoparticles offers opportunities for both cancer treatment and diagnosis. To this end, MDs utilize theranostic nanoparticles (29) to monitor aspects like drug transport, drug release, treatment efficacy, tumor identification, and targeted drug delivery (30).

MD provides platforms for modeling crucial cancer processes, including apoptosis, wound healing, invasion, and metastasis. For instance, in breast cancer combination therapy, a polymeric nanoparticle drug delivery system loaded with paclitaxel and lonidamine targets EGFR (31). Another investigation by Han et al. (32) employed doxorubicin (DOX)-loaded mesoporous silica nanoparticles to create redox- and pH-sensitive devices to combat drug resistance in breast cancer. An inhalation regimen featuring cisplatin and DOX-loaded mesoporous nanoparticles, along with siRNA targeting MRP1 and BCL2, was designed to enhance lung cancer cell apoptosis and reduce resistance to lung cancer treatment (33).

Microfluidic technology facilitates the automated culture of tumor cells and has fostered the development of multicellular co-cultures and the utilization of organoids to simulate tumors (34). Notably, various MDs designed to mimic lung cancer can replicate the metastatic process (35). Additionally, through a 3D matrix MD, Nguyen et al. have harnessed electrical impedance to detect the motion of individual cancer cells (36).

11.2.3 Respiratory Infection Detection (SARS-CoV-2)

Throughout the COVID-19 pandemic, numerous microfluidics-based point-of-care (POC) detection techniques for the disease have emerged. These methods encompass various categories, including nucleic acid detection, anti-SARS-CoV-2 antibody detection, and antigen detection within MDs(37).

In a distinct research study, Ho et al. (38) devised a disposable POC digital microfluidic cartridge for real-time quantitative polymerase chain reaction (qPCR) to identify the N gene in SARS-CoV-2. This study revealed that the digital microfluidic (DMF) cartridge exhibited uniform droplet generation, consistent temperature control, and an appropriate fluorescence readout, enabling qPCR POCT. Paper-based MDs have also made recent appearances in this context. Akarapipad et al. (39) employed a paper-based MD for the convenient and straightforward detection of SARS-CoV-2 in saliva samples. Flow profile analysis provided a means to assess the infection level. A smartphone was utilized to measure particle-target immunoagglutination within the channel, enabled by changes in capillary flow velocity and surface tension. Similarly, Kim et al. (40) demonstrated the direct capture of airborne droplets on a paper MD in less than 30 minutes, from collection to assay, without requiring additional equipment. This innovative approach was based on aerosolizing 10% of human saliva samples infected with SARS-CoV-2 to create liquid droplets and aerosols. The quantification of immunoagglutinated particles on the paper microchip was achieved through a smartphone-based fluorescence microscope, after introducing antibody-conjugated particles into the paper channel. Consequently, a portable and cost-effective method for detecting SARS-CoV-2 directly from the air was established.

11.2.4 GENETIC DISORDERS DETECTION

The link between local irregularities or mutations within the nucleotide sequence encoded in an organism's DNA and a wide range of diseases and disorders is growing increasingly evident. Even a minor alteration in the sequence can have a significant impact on the structure and function of the resulting expressed proteins, often leading to adverse effects on health. Identifying the pathways through which genomics can contribute to disease offers the potential for a revolution in medicine by enabling the rapid and cost-effective detection of these sequence changes using small samples and reagent volumes (41, 42).

These ambitious goals are becoming more feasible due to ongoing advancements in microfluidic technology, which leverages various photolithography-based fabrication techniques originally developed for the semiconductor industry. These processes enable the creation of miniature lab-on-a-chip (LOC) systems capable of conducting a variety of chemical and biological analytical assays precisely where the data are most needed. The ability to produce hundreds or even thousands of these devices simultaneously enhances the potential for transformative developments in the field of medicine.

11.2.4.1 Scanning Techniques for Mutation Analysis Using MDs

11.2.4.1.1 Analysis of Single-Strand Conformations

Tian and their research team employed capillary electrophoresis (CE) microchips to investigate mutations linked to the human *BRCA1* and *BRCA2* genes associated with breast cancer (43). The process involved amplifying 60–80 ng of genomic DNA using primers labeled with fluorescence and targeting three mutations. This was followed by testing the amplified product using microchip capillary electrophoresis. The amplification was conducted through 35 cycles off-chip using a benchtop thermal cycler with a reaction volume of 50 µl, and 1 µl of the product was introduced into the gel of a CE wafer loaded with 2% hydroxyethylcellulose (HEC). Fragment observation occurred within 120 seconds, focusing on fragments with lengths between 200 and 400 bp.

11.2.4.1.2 Assessment of Heteroduplexes

Tian and colleagues also explored six heterozygous mutations through microchip-based electrophoresis (44). In this approach, 40–80 ng of genomic template DNA was subjected to off-chip PCR using reaction volumes of 50 µl. Subsequently, the results were loaded into glass electrophoresis chips equipped with an HEC sieving matrix. The fragments produced were efficiently separated in less than 8 minutes and ranged in size from 100 to 400 bp. In later research, efforts were made to optimize the sieving matrix to enhance separation performance (45).

11.3 MDS FOR RAPID AND POC DIAGNOSTICS

The development of rapid POC diagnostic devices is certainly required for different types of life-threatening diseases, which can either be transmittable (HIV, influenza, hepatitis, etc.) or nontransmittable (CVD, diabetes, cancer, etc.). Conventional diagnostic techniques such as enzyme-linked immunosorbent assay (ELISA), PCR, and other immunoassays are involved with the cell culturing of pathogens and a large number of sample preparation processes, etc. with the consumption of too much time. Modern technology can help to avoid such problems in the diagnostic process by microfluidic techniques which include all the steps of sample preparation, assay procedure, identification, and analytical work in a single chip (46–48). The different types of MD are depicted in Figure 11.1.

11.3.1 PDMS-Based MD

PDMS is a low-price polymer, largely used for the development of MD. In this, patterns of channel carving are done by the soft lithography method (49). The initial template of PDMS MD made in a dust-free area makes it inexpensive and convenient to manufacture by unceasing copy and production. Its 2D structures made it limited

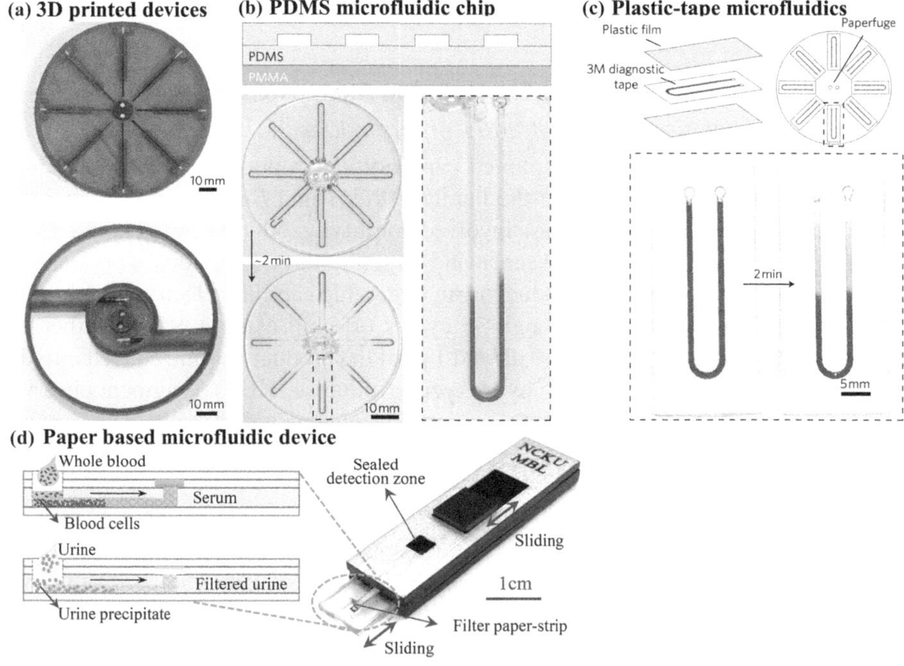

FIGURE 11.1 Different types of MD. Adopted with permission from (58, 59).

to use, where fluid is required to flow in stereoscopic space (50). Nowadays, the thermoplastic elastomer is used to make microchannels over PDMS, since elastomer is cheap and convenient for large-scale production of MDs (51).

11.3.2 Paper-Based MDs

Due to its low cost, rapid and easy analytical operation, it has become a popular diagnostic tool in medium- and low-resource areas (52). The microchannels drawn with wax printing on paper-based microfluidics give it good fluid flow control over the other MDs. The various biological fluids (viz. urine, blood plasma, saliva, etc.) base analysis makes a useful POC diagnostic tool for different diseases. Diagnosis of acute myocardial infarction with the help of cardiac biomarker detection (19) and dry-eye problems by the detection of electrolytes in tears (53) are some useful examples to prove the significance of paper-based MD. However, the detection of complex samples is difficult to analyze with precision by this technique.

11.3.3 3D-Printed MDs

These technologies are more automated which helps to eliminate the manual errors that may occur in the manufacturing MDs by other technologies. The scientific community has confidence in this technology to develop MDs since it simulates the actual flow of fluid and has a wide range of advantages, including low cost, quick production, high resolution, and huge commercial potential (54–56). A prototype device inbuilt MD developed by the 3D-printing method is already in the market to detect the Zika virus, which is based on the saliva sample-based reverse-transcription loop-mediated isothermal amplification technology (57). Three-dimensional-printing-based MDs would revolutionize underdeveloped areas around the world in the field of diagnostic tool development.

11.3.4 Mobile Sensors Based on Integrated MD and Smartphones

The combination of MD and smartphones is an inclusive idea for the use of mobile sensing methods. This technology is known as MS^2. In underdeveloped and remote areas, this technique could play a noteworthy role in the diagnosis of therapeutic ailments (60–62) For example, different markers present in urine are useful for the detection of diseases. These markers develop color complexes with reagent paper combined with MDs. The smartphone camera detects the color change in the complex of reagents and urine markers, which are properly identified by specifically designed algorithms in smartphones (63). Besides the promising values, reliability, and reproducible results of MS^2 technology, many challenges are ahead with complex detection methods that need the additional contribution of other equipment with MS^2 techniques.

11.3.5 Based on Dielectrophoresis Technology

Dielectrophoresis (DEP) is an electrical phenomenon-based technology that consumes very small samples (micro or nano L) and reagents for detection or diagnosis. Both the bacteria and cells like dielectric and charged particles are processed at the same time in DEP. In this technology suspension and medium are in relative motion under uneven electric field. This motion is forced by dielectrophoretic force (64). From the point of view of a blood sample–based diagnosis, DEP is a very useful technique as the dielectric electrophoresis differentiator has been developed for the separation of blood cells (65).

11.4 DEVELOPMENT OF OOAC DEVICES FOR DRUG SCREENING, TOXICITY TESTING, AND PERSONALIZED MEDICINE

In vitro cell-culture platforms and in vivo animal models are frequently employed in current physiological and pathological research. In vivo, animal models do, however, have drawbacks, including challenging analysis, problematic usage, and doubts regarding their biological applicability to individuals. Platforms for in vitro cell culture are not able to effectively predict physiological responses because they are unable to mimic organ–organ and tissue–tissue interactions. The use of the current in vitro and in vivo models is constrained by these drawbacks. Therefore, as low-cost replacements to these earlier models, OOAC platforms that combine 3D tissue-engineered constructions with microfluidic network systems are being proposed (66, 67). When biophysical and biological signals are included, the micro-scale system more accurately simulates in vivo cell–microenvironment communications in vitro than two-dimensional cell culture models. Owing to the ethical issues and poor replication of human pathophysiology in two-dimensional cell culture and animal models, OOAC systems can replace these methods (68). OOAC systems have been widely used in the past few decades to mimic the physiological microenvironment of numerous organs, including the liver (69, 70), lung (71, 72), gut (73–75), kidney (76, 77), heart (78, 79), brain (80, 81), and bone (82–84). Various OOAC systems have been discussed as follows.

11.4.1 LIVER-ON-A-CHIP

Non-alcoholic fatty liver disease (NAFLD), one of the illnesses with the greatest rate of growth in the world, makes the liver-on-a-chip model urgently necessary (85). In order to accurately research NAFLD, Du et al. created a microfluidic-based liver lobule chip (LC), which offered a platform for the co-culturing of hepatic cells (86). The LC platform used a dual blood supply from the hepatic artery (HA) and hepatic portal vein (HPV) to produce liver microtissue that mimics in vivo organs. For the early stages of NAFLD progression, the lipid zonation was changed while the NAFLD was exposed to nutritional sources. A research work conducted by Lee et al. (87) resulted in the fabrication of a gut-liver chip to mimic hepatic steatosis. In a different study, the OOAC platforms were put to the test to look into the toxicological profile of the medicinal agent and its metabolites in the process of developing new drugs. A pumpless heart/liver-on-a-chip (HLC) MD was designed by Soltantabar et al. to investigate the cardiotoxicity of the drug DOX (88). The remarkable vitality of HepG2 hepatocellular carcinoma cells and H9c2 rat cardiomyocytes was explained by the HLC platform. In comparison to three-dimensional static culture, this system was particularly effective at monitoring the damage to heart cells. As a result, the established HLC platform may prove to be a useful tool for researching cardiotoxicity in the heart. A unique adipose-on-chip (AOC) disease model was created by Leung et al. to replicate adipose tissue hypertrophy and inflammation in the presence of high levels of free fatty acid (FFA) (89). Oleic and palmitic acids were used to start inflammation in adipocytes via hypertrophic lipid droplets, replicating the disease model. The created model provided a fresh approach to researching metabolic illnesses linked to obesity.

11.4.2 LUNG-ON-A-CHIP

The alveoli network is essential for accurately simulating the physiological characteristics of the lung in vitro since it is challenging to replicate the air-blood barrier in lung-on-a-chip platforms. In order to duplicate an array of alveoli, Zamprogno et al. created a lung-on-a-chip platform. Because the lung extracellular matrix (ECM) contains proteins like collagen, elastin, and others, this system has the advantages of elasticity and biodegradability in the biological membrane (90). Utilizing alveolar epithelial cells and primary human lung endothelial, the platform displayed an effective model demonstration for prolonged air-blood barrier functioning and proposed a cutting-edge method to recreate biological barriers of the organs. Additionally, the lung-on-a-chip platform investigated by Zhu et al. (91) demonstrated favorable biomimetic breathing of human lungs with microphysiological breathing monitoring.

11.4.3 GUT-ON-A-CHIP

In order to accurately research the physiology and pathophysiology of the gut milieu and to dynamically imitate it, three-dimensional models are needed. By using multiple intestinal cell types to imitate the in vivo architecture of the gut and consistently perfused microchannels, gut-on-a-chip (GoC) devices are advantageous for simulating gut dynamics (75). In order to better understand pathogenic disorders, an effective examination of microbial pathogenicity mechanisms in the immunocompetent intestinal microenvironment was conducted. To study intestinal permeability outside of the body, Amirabadi and his associates developed the intestinal explant barrier chip (IEBC) (92). In order to explore the intestinal absorption of therapies in a dynamic milieu with tiny nonspecific binding of therapeutic molecules, the innovative platform included explants of human and pig intestinal colon tissue in separate microchannels. The aforementioned MD might be modified for use in drug testing on the skin or in the liver, among other organs. To research epithelial cell differentiation in vitro, Jeon et al. created the GoC platform (93). Additionally, the functioning of the intestinal epithelial barrier was examined while the injured epithelium layer was co-cultured, and probiotics that subsequently encouraged the restoration of barrier functioning were observed with the aid of the human microbiome without bacterial overgrowth. By simulating the intestinal lumen's immunological tolerance with characteristics of mucosal macrophages and dendritic cells, Maurer et al. created an intestine-on-a-chip platform to explore microbial interactions in the gut microbiota (94).

11.4.4 Kidney-on-a-Chip

The most important component of a kidney is the glomerulus, which filters blood on a regular basis by utilizing a capillary network and unique cells known as podocytes. Therefore, it is essential to imitate the glomerulus in order to study kidney physiology and disorders. In order to obtain a genetically matched tissue profile, Roye et al. conceived and demonstrated a personalized glomerulus chip that uses human-induced pluripotent stem cells (hiPSCs)-differentiated nephron progenitor cells and vascular endothelial cells (VECs) from a single patient to mimic glomerulus barrier function (95). In another instance, Lee et al. (96) developed the kidney OOAC platform to examine the biochemical impact on the in vitro development of human kidney organoids produced from human pluripotent stem cells (hPSCs). The results showed that the glomerulus chip generated potential outcomes to reproduce functional glomerulus and glomerulus-related disorders. A disease model was also developed to study the glomerulus injury.

11.4.5 Heart-on-a-Chip

The foundational components for developing heart-on-chip devices are differentiated cardiomyocytes (CMs) from hPSCs. However, the adult myocardium claims that the immaturity of hPSC CMs makes it tough to replicate cardiac disease and physiology precisely (97). A unique heart-on-chip platform was created by Zhang et al. (98) to address the immaturity of hPSCs and CMs. The long-term dynamic culture of hPSCs-CMs was made possible by the MD, and the development of CMs to mimic native heart tissue was monitored in real time while being electrically stimulated.

11.4.6 Brain-on-a-Chip

Many scientists have attempted to replicate the physiology of human tissue on an artificial platform ever since the development of OOAC. Brain function depends on structural connections and cell-cell interactions in the case of brain tissue. Brain-on-a-chip is a recently developed technology that aims to replicate the anatomical and functional characteristics of brain tissue on a miniature constructed substrate (99). In order to distinguish seizure-like activity, Pelkonen et al. introduced a microfluidic platform for epilepsy modeling (100). This platform includes a microelectrode array (MEA). hPSCs and differentiated neurons were used to create functioning neural networks, and kainic acid (KA) therapy on neuronal networks was used to replicate seizure-like behavior. Numerous studies have shown that the gut environment might affect the brain's neurocognitive capabilities, and exosomes may also be able to control signaling in the gut–brain axis (GBA). To research the communication between the stomach and the brain, Kim et al. created a GBA-on chip (101). These microchips replicated the co-culture of brain endothelial and gut endothelial cells by including the blood–brain barrier (BBB) and gut barrier. Trans-endothelial/epithelial electrical resistance (TEER) was used to test the integrity of the barriers, and after treatment with lipopolysaccharides (LPSs) or butyrate which ultimately led to an inflammatory response in the gut-brain axis and affected the permeability of the BBB changes in the barriers were seen.

11.5 ENGINEERING OF FUNCTIONAL TISSUES AND SCAFFOLDS FOR REGENERATIVE MEDICINE

The restoration or improvement of tissue function is the main interest of tissue engineering which is an amalgamation of life science and engineering principles (102). This technique uses cells with the ability to tissue formation, scaffolds to fill tissue voids, and growth-responsible factors to regenerate tissues or supplant damaged tissues, while other techniques like immunomodulation, cellular therapy, or gene therapy when matched with tissue engineering are known as regenerative medicine (103–105). This technique mainly focuses on the usage of porous scaffolds that are suited to serve the tissue or organ regeneration condition. Scaffold matrices are a kind of template for growing tissues with the help of cell seeds and different growth factors. Sometimes bioreactors or other chemical and mechanical stimulus devices can also be used (106). These cultured scaffolds are rooted in injured tissue sites or can be used in vitro for synthetic tissues.

11.5.1 PROPERTIES REQUIRED FOR THE DESIGN OF SCAFFOLDS

11.5.1.1 Biocompatibility

The biocompatibility of a scaffold is an essential property. The adherence of the cell and its normal biological function after reaching to surface for proliferation is a characteristic of the scaffold matrix. The incompatibility of the scaffold may induce an immunological inflammatory response, which may lead to the rejection of the scaffold before its normal function.

11.5.1.2 Biodegradability

After the start of the development of normal body cells, the scaffold implants must be replaced, and the by-product should undergo degradation without causing any toxicity followed by excretion from the body. The presence of immunological compatibility and macrophage scavenging properties help the tissue-engineered construct to be used clinically in a more generous way (107, 108).

11.5.1.3 Mechanical Property

The scaffold must be mechanically strong enough so that during complicated procedures like orthopedics or cardiovascular surgery, it retains its integrity up to the remodeling (109). The in-vitro successful scaffolds are still struggling for their *in-vivo* reliability due to inconsistent vascularization. The permeable structure and mechanical strength equilibrium can serve suitability to vascularization that occurs after cell infiltration.

11.5.1.4 Structure of Scaffold

The highly interconnected porous structure of cell-cultured scaffold allows the penetration of nutrition to extracellular matrix formed by as well as their waste disposal. Regarding the design of the scaffold, the issue of degradation of the core, which occurs due to the absence of blood vessels and waste clearance from the center of tissue-produced constructions, is a major hurdle. The surface modification by various techniques generates the different chemical ligands peripherally and facilitates the binding of different cell structures to the scaffold. The accessible surface inside a pore to which cells can cling governs the density of the ligand. It depends on the mean pore size of the scaffold. Hence, the size of the pores should be large enough to permit the migration of the cell into the structure, and tiny enough to exhibit a low ligand density and high specific surface that leads to significant binding of a required number of cells to the scaffold (110).

11.5.2 CELLS USED IN TISSUE ENGINEERING

The cells used for the in vitro matrices development which meet the inherent tissue property of the host are very important to avoid the rejection of the scaffold. The ideal cell source can be targeted patients for implantation, which has certain limitations of invasion of disease with the cells used for seeding of the scaffold. To avoid such risk other sources of cells have been considered nowadays.

11.5.2.1 Embryonic Stem Cells

The embryonic stem (ES) cell bank or cloning can be a useful source for populating tissues of required properties. The advantage of ES cells is the survival for a prolonged cultural period that also helps grow the large population of cells to develop tissues. The major challenge in the selection of ES cells is to control their differentiating property, which has been already proved in ES cells of teratoma, to manage the differentiation of cells to the required tissue lineage (111). The bone marrow–mesenchymal stem cells (BM-MSC) protocols are normally used for the differentiation of ES cells that can be expressed for the feature of mineral collection in bone (112).

11.5.2.2 Bone Marrow–Derived Mesenchymal Stem Cells

For the development of osteogenic lineage, BM-MSC-type stem cells are used, which accelerate the repair of bone and cartilage. These cells can be isolated from the fibroblastic units containing bone marrow-associated colonies. The bone marrow cells of the required group can be isolated by different antibody selection procedures, such as Endoglin (113) and STRO-1 (114). Thus, the cells separated from the marrow used as filler for some critical bone defects, which are normally considered difficult to heal.

11.5.2.3 Cord-Derived Mesenchymal Stem Cells

The umbilical cord blood mesenchymal stem cells (UC-MSCs) are presently having great research interest for their gene expression. During the research, it was found the similarity of UC-MSCs similarity with BM-MSCs in gene expression profiles for differentiating in osteoblasts, hepatocytes, and adipocytes (115–117).

11.5.3 TECHNIQUES USED IN TISSUE ENGINEERING AND REGENERATIVE MEDICINE

The progression of tissue engineering and different newer techniques like 3D printing and microfluidics are milestones in designing scaffolds. Genomic engineering is very often used to generate cells for tissue engineering. Further, the development of whole organs and different types of bioreactors are some useful options along with the OOAC and microfluidics technique.

11.5.3.1 3D Printing

For the construction of tissue-engineered material like skin tissue, bioprinting is an efficient technique. It uses biomolecules and pattern cells for designing copies of tissue constructs. Extrusion and laser droplet bioprinting are some methods used for the 3D printing of hydrogels, cells, and growth factors. By using bioink, stem cells like MSCs with significant osteogenic activity have been developed. Furthermore, the human skin model associated with polycaprolactone (PCL)construct to develop proper mature skin is a good example of bio-printing (118).

11.5.3.2 Genome Engineering

Advancements in genomic engineering have given the opportunity for the alteration of gene sequences in cells. Direct genomic alteration was now possible through the CRISPR/Cas system (119). Through this technique, functional genetic variants of benefit can be systemically dissected. The Cas9 system was considered very precise for multiple gene activation and noncoding RNA activation. The unpredicted mutation and physiological changes could be life-threatening for the patient, which is a major concern with the CRISPR/Cas system. To improve safety, CRISPR/Cas9 delivery system comprising PEGylated nanoparticles based on poly (g-4-((2-(piperidin-1-yl) ethyl)aminomethyl)benzyl-L-glutamate) for delivering Cas9 expression plasmid and sgRNA was reported (120).

11.5.3.3 Microfluidics

The variety of microfluidic techniques allows the encapsulation of the cell in microfibers, or microcapsules, as in MDs, different structures like hollows, grooves, and others are available. A group of scientists has developed microfibers by injection capillary microfluidics or spindle-knot-structured microfibers by the same technique (121). Capillary array microfluidic technique, used for the construction of controlled macropores and heterogeneous microstructure. Thus, the micro-carrier with cell encapsulations may be used for similar acts as natural tissues. Some examples like alginate-based hydrogel microfiber as blood-vessel-on-chip to copy the natural swirling blood flow or E. coli encapsulation by micro-droplets are some effective examples of microfluidic technique in tissue engineering.

11.5.4 OOAC

It has proven difficult to bridge the knowledge gap between 3D tissue culture conditions in vivo and discoveries in 2D cell culture in vitro. OOAC is now possible by using MDs and 3D printing. Many organs got mimicked like the BBB, umbilical vein endothelial cells, neural cells, and so on by microfluidic technique. In a different study, scientists used a microfluidic platform to replicate natural biological processes. With this platform, they were able to spatially manage the co-culture of endothelial cells with stromal fibroblasts or cancer cells. Furthermore, a group of scientists has developed a vascular structure with a macrochannel based on 3D hydrogel using OOAC devices (122–124).

11.5.4.1 Design and Manufacturing of Scaffold

It is important to develop some reproducible methods for the fabrication of scaffolds. Biodegradable polymers, such as polylactic acid (PLA), are commonly used, however, the final scaffold properties may be tailored based on how these polymers are handled and what additives are applied during manufacture. Here, some scaffold types are discussed. For tissue engineering methods, hydrolyzable polymers that offer a controlled drug release and degradation, such as poly-hydroxyl acids like PLA and poly lactic-co-glycolic acid (PLGA) are often used. Materials having specialized properties suitable for use in tissue engineering matrices may be developed by the careful use of molecular weights, cross-links, and side chains.

11.5.4.2 Injectable Materials Used in TERM

The "Injectabone," a biodegradable novel scaffold useful in bone trauma, is injected into the site (125). Using two different types of PLGA, a dynamic scaffold was designed that permits the injected scaffold to solidify at body temperature to cure non-union bone deformity with a noninvasive delivery form. The adherent or temperature and moisture-sensitive systems are some options that make microparticles a good candidate for delivering injectable scaffolds. Apart from the incorporation of drugs, live cells can also be uploaded into this system for making injectable scaffolds with homogenously distributed cells.

11.5.4.3 Growth Factor Inclusion Into Scaffolds

The scaffolds can be utilized to distribute drugs or growth factors to the areas that need repair to accelerate the healing process. Some of the factors, namely, the kinetics of growth factor release from scaffold matrices, function, and conformation of protein within scaffold construction; need to be considered during the scaffold design. Kanczler et al. attempted the inclusion of vascular endothelial growth factor in PLA constructs for angiogenic signal's control release from scaffold construct. The attachment of basic fibroblastic growth factors (bFGFs) with the anime group on the surface of alginate beads; is an example of another approach for incorporation of growth factor. Thus, the surface attachment of bFGFs serves as the microenvironment facility for culturing and proliferation of human neuronal stem cells in scaffolds before its use in tissue engineering. Incorporating DNA plasmids encoding a gene and a mammalian promoter into the polymer is an alternative to growth factor incorporation, thus transfection of DNA, facilitating the growth of their factors (126).

11.5.4.4 Custom Scaffolds Production

Custom 3D printing utilizing a laser stereolithography technique has built scaffolds for specific persons. This makes it possible to construct the scaffold using computed 3D data obtained from patient scans or computer simulations (127). This method is a prototype procedure in which particles are layered by sintered fusion to produce a custom scaffold. Other than the sintered procedure, gel fusion and cell bead systems can also be used for 3D printing (128). A flexible polymer, poly(1,8-octanediolco-citric acid), incorporated scaffold is suitable to mimic the inherent quality like flexibility for the mode of action of host tissues (129).

11.5.4.5 Scaffold Surface Modification

By using the charged gas plasma polymerization deposition technique, surface modification of the scaffold can be done which allows the control areas where cells will attach and proliferate. The chemical manipulation involves the plasma polymerized allyl amine deposition giving significant adherence property to the scaffold surface for the cell. As 3D materials like tissue engineering scaffolds are easily penetrated by plasma, it is possible to alter the characteristics of the scaffolds or the attachment of cells by creating gradients of surface chemistries by putting down low to high cell adhesion zones. The plasma polymerized hexane, which is a kind of cell adhesion repellent, may be used on the surface which facilitates the cell transfer from the less-adherent outer layer to the more-adherent inner core This allows some rectification of the conventional cell attachment that occurs largely to the surface of scaffolds (130).

11.6 MICROFLUIDIC PLATFORMS FOR HIGH-THROUGHPUT SCREENING

The amalgamation of microfluidics and high throughput screening (HTS) has revolutionized the landscape of scientific research and technological innovation. Microfluidics, rooted in the manipulation of minute fluid volumes within microscale channels, offers a powerful platform for conducting experiments with enhanced precision, reduced reagent consumption, and unprecedented levels of control (131). HTS, by comparison, entails the rapid and systematic screening of large compound libraries or biomolecules to identify candidates with desired properties (132). The integration of microfluidics and HTS yields a synergistic synergy, enabling the seamless exploration of diverse assays and an array of applications that transcend traditional boundaries.

11.6.1 Microfluidic Platforms for Enhanced HTS

Diverse microfluidic platforms serve as the canvas upon which high throughput screening endeavors unfold. These platforms encompass microchips, droplet-based systems, micro-well arrays, and more, each offering unique advantages and tailored functionalities (133–137). Different types of microfluidic platforms are nicely discussed by Zhou et al. (133) and represented in Figure 11.2.

11.6.1.1 Microarray

Microarray is a key microfluidic technology that incorporates a large number of separate reactors on a single substrate. Furthermore, each reactor is micro-scaled, with capacities ranging from nanoliters to picoliters. It enables the simultaneous testing of numerous parameters by running tens to hundreds of thousands of tests. Each batch contains thousands of trials. Zhang and colleagues created a hydrogel microarray (Figure 11.2a) in which 2000 unique microgels with varied bioactivities were routinely printed on a typical microscope slide, resulting in a high-throughput

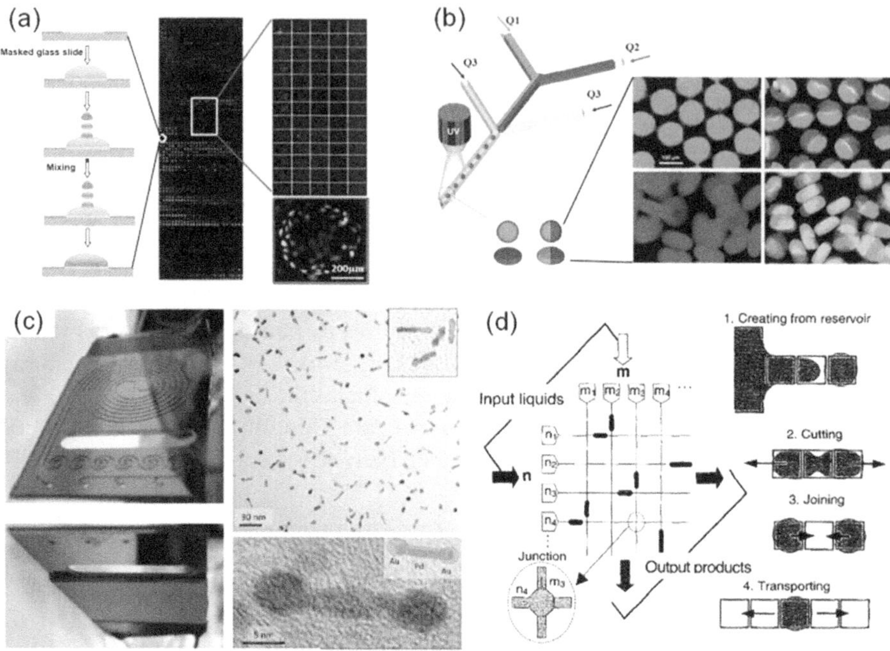

FIGURE 11.2 (a) A typical microarray-based high-throughput platform (HTP). (b) A microdroplet-based HTP representation. (c) Au-Pd dumbbell nanoparticles were created using a typical continuous-flow microfluidic setup. (d) A digital microfluidic circuit, as well as the four basic droplet activities of producing, cutting, joining, and transporting. (Adopted from (133).)

platform (HTP) for rapidly screening desirable polymers with thermal-responsive characteristics (134).

11.6.1.2 Microdroplet

Despite the increase in throughput, microarray-based HTPs remain restricted in many applications where improved screening efficiency is required. To solve the problem, microdroplet technology has gained popularity and has been developed for high-throughput screens (138). Microfluidic droplet chips are classified as either continuous (Figure 11.2b, Figure 11.2c) (139–143) or digital (Figure 11.2d) (144–146). Shepherd's group developed a continuous MD (Figure 11.2b) for producing monodisperse colloid-filled hydrogel particles of various shapes and compositions (135). Jensen et al. have developed a novel technique for producing Au-Pd dumbbell-like nanostructures with good electrocatalytic activity (136). To regulate the development of Au on both sides of Pd nanorods, this device was combined with a sequential-addition microfluidic reactor and an ultrasonic (Figure 11.2c). The continuous microfluidic chip, as the primary platform of microdroplet technology, can manufacture monodisperse droplets (typically nano- or picoliters) at extremely high rates (tens to thousands of droplets per second;147, 148).

11.6.2   APPLICATIONS OF MICROFLUIDICS IN **HTS**

Microfluidic HTS transcends a multitude of applications spanning drug discovery, genomics, proteomics, and beyond (149). Detailed applications are tabulated in Table 11.1.

TABLE 11.1

Applications of Microfluidics in HTS

S.No.	Application	Key Features	References
1	Drug Discovery	Miniaturized assays, High throughput screening of compound libraries, Reduced reagent consumption, Precise control of reaction conditions	(150–152)
2	Cell-Based Assays	High content analysis on a single chip, Parallel screening of cellular responses, Real-time observation of cell behavior	(153, 154)
3	Genomic Analysis	Parallel analysis of DNA/RNA samples, Single-cell analysis capabilities, Efficient amplification and analysis of genetic material	(149)
4	Proteomic Profiling	Multiplexed assays for protein analysis, Enhanced sensitivity and resolution, Reduction in sample volume	(132)
5	Diagnostics	Rapid and sensitive detection of biomarkers, POCT applications, and Integration with sensors for real-time monitoring	(131, 152)
6	Pharmacokinetics Studies	Rapid evaluation of drug metabolism, Analysis of pharmacokinetic parameters, Reduced sample requirement	(151)
7	Pathogen Detection	High sensitivity and specificity, Multiplexed detection of pathogens, Integration with nucleic acid amplification	(155)
8	Enzyme Assays	Precise control over reaction conditions, High-throughput enzyme activity screening, Accurate kinetic measurements	(153)
9	Toxicity Screening	Assessment of compound toxicity, Real-time monitoring of cellular responses, Integration with viability assays	(150)
10	Phenotypic Screening	Parallel analysis of cellular phenotypes, High-resolution imaging within microchannels, Real-time tracking of phenotypic changes	(154)
11	Biomolecular Interaction Studies	Label-free analysis of biomolecular interactions, Real-time monitoring of binding kinetics, High sensitivity and throughput	(156)
12	Chemical Library Screening	High throughput analysis of chemical libraries, Screening for drug candidates and compounds, Rapid identification of bioactive molecules	(157)

(Continued)

TABLE 11.1
(Continued)

S.No.	Application	Key Features	References
13	Personalized Medicine	Patient-specific diagnostic and therapeutic approaches, Tailored treatment strategies, Precision medicine advancements	(158)
14	Biochemical Assays	Study of enzymatic reactions and kinetics, Quantitative analysis of biochemical processes, High sensitivity and reduced reagent consumption	(159)
15	Stem Cell Research	Manipulation and analysis of stem cells, Investigation of differentiation pathways, High-throughput screening of stem cell behavior	(160)
16	Neuroscience Studies	Analysis of neuronal activity and connectivity, High-resolution imaging of neuronal processes, Drug screening for neurological disorders	(161)
17	Environmental Monitoring	Detection of pollutants and contaminants, On-chip analysis of environmental samples, Real-time monitoring of water and air quality	(162)

11.7 CONTROLLED DRUG DELIVERY SYSTEMS USING MD

The development of drug delivery techniques, an area of critical importance to clinical treatment and healthcare, has received a lot of attention in recent years. These approaches are designed to increase the drug's specificity and bioavailability, lessen its cytotoxicity, and provide patient compliance. Numerous drug carriers have been developed utilizing advances in nanotechnology to encapsulate pharmaceuticals and therapeutic biomolecules for controlled and targeted drug delivery (163). These carriers ought to be stimuli-responsive, targeted, biocompatible, and degradable. Additionally, they must prevent early degradation, regulate the rate of release, improve absorption and bioavailability, and minimize side effects (164). For dependable and manageable drug delivery, monodispersed drug carriers with regulated physical and chemical properties are crucial.

To produce particles of a specific size, the layer-by-layer assembly utilizes the benefits of the electrostatic interaction of polyelectrolytes with opposing charges (165). However, since the particles and emulsified-droplet size can be quite heterogeneous with bulk mixing, drug carriers produced using these procedures have substantial polydispersity and batch-to-batch variance. These techniques also have strict processing requirements and are ineffective in continuous manufacturing, both of which severely restrict their use. Microfluidic technologies are now being used as an alternative for developing monodispersed and multifunctional drug carriers with regulated physical and chemical properties. These technologies provide the advantages of a homogeneous reaction environment, reliable and precise fluid control, high surface-to-volume ratios, improved mass and heat transfer, and miniaturization (166). Furthermore, they allow for real-time process control and fine-tuning, which improves processing precision and effectiveness. Self-assembled carriers and droplet-based particle carriers are only two examples of the numerous drug carriers that have been fabricated, all with different dimensions and shapes.

Self-assembled carriers are typically produced utilizing microfluidic hydrodynamic flow-focusing devices. The continuous phase of a miscible buffer concentrates the surfactant mixture-containing dispersed phase. Diffusive mixing at the boundary between the two miscible phases produces nanoscale carriers, which precipitate downstream of the channel (167). The geometry of the microchannels, the fluids' diffusivity, and their flow rates all influence the diffusive mixing time, which controls the size of the carriers (168). Self-assembly has been used to synthesize lipid-based nanocarriers (169, 170), polymeric carriers (171), and lipid–polymer hybrid carriers (172). Additionally, DNA nanocomplexes like lipoplex or polyplex have been developed for siRNA or DNA gene delivery (173). Self-assembled carriers produced by flow-focusing MD are more effectively transfected than bulk-mixed carriers because of their highly homogeneous size distribution (174).

Due to their clear advantages in precisely controlling and reliably producing monodisperse single- or multiple-emulsion droplets, micro/nanoparticles produced through MD become great choices for DDSs (175). Monodispersed particles from a variety of biocompatible materials have been developed by microfluidics with the appropriate characteristics and capabilities for the delivery of both hydrophilic and hydrophobic drugs. The biocompatible materials include polymers (e.g., PLGA, poly(N-isopropylacrylamide) [PNIPAAm]), poly(ethylene glycol) (PEG), PLA, chitosan, alginate, and pectin.

Nanoparticles with PLGA cores and lipid shells have been fabricated with the aid of a multistage co-flow microfluidic system (176). Due to the presence of the lipid shells, which improve cellular uptake of the resulting core–shell nanoparticles, a hydrophobic drug is successfully loaded into the nanoparticles. In addition, hydrophilic drugs like siRNA and DOX can be effectively entrapped and then delivered to target cells for particular therapeutic applications. These nanoparticles are uniform and rigid and have more complex structures (water core/PLGA shell/lipid outer layer) that have been successfully produced by microfluidics (177). New all-aqueous multiphase microfluidics techniques have been researched for the preparation of polyelectrolyte microcapsules, liposome, and protein fibril microcapsules without the use of organic solvents, allowing for high-efficiency encapsulation and bioactivity retention of the encapsulated biomolecules (178, 179). As a result of molecular diffusion and matrix swelling/degradation, the majority of existing DDSs typically exhibit either burst or sustained drug release characteristics; nevertheless, for certain therapeutic applications, programmable on-demand release becomes essential. Functional DDSs, such as core–shell nanoparticles with pH-sensitive Eudragit shell and microcapsules of PLGA that have distinct degradation rates and varying shell thickness, have been formulated by microfluidics to meet these requirements, realizing pH- and mechano-responsive releases of drugs for the enhanced repair of musculoskeletal tissues and oral delivery of chemotherapeutics to colons, respectively (180). Moreover, utilizing water-oil-water-oil-water (W/O/W/O/W) quadruple-emulsion droplets as templates, numerous medicines can be controllably released from multicompartment microcapsules created on an MD (181). Ultra-thin polymer shells separate the several water-phased compartments of the microcapsules. The programmed release of the many drugs that are enclosed can be managed by adjusting the various compositions of the polymeric shells. Multiphase microfluidics can be used to produce hydrogel microfibers that allow for the controlled encapsulation and release of pharmaceuticals, such as antibacterial metal–organic frameworks (MOFs). The locally controlled releasing MOFs in the hydrogel microfibrous scaffolds have demonstrated superior efficacy in promoting wound healing (182).

11.8 CHALLENGES IN SCALING UP THE MICROFLUIDIC TECHNOLOGIES FOR COMMERCIAL USE

In spite of numerous published publications showcasing the potential and distinctive features of microfluidic-generated materials, the technology's transfer from academic labs to industry has been difficult, mostly due to fundamental challenges. The physics guiding the flow of immiscible fluids contained within micrometer-scale channels limits the throughput of microfluidic materials development, and this performance typically is several orders of magnitude less than what ought to be required for clinical and commercial applications (183).

Contrary to the early stages of the development of microfluidics, where the majority of researchers concentrated primarily on a basic understanding of fluidic design concepts and the operation of biological particles, as well as other inventions, an increasing number of researchers have been creating practical devices toward commercialization to address particular market requirements (184). In this regard, manufacturing processes might vary greatly between large-scale production in industry and prototype development in the academy. The roadmap toward commercialization will present many difficulties, and these are emphasized in order to move from laboratory development to microfluidics for commercialization.

11.8.1 MATERIALS FOR THE SCALE-UP OF MD FABRICATION

Currently, soft lithography is used by most research facilities to create MD using PDMS (185, 186). The desirable characteristics of PDMS include (1) it is optically transparent; enabling the imaging of samples across a device. (2) Its surface can be sealed and treated. (3) Due to its consistency, it can be removed from molds with ease and can adhere to or contact other surfaces in a uniform manner. (4) Its permeability for gases and many liquid vapors makes it suitable for creating an oxygen-rich environment for cell growth but not suitable for preventing excessive water evaporation from aqueous solutions (187). Contrary to these features, its limitations include (1) time-intensive processing. It is challenging to seal (188). It expands with various non-polar organic solvents, which restricts the hydrophobic compounds that may be utilized with it (189). It selectively removes hydrophobic compounds from aqueous streams (131), and it is challenging to maintain its surface treatment. Due to these drawbacks, scaling up the manufacture of MDs provides substantial difficulty in finding reasonable materials and methods that can be used easily and affordably in both research and industrial contexts.

11.8.2 Complex Manufacturing Process and High Failure Rate

As shown in Figure 11.3, several strategies are utilized in various processes and process phases for production scaling up and will experience prototyping. In addition to being scalable with minimal effort for scale-up redevelopment, a successful prototyping process should also have strong material compatibility and acceptable manufacturing precision. Additionally, the failure rate may be considerable since the production of microfluidic chips necessitates the integration of numerous materials and numerous micro-manufacturing techniques (190). This is especially true for techniques that are not frequently used in mass production, including reagent integration, chip bonding, metallization, surface treatment, and others, where standard protocols are not available like injection molding. The production process may fail more frequently as a result of this. Hence, process optimization and quality control may require a lot of work.

11.8.3 Programmability of Microfluidic Chips and Cartridge

Microfluidic chips are different from microelectronic processors in that the former may be programmed and frequently have designs that are tailored to a particular use. Researchers have made an effort to shift this paradigm and create programmable microfluidic chips, but development has been sluggish, and prevalent commercial acceptance has been hindered by problems with generalizability, pricing, and reliability (191). Instead, integrating discrete MDs, each of which has a unique purpose,

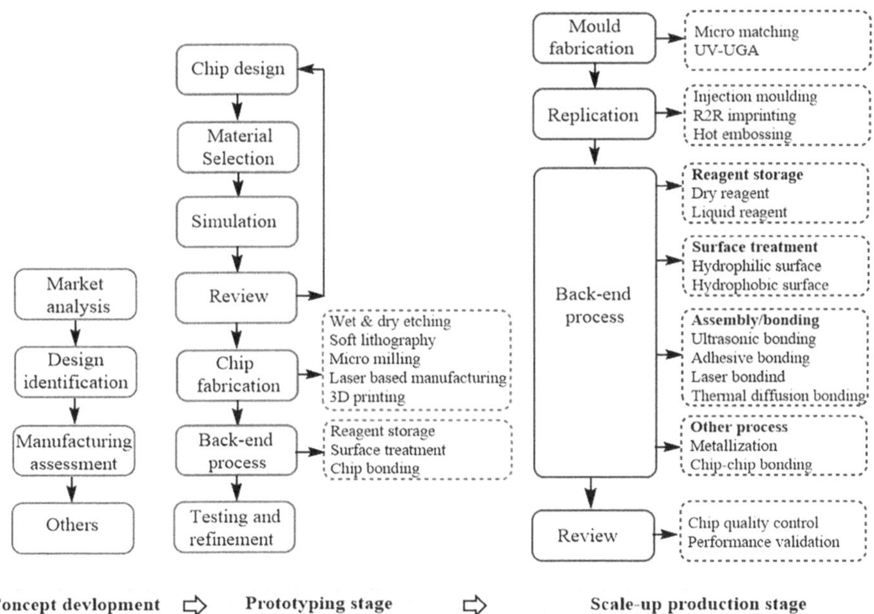

FIGURE 11.3 Development process of MD in prototyping and scale-up production stages.

into a single system poses the most immediate practical obstacle. Instead, integrating discrete MDs, each of which has a unique purpose, into a single system poses the most immediate practical obstacle. Each component is reliable when used alone, but because of its distinct flow needs, geometrical features, and actuation modes, connecting it to other components with various and occasionally incompatible specifications can be challenging (192). Component chip designs should be improved to render them suitable for larger-scale systems. The microfluidic chip is further improved to become a microfluidic cartridge that may be used with the microfluidic instrument for large-scale manufacturing. The importance of low-cost scale-up production is growing. There is a need for more than 10,000 segments, a brief production cycle, strict quality standards, and uniformity. Automation may be necessary when the quantity is grown to more than 20,000 segments in order to obtain high uniformity and reduced expenses. Along with the production of the reagent and the instrument, this process can take three to five years. A complete MD requires a considerable amount of time, plus extra effort for system optimization and audit/ inspection. Given the length of the development phase, a production strategy should be developed.

11.8.4 Lack of Standardization

Microfluidic researchers sometimes fail to reference repeatability and reproducibility data and measure batch-to-batch (chip-to-chip) variations within a specific fabrication or prototype approach. Due to the absence of industry standards, novel microfluidic tests for a given application, including the protocols, tools, and materials, frequently do not work with already available technology. For instance, PDMS is the most popular material used for constructing MDs in the lab. However, because of problems with scaling up and manufacturability, the majority of businesses in the microfluidic industry, except for Fluidigm, avoid utilizing PDMS (184, 193). A well-established standardization system will save time and money on development and manufacture. Once agreed standards on areas ranging from interface dimensions to testing methodologies have been defined, more resources and effort might be directed toward other elements such as creative chip design. This would hasten development at both the chip and system levels, as well as regulatory clearances (194, 195).

11.8.5 Lack of Integration

Researchers need to guarantee that each component is compatible with one another and take the final commercial use into account during the early design stages of LOC devices in order to fully realize their potentiality. For instance, many devices need pumps or voltage supplies to function and the user needs to learn specialized computer software to analyze and understand the findings. Furthermore, sample preparation is necessary for many biological experiments. Customers would be reluctant to utilize the device if the preparation of samples is the rate-limiting phase and must be performed off-chip. Therefore, simultaneous operation of the procedures with seamless transition between steps is necessary for the successful performance of technically complicated analyses on-chip. A further need is that the integrated product be self-contained and, ideally, not require any prior sample processing, preparation, or amplification. To minimize mistakes and make use easier for operators without microfluidics knowledge, it should be totally automated. To reduce the need for arbitrary user interpretation, the results should be presented unambiguously (184).

11.8.6 High Cost

The cost of manufacturing MD could be considerable due to the intricate process of manufacturing, substantial failure rate, and initial low production volume. When the price of reagents is reasonably stable for POCT, the cost of a cartridge might affect the overall cost per test and ultimately the cost-effectiveness of the POCT product (196). Adequacy of professionals with cross-disciplinary expertise, unsatisfactory outcomes as a result of tailoring the protocols from prototyping to mass manufacturing, and challenges in maintaining the cartridge's long-term performance (particularly reagent performance) may all be problems in addition to those already mentioned.

It is additionally pertinent to note that a large manufacturing company is less interested in assisting researchers in taking their design to the stage of preclinical and clinical studies because of the lengthy development period and numerous skill requirements in micro manufacturing, especially for small-scale production. Therefore, to reduce the risk of failure in cartridge development, researchers who are driven by future commercialization should have a deeper understanding of the manufacturing process chains of microfluidics.

11.9 EMERGING TRENDS AND PROSPECTS IN BIOMEDICAL MICROFLUIDIC RESEARCH

Over the last 30 years, microfluidics has quickly developed from the idea of "µTAS" (miniaturized Total Analysis System) into an emergent field with huge commercial potential (197). This technology is developed through the fundamental study of microfluidics, making it fit for commercial application. In order to see a tangible return on their investment, funding organizations are also more interested in initiatives with a higher likelihood of translation or collaboration of research with industry (184). To address issues that arise in the real world, researchers are being motivated by the commercialization culture in academia to bring to market microfluidic solutions developed in the lab, like the fast diagnosis of the SARS-CoV-2 virus. Many academic sequels, including Blu Sense Diagnostics from the Technical University of Denmark; Stilla Technologies from the laboratory of hydrodynamics (LadHyX) at EcolePolytechnique; and Fluid-Screen from Yale University, have all been developed as a result of the creative potential of their technologies.

Despite rapid progress in MFs, several technological obstacles remain, such as commercialization, an improved signal-to-noise ratio due to miniaturization, the need for a complex external system to function effectively, and human ethics and behavior related to the possibility of unskilled public diagnosis. The applications of

MFs and microsystems technologies in agriculture, plant sciences, and environmental monitoring, which have substantial social and economic implications, are currently understudied compared to other biological devices. Future-looking techniques include smart contact lens sensors, tattoo-based sensors, and noninvasive physiological parameter diagnosis from tear fluid for real-time monitoring. Due to a mass reduction in the advantages of the microscale, space science is another prospective field of MF usage. As astronauts need to be diagnosed quickly when in space, the LOC gadget, which can estimate blood sugar, liver function, and renal function, will keep them safer. The "LOC revolution"is anticipated to happen within the next two decades, and the commercialization of MFs-based technology will result in an expansion of MFDs from molecular diagnostics to various other fields (4). This will further demonstrate the growing acceptance of academic entrepreneurship across higher education institutions around the world (198).

11.10 CONCLUSION

Microfluidics devices, which are employed in many applications, from disease modeling to diagnostics, have undergone tremendous advancements over the past few decades. This book chapter describes and discusses developments in microfluidics for biomedical engineering, with a focus on the fundamental ideas and current research trends in the field. These developments include their application to bioassays, biofabrication, and tissue engineering. There are several advantages that microfluidic platforms have over traditional technologies, making it feasible to develop newer approaches for biomedical applications. The most promising bioassays are those that provide miniaturized, high-throughput, and automated biochemical analysis, which can be performed on MD coupled with well-established detection technologies. They are also effective tools for creating innovative functional biomaterials with intricate architectures and predetermined features for enhanced therapies, drug delivery, tissue engineering, and high-throughput drug screening. Furthermore, although they are still in their infancy, microfluidics-based OOAC systems are gaining ground as an alternative to developing artificially engineered in vitro cell cultures and in vivo animal testing models. Research in this area has mainly focused on developing defined 3D microarchitectures and physiologically normal microenvironments for cell cultures that simulate the responses produced by stimuli and the functioning of single or multiple organs. The first issue that needs to be addressed in the future development of microfluidics-based technology is the change from lab to industry and moving from academic reporting to successful commercialization. Future development of microfluidics-based platforms should also focus on clinical diagnosis and trials, including developing bioassays for patient clinical indices, POCT, and organ regeneration. In conclusion, microfluidics is anticipated to have a promising future in medical and biomedical applications with advancements in associated technologies.

ACKNOWLEDGMENTS

The authors express their sincere gratitude to the host institutions for generously providing all the necessary facilities throughout the course of this study.

FUNDING

None.

CONFLICT OF INTEREST

None.

REFERENCES

1. Zhong Q, Ding H, Gao B, He Z, Gu Z. Advances of microfluidics in biomedical engineering. *Adv Mater Technol* 2019 Jun;4(6):1800663.
2. Gharib G, Bütün I, Muganlı Z, Kozalak G, Namlı I, Sarraf SS, Ahmadi VE, Toyran E, Van Wijnen AJ, Koşar A. Biomedical applications of MD: A review. *Biosensors* 2022 Nov 16;12(11):1023.
3. Van Den Berg A, Craighead HG, Yang P. From microfluidic applications to nanofluidic phenomena. *ChemSoc Rev* 2010;39(3):899–900.
4. Solanki S, Pandey CM, Gupta RK, Malhotra BD. Emerging trends in microfluidics based devices. *Biotechnol J* 2020 May;15(5):1900279.
5. Meijer HE, Singh MK, Kang TG, Den Toonder JM, Anderson PD. Passive and active mixing in MD. In *Macromolecular symposia 2009 May* (Vol. 279, No. 1, pp. 201–209). Weinheim: WILEY-VCH Verlag.
6. Zhang Y, Zheng T, Wang L, Feng L, Wang M, Zhang Z, Feng H. From passive to active sorting in microfluidics: A review. *Rev Adv Mater Sci* 2021 Dec 31;60(1):313–24.
7. Tian C, Tu Q, Liu W, Wang J. Recent advances in microfluidic technologies for organ-on-a-chip. *TrAC Trends Analyt Chem* 2019 Aug 1;117:146–56.
8. Ahmed T. Organ-on-a-chip microengineering for bio-mimicking disease models and revolutionizing drug discovery. *BiosensBioelectron X* 2022 Jul 15:100194.
9. Yokoi F, Deguchi S, Takayama K. Organ-on-a-chip models for elucidating the cellular biology of infectious diseases. *BiochimBiophysActaMol Cell Res* 2023 May 26:119504.
10. Akgönüllü S, Bakhshpour M, Pişkin AK, Denizli A. Microfluidic systems for cancer diagnosis and applications. *Micromachines* 2021 Oct 31;12(11):1349.
11. Wang X, Hong XZ, Li YW, Li Y, Wang J, Chen P, Liu BF. Microfluidics-based strategies for molecular diagnostics of infectious diseases. *Mil Med Res* 2022 Dec;9(1):1–27.
12. Lakhera P, Chaudhary V, Bhardwaj B, Kumar P, Kumar S. Development and recent advancement in microfluidics for point of care biosensor applications: A review. *BiosensBioelectron X* 2022 Sep 1;11:100218.
13. Li X, Valadez AV, Zuo P, Nie Z. Microfluidic 3D cell culture: Potential application for tissue-based bioassays. *Bioanalysis* 2012 Jun;4(12):1509–25.
14. Sapp PA, Riley TM, Tindall AM, Sullivan VK, Johnston EA, Petersen KS, Kris-Etherton PM. Nutrition and Atherosclerotic Cardiovascular Disease. In *Present Knowledge in Nutrition* 2020 Jan 1 (pp. 393–411). Academic Press.
15. Roth GA, Mensah GA, Johnson CO, Addolorato G, Ammirati E, Baddour LM, Barengo NC, Beaton AZ, Benjamin EJ, Benziger CP, Bonny A. Global burden of cardiovascular diseases and risk factors, 1990–2019: Update from the GBD 2019 study. *J Am CollCardiol* 2020 Dec 22;76(25):2982–3021.
16. Maruyama K, Iso H. Overview of the Role of Antioxidant Vitamins as Protection Against Cardiovascular Disease: Implications for Aging. In *Aging* 2014 Jan 1 (pp. 213–224). Academic Press.

17. Shi C, Xie H, Ma Y, Yang Z, Zhang J. Nanoscale technologies in highly sensitive diagnosis of cardiovascular diseases. *Front BioengBiotechnol* 2020 Jun 5;8:531.

18. Ma Q, Ma H, Xu F, Wang X, Sun W. Microfluidics in cardiovascular disease research: State of the art and future outlook. *MicrosystNanoeng* 2021 Mar 3;7(1):19.

19. Lim WY, Thevarajah TM, Goh BT, Khor SM. Paper microfluidic device for early diagnosis and prognosis of acute myocardial infarction via quantitative multiplex cardiac biomarker detection. *BiosensBioelectron* 2019 Mar 1;128:176–85.

20. Cheng HL, Fu CY, Kuo WC, Chen YW, Chen YS, Lee YM, Li KH, Chen C, Ma HP, Huang PC, Wang YL. Detecting miRNA biomarkers from extracellular vesicles for cardiovascular disease with a microfluidic system. *Lab Chip* 2018;18(19):2917–25.

21. Mohammed MI, Desmulliez MP. Autonomous capillary microfluidic system with embedded optics for improved troponin I cardiac biomarker detection. *BiosensBioelectron* 2014 Nov 15;61:478–84.

22. Dinter F, Burdukiewicz M, Schierack P, Lehmann W, Nestler J, Dame G, Rödiger S. Simultaneous detection and quantification of DNA and protein biomarkers in spectrum of cardiovascular diseases in a microfluidic microbead chip. *Anal Bioanal Chem* 2019 Nov;411:7725–35.

23. Qiu J, Jiang P, Wang C, Chu Y, Zhang Y, Wang Y, Zhang M, Han L. Lys-AuNPs@ MoS2 nanocomposite self-assembled microfluidic immunoassay biochip for ultrasensitive detection of multiplex biomarkers for cardiovascular diseases. *Anal Chem.* 2022 Mar 8;94(11):4720–8.

24. Sinha A, Tai TY, Li KH, Gopinathan P, Chung YD, Sarangadharan I, Ma HP, Huang PC, Shiesh SC, Wang YL, Lee GB. An integrated microfluidic system with field-effect-transistor sensor arrays for detecting multiple cardiovascular biomarkers from clinical samples. *BiosensBioelectron* 2019 Mar 15;129:155–63.

25. Beck F, Horn C, Baeumner AJ. Dry-reagent microfluidic biosensor for simple detection of NT-proBNP via Ag nanoparticles. *Anal ChimActa* 2022 Jan 25;1191:339375.

26. Yin B, Wan X, Qian C, Sohan AM, Wang S, Zhou T. Point-of-care testing for multiple cardiac markers based on a snail-shaped microfluidic chip. *Front Chem* 2021 Oct 4;9:741058.

27. Sung H, Ferlay J, Siegel RL, Laversanne M, Soerjomataram I, Jemal A, Bray F. Global cancer statistics 2020: GLOBOCAN estimates of incidence and mortality worldwide for 36 cancers in 185 countries. *CA Cancer J Clin* 2021 May;71(3):209–49.

28. Wu J, Hu S, Zhang L, Xin J, Sun C, Wang L, Ding K, Wang B. Tumor circulome in the liquid biopsies for cancer diagnosis and prognosis. *Theranostics* 2020;10(10):4544.

29. Patra JK, Das G, Fraceto LF, Campos EV, Rodriguez-Torres MD, Acosta-Torres LS, Diaz-Torres LA, Grillo R, Swamy MK, Sharma S, Habtemariam S. Nano based drug delivery systems: Recent developments and future prospects. *J Nanobiotechnol* 2018 Dec;16(1):1–33.

30. Swierczewska M, Han HS, Kim K, Park JH, Lee S. Polysaccharide-based nanoparticles for theranostic nanomedicine. *Adv Drug Deliv Rev* 2016 Apr 1;99:70–84.

31. Milane L, Duan Z, Amiji M. Development of EGFR-targeted polymer blend nanocarriers for combination paclitaxel/lonidamine delivery to treat multi-drug resistance in human breast and ovarian tumor cells. *Mol Pharm* 2011 Feb 7;8(1):185–203.

32. Han N, Zhao Q, Wan L, Wang Y, Gao Y, Wang P, Wang Z, Zhang J, Jiang T, Wang S. Hybrid lipid-capped mesoporous silica for stimuli-responsive drug release and overcoming multidrug resistance. *ACS Appl Mater Interfaces* 2015 Feb 11;7(5):3342–51.

33. Taratula O, Garbuzenko OB, Chen AM, Minko T. Innovative strategy for treatment of lung cancer: Targeted nanotechnology-based inhalation co-delivery of anticancer drugs and siRNA. *J Drug Target* 2011 Dec 1;19(10):900–14.

34. Guo QR, Zhang LL, Liu JF, Li Z, Li JJ, Zhou WM, Wang H, Li JQ, Liu DY, Yu XY, Zhang JY. Multifunctional microfluidic chip for cancer diagnosis and treatment. *Nanotheranostics* 2021;5(1):73.

35. Xu Z, Li E, Guo Z, Yu R, Hao H, Xu Y, Sun Z, Li X, Lyu J, Wang Q. Design and construction of a multi-organ microfluidic chip mimicking the in vivo microenvironment of lung cancer metastasis. *ACS Appl Mater Interfaces* 2016 Oct 5;8(39):25840–7.

36. Nguyen TA, Yin TI, Reyes D, Urban GA. Microfluidic chip with integrated electrical cell-impedance sensing for monitoring single cancer cell migration in three-dimensional matrixes. *Anal Chem* 2013 Nov 19;85(22):11068–76.

37. Jamiruddin MR, Meghla BA, Islam DZ, Tisha TA, Khandker SS, Khondoker MU, Haq MA, Adnan N, Haque M. Microfluidics technology in SARS-CoV-2 diagnosis and beyond: A systematic review. *Life* 2022 Apr 27;12(5):649.

38. Ho KL, Liao HY, Liu HM, Lu YW, Yeh PK, Chang JY, Fan SK. Digital microfluidic qPCR cartridge for SARS-CoV-2 detection. *Micromachines* 2022 Jan 27;13(2):196.

39. Akarapipad P, Kaarj K, Breshears LE, Sosnowski K, Baker J, Nguyen BT, Eades C, Uhrlaub JL, Quirk G, Nikolich-Žugich J, Worobey M. Smartphone-based sensitive detection of SARS-CoV-2 from saline gargle samples via flow profile analysis on a paper microfluidic chip. *Biosens Bioelectron* 2022 Jul 1;207:114192.

40. Kim S, Akarapipad P, Nguyen BT, Breshears LE, Sosnowski K, Baker J, Uhrlaub JL, Nikolich-Žugich J, Yoon JY. Direct capture and smartphone quantification of airborne SARS-CoV-2 on a paper microfluidic chip. *Biosens Bioelectron* 2022 Mar 15;200:113912.

41. Collins FS, Green ED, Guttmacher AE, Guyer MS, US National Human Genome Research Institute. A vision for the future of genomics research. *Nature* 2003 Apr 24;422(6934):835–47.

42. Syvänen AC. Toward genome-wide SNP genotyping. *Nat Genet* 2005 Jun;37(Suppl 6):S5–10.

43. Tian H, Jaquins-Gerstl A, Munro N, Trucco M, Brody LC, Landers JP. Single-strand conformation polymorphism analysis by capillary and microchip electrophoresis: A fast, simple method for detection of common mutations in BRCA1 and BRCA2. *Genomics* 2000 Jan 1;63(1):25–34.

44. Tian H, Brody LC, Landers JP. Rapid detection of deletion, insertion, and substitution mutations via heteroduplex analysis using capillary-and microchip-based electrophoresis. *Genome Res* 2000 Sep 1;10(9):1403–13.

45. Tian H, Landers JP. Hydroxyethylcellulose as an effective polymer network for DNA analysis in uncoated glass microchips: Optimization and application to mutation detection via heteroduplex analysis. *Anal Biochem* 2002 Oct 15;309(2):212–23.

46. Rissin DM, Kan CW, Song L, Rivnak AJ, Fishburn MW, Shao Q, Piech T, Ferrell EP, Meyer RE, Campbell TG, Fournier DR. Multiplexed single molecule immunoassays. *Lab Chip* 2013;13(15):2902–11.

47. Myers FB, Lee LP. Innovations in optical microfluidic technologies for point-of-care diagnostics. *Lab Chip* 2008;8(12):2015–31.

48. Iha K, Inada M, Kawada N, Nakaishi K, Watabe S, Tan YH, Shen C, Ke LY, Yoshimura T, Ito E. Ultrasensitive ELISA developed for diagnosis. *Diagnostics*. 2019 Jul 18;9(3):78.

49. Mohd Fuad N, Carve M, Kaslin J, Wlodkowic D. Characterization of 3D-printed moulds for soft lithography of millifluidic devices. *Micromachines* 2018 Mar 8;9(3):116.

50. Boffetta G, Ecke RE. Two-dimensional turbulence. *Annu Rev Fluid Mech* 2012 Jan 21;44:427–51.

51. Ren K, Zhou J, Wu H. Materials for microfluidic chip fabrication. *Acc Chem Res* 2013 Nov 19;46(11):2396–406.

52. Nnachi RC, Sui N, Ke B, Luo Z, Bhalla N, He D, Yang Z. Biosensors for rapid detection of bacterial pathogens in water, food and environment. *Environ Int* 2022 Aug 1;166:107357.

53. Li Q, Cao Y, Wang P. Recent advances in hydrogels for the diagnosis and treatment of dry eye disease. *Gels* 2022 Dec 11;8(12):816.

54. Zoupanou S, Chiriacò MS, Tarantini I, Ferrara F. Innovative 3D microfluidic tools for on-chip fluids and particles manipulation: From design to experimental validation. *Micromachines* 2021 Jan 21;12(2):104.

55. Waheed S, Cabot JM, Macdonald NP, Lewis T, Guijt RM, Paull B, Breadmore MC. 3D printed MD: Enablers and barriers. *Lab Chip* 2016;16(11):1993–2013.

56. Chan HN, Tan MJ, Wu H. Point-of-care testing: Applications of 3D printing. *Lab Chip* 2017;17(16):2713–39.

57. Song J, Mauk MG, Hackett BA, Cherry S, Bau HH, Liu C. Instrument-free point-of-care molecular detection of Zika virus. *Anal Chem* 2016 Jul 19;88(14):7289–94.

58. Bhamla MS, Benson B, Chai C, Katsikis G, Johri A, Prakash M. Hand-powered ultralow-cost paper centrifuge. *Nat Biomed Eng* 2017 Jan 10;1(1):0009.

59. Laurenciano CJ, Tseng CC, Chen SJ, Lu SY, Tayo LL, Fu LM. Microfluidic colorimetric detection platform with sliding hybrid PMMA/paper microchip for human urine and blood sample analysis. *Talanta* 2021 Aug 15;231:122362.

60. Wojtczak J, Bonadonna P. Pocket mobile smartphone system for the point-of-care submandibular ultrasonography. *Am J Emerg Med* 2013 Mar 1;31(3):573–7.

61. Gallegos D, Long KD, Yu H, Clark PP, Lin Y, George S, Nath P, Cunningham BT. Label-free biodetection using a smartphone. *Lab Chip* 2013;13(11):2124–32.

62. Xu X, Akay A, Wei H, Wang S, Pingguan-Murphy B, Erlandsson BE, Li X, Lee W, Hu J, Wang L, Xu F. Advances in smartphone-based point-of-care diagnostics. *Proc IEEE* 2015 Feb;103(2):236–47.

63. Jalal UM, Jin GJ, Shim JS. Paper–plastic hybrid microfluidic device for smartphone-based colorimetric analysis of urine. *Anal Chem* 2017 Dec 19;89(24):13160–6.

64. Pohl HA. The motion and precipitation of suspensoids in divergent electric fields. *J Appl Phys* 1951 Jul;22(7):869–71.

65. Demircan Y, Özgür E, Külah H. Dielectrophoresis: Applications and future outlook in point of care. *Electrophoresis* 2013 Apr;34(7):1008–27.

66. Bédard P, Gauvin S, Ferland K, Caneparo C, Pellerin È, Chabaud S, Bolduc S. Innovative human three-dimensional tissue-engineered models as an alternative to animal testing. *Bioengineering* 2020 Sep 17;7(3):115.

67. Ingber DE. Human organs-on-chips for disease modelling, drug development and personalized medicine. *Nat Rev Genet* 2022 Aug;23(8):467–91.

68. Shyam R, Reddy LV, Palaniappan A. Fabrication and Characterization Techniques of In Vitro 3D Tissue Models *Int J Mol Sci*. 2023 Jan 18;24(3):1912.

69. Messelmani T, Morisseau L, Sakai Y, Legallais C, Le Goff A, Leclerc E, Jellali R. Liver organ-on-chip models for toxicity studies and risk assessment. *Lab Chip* 2022;22(13):2423–50.

70. Fu J, Qiu H, Tan CS. Microfluidic liver-on-a-chip for preclinical drug discovery. *Pharmaceutics* 2023 Apr 21;15(4):1300.

71. Francis I, Shrestha J, Paudel KR, Hansbro PM, Warkiani ME, Saha SC. Recent advances in lung-on-a-chip models. *Drug Discov Today* 2022 Sep 1;27(9):2593–602.

72. Tavares-Negrete JA, Das P, Najafikhoshnoo S, Zanganeh S, Esfandyarpour R. Recent advances in lung-on-a-chip technology for modeling respiratory disease. *Bio-Des Manuf* 2023 Jun 13:1–23.

73. Marrero D, Pujol-Vila F, Vera D, Gabriel G, Illa X, Elizalde-Torrent A, Alvarez M, Villa R. Gut-on-a-chip: Mimicking and monitoring the human intestine. *Biosens Bioelectron* 2021 Jun 1;181:113156.

74. De Haan P, Santbergen MJ, van der Zande M, Bouwmeester H, Nielen MW, Verpoorte E. A versatile, compartmentalised gut-on-a-chip system for pharmacological and toxicological analyses. *Sci Rep* 2021 Mar 1;11(1):4920.

75. Xian C, Zhang J, Zhao S, Li XG. Gut-on-a-chip for disease models. *J Tissue Eng* 2023 Jan;14:20417314221149882.

76. Wang D, Gust M, Ferrell N. Kidney-on-a-chip: Mechanical stimulation and sensor integration. *Sensors* 2022 Sep 13;22(18):6889.

77. Nguyen VV, Gkouzioti V, Maass C, Verhaar MC, Vernooij RW, van Balkom BW. A systematic review of kidney-on-a-chip-based models to study human renal (patho-) physiology. *Dis Model Mech* 2023 Jun 1;16(6).

78. Jastrzebska E, Tomecka E, Jesion I. Heart-on-a-chip based on stem cell biology. *Biosens Bioelectron* 2016 Jan 15;75:67–81.

79. Yang Q, Xiao Z, Lv X, Zhang T, Liu H. Fabrication and biomedical applications of heart-on-a-chip. *Int J Bioprint* 2021;7(3).

80. Amirifar L, Shamloo A, Nasiri R, de Barros NR, Wang ZZ, Unluturk BD, Libanori A, Ievglevskyi O, Diltemiz SE, Sances S, Balasingham I. Brain-on-a-chip: Recent advances in design and techniques for microfluidic models of the brain in health and disease. *Biomaterials* 2022 Jun 1;285:121531.

81. Zhao C, Wang Z, Tang X, Qin J, Jiang Z. Recent advances in sensor-integrated brain-on-a-chip devices for real-time brain monitoring. *Colloids Surf B Biointerfaces* 2023 Jun 28:113431.

82. Zhang Y, Yu T, Ding J, Li Z. Bone-on-a-chip platforms and integrated biosensors: Towards advanced in vitro bone models with real-time biosensing. *Biosens Bioelectron* 2023 Jan 1;219:114798.

83. Galván-Chacón VP, Zampouka A, Hesse B, Bohner M, Habibovic P, Barata D. Bone-on-a-chip: A microscale 3D biomimetic model to study bone regeneration. *Adv Eng Mater* 2022 Jul;24(7):2101467.

84. Alamán-Díez P, García-Gareta E, Arruebo M, Pérez MÁ. A bone-on-a-chip collagen hydrogel-based model using pre-differentiated adipose-derived stem cells for personalized bone tissue engineering. *J Biomed Mater Res A* 2023 Jan;111(1):88–105.

85. Hassan S, Sebastian S, Maharjan S, Lesha A, Carpenter AM, Liu X, Xie X, Livermore C, Zhang YS, Zarrinpar A. Liver-on-a-chip models of fatty liver disease. *Hepatology* 2020 Feb 1;71(2):733–40.

86. Du K, Li S, Li C, Li P, Miao C, Luo T, Qiu B, Ding W. Modeling nonalcoholic fatty liver disease on a liver lobule chip with dual blood supply. *Acta Biomater* 2021 Oct 15;134:228–39.

87. Lee SY, Sung JH. Gut–liver on a chip toward an in vitro model of hepatic steatosis. *Biotechnol Bioeng* 2018 Nov;115(11):2817–27.

88. Soltantabar P, Calubaquib EL, Mostafavi E, Ghazavi A, Stefan MC. Heart/liver-on-a-chip as a model for the evaluation of cardiotoxicity induced by chemotherapies. *Organs Chip* 2021 Nov 1;3:100008.

89. Leung CM, Ong LJ, Kim S, Toh YC. A physiological adipose-on-chip disease model to mimic adipocyte hypertrophy and inflammation in obesity. *Organs Chip* 2022 Dec 1;4:100021.

90. Zamprogno P, Wüthrich S, Achenbach S, Thoma G, Stucki JD, Hobi N, Schneider-Daum N, Lehr CM, Huwer H, Geiser T, Schmid RA. Second-generation lung-on-a-chip with an array of stretchable alveoli made with a biological membrane. *Commun Biol* 2021 Feb 5;4(1):168.

91. Zhu Y, Sun L, Wang Y, Cai L, Zhang Z, Shang Y, Zhao Y. A biomimetic human lung-on-a-chip with colorful display of microphysiological breath. *Adv Mater* 2022 Apr;34(13):2108972.

92. Amirabadi HE, Donkers JM, Wierenga E, Ingenhut B, Pieters L, Stevens L, Donkers T, Westerhout J, Masereeuw R, Bobeldijk-Pastorova I, Nooijen I. Intestinal explant barrier chip: long-term intestinal absorption screening in a novel microphysiological system using tissue explants. *Lab Chip* 2022;22(2):326–42.

93. Jeon MS, Choi YY, Mo SJ, Ha JH, Lee YS, Lee HU, Park SD, Shim JJ, Lee JL, Chung BG. Contributions of the microbiome to intestinal inflammation in a gut-on-a-chip. *Nano Converg* 2022 Feb 8;9(1):8.

94. Maurer M, Gresnigt MS, Last A, Wollny T, Berlinghof F, Pospich R, Cseresnyes Z, Medyukhina A, Graf K, Groeger M, Raasch M. A three-dimensional immunocompetent intestine-on-chip model as in vitro platform for functional and microbial interaction studies. *Biomaterials* 2019 Nov 1;220:119396.

95. Roye Y, Bhattacharya R, Mou X, Zhou Y, Burt MA, Musah S. A personalized glomerulus chip engineered from stem cell-derived epithelium and vascular endothelium. *Micromachines* 2021 Aug 16;12(8):967.

96. Lee HN, Choi YY, Kim JW, Lee YS, Choi JW, Kang T, Kim YK, Chung BG. Effect of biochemical and biomechanical factors on vascularization of kidney organoid-on-a-chip. *Nano Converg* 2021 Dec;8:1–10.

97. Andrysiak K, Stępniewski J, Dulak J. Human-induced pluripotent stem cell-derived cardiomyocytes, 3D cardiac structures, and heart-on-a-chip as tools for drug research. *Pflugers Arch PFLUG ARCH EUR J PHY* 2021 Jul;473:1061–85.

98. Zhang F, Qu KY, Zhou B, Luo Y, Zhu Z, Pan DJ, Cui C, Zhu Y, Chen ML, Huang NP. Design and fabrication of an integrated heart-on-a-chip platform for construction of cardiac tissue from human iPSC-derived cardiomyocytes and in situ evaluation of physiological function. *Biosens Bioelectron* 2021 May 1;179:113080.

99. Bang S, Jeong S, Choi N, Kim HN. Brain-on-a-chip: A history of development and future perspective. *Biomicrofluidics* 2019 Sep 1;13(5).

100. Pelkonen A, Mzezewa R, Sukki L, Ryynänen T, Kreutzer J, Hyvärinen T, Vinogradov A, Aarnos L, Lekkala J, Kallio P, Narkilahti S. A modular brain-on-a-chip for modelling epileptic seizures with functionally connected human neuronal networks. *Biosens Bioelectron* 2020 Nov 15;168:112553.

101. Kim MH, Kim D, Sung JH. A gut-brain axis-on-a-chip for studying transport across epithelial and endothelial barriers. *J Ind Eng Chem* 2021 Sep 25;101:126–34.

102. Vacanti JP, Langer R. Tissue engineering: The design and fabrication of living replacement devices for surgical reconstruction and transplantation. *Lancet* 1999 Jul 1;354:S32–4.

103. Lysaght MJ, Crager J. Origins. *Tissue Eng Part A* 2009 Jul 1;15(7):1449–51.

104. Lindroos B, Suuronen R, Miettinen S. The potential of adipose stem cells in regenerative medicine. *Stem Cell Rev Rep* 2011 Jun;7:269–91.

105. Salgado AJ, Oliveira JM, Martins A, Teixeira FG, Silva NA, Neves NM, Sousa N, Reis RL. Tissue engineering and regenerative medicine: Past, present, and future. *Int Rev Neurobiol* 2013 Jan 1;108:1–33.

106. Martin I, Wendt D, Heberer M. The role of bioreactors in tissue engineering. *TRENDS in Biotechnol* 2004 Feb 1;22(2):80–6.

107. Brown BN, Valentin JE, Stewart-Akers AM, McCabe GP, Badylak SF. Macrophage phenotype and remodeling outcomes in response to biologic scaffolds with and without a cellular component. *Biomaterials* 2009 Mar 1;30(8):1482–91.

108. Lyons FG, Al-Munajjed AA, Kieran SM, Toner ME, Murphy CM, Duffy GP, O'Brien FJ. The healing of bony defects by cell-free collagen-based scaffolds compared to stem cell-seeded tissue engineered constructs. *Biomaterials* 2010 Dec 1;31(35):9232–43.

109. Hutmacher DW. Scaffolds in tissue engineering bone and cartilage. *Biomaterials* 2000 Dec 15;21(24):2529–43.

110. Murphy CM, Haugh MG, O'Brien FJ. The effect of mean pore size on cell attachment, proliferation and migration in collagen–glycosaminoglycan scaffolds for bone tissue engineering. *Biomaterials* 2010 Jan 1;31(3):461–6.

111. Hewitt Z, Priddle H, Thomson AJ, Wojtacha D, McWhir J. Ablation of undifferentiated human embryonic stem cells: Exploiting innate immunity against the gal α1-3Galβ1-4GlcNAc-R (α-Gal) epitope. *Stem Cells* 2007 Jan 1;25(1):10–8.

112. Buttery LD, Bourne S, Xynos JD, Wood H, Hughes FJ, Hughes SP, Episkopou V, Polak JM. Differentiation of osteoblasts and in vitro bone formation from murine embryonic stem cells. *Tissue Eng* 2001 Feb 1;7(1):89–99.

113. Haynesworth SE, Barer MA, Caplan AI. Cell surface antigens on human marrow-derived mesenchymal cells are detected by monoclonal antibodies. *Bone* 1992 Jan 1;13(1):69–80.

114. Simmons PJ, Torok-Storb B. Identification of stromal cell precursors in human bone marrow by a novel monoclonal antibody, STRO-1. *Blood* 1991:78:55–62.

115. Lee OK, Kuo TK, Chen WM, Lee KD, Hsieh SL, Chen TH. Isolation of multipotent mesenchymal stem cells from umbilical cord blood. *Blood* 2004 Mar 1;103(5):1669–75.

116. Kang XQ, Zang WJ, Bao LJ, Li DL, Xu XL, Yu XJ. Differentiating characterization of human umbilical cord blood-derived mesenchymal stem cells in vitro. *Cell Biol Int* 2006 Jul;30(7):569–75.

117. Jeong JA, Hong SH, Gang EJ, Ahn C, Hwang SH, Yang IH, Han H, Kim H. Differential gene expression profiling of human umbilical cord blood–derived mesenchymal stem cells by DNA microarray. *Stem Cells* 2005 Apr 1;23(4):584–93.

118. Kim BS, Kwon YW, Kong JS, Park GT, Gao G, Han W, Kim MB, Lee H, Kim JH, Cho DW. 3D cell printing of in vitro stabilized skin model and in vivo pre-vascularized skin patch using tissue-specific extracellular matrix bioink: A step towards advanced skin tissue engineering. *Biomaterials* 2018 Jun 1;168:38–53.

119. Komor AC, Badran AH, Liu DR. CRISPR-based technologies for the manipulation of eukaryotic genomes. *Cell* 2017 Jan 12;168(1):20–36.

120. Wang HX, Song Z, Lao YH, Xu X, Gong J, Cheng D, Chakraborty S, Park JS, Li M, Huang D, Yin L. Nonviral gene editing via CRISPR/Cas9 delivery by membrane-disruptive and endosomolytic helical polypeptide. *Proc Natl Acad Sci.* 2018 May 8;115(19):4903–8.

121. Wang J, Zou M, Sun L, Cheng Y, Shang L, Fu F, Zhao Y. Microfluidic generation of Buddha beads-like microcarriers for cell culture. *Sci China Mater* 2017 Sep 1;60(9):857–65.

122. Bang S, Lee SR, Ko J, Son K, Tahk D, Ahn J, Im C, Jeon NL. A low permeability microfluidic blood-brain barrier platform with direct contact between perfusable vascular network and astrocytes. *Sci Rep* 2017 Aug 14;7(1):8083.

123. Kim S, Lee H, Chung M, Jeon NL. Engineering of functional, perfusable 3D microvascular networks on a chip *Lab Chip* 2013;13(8):1489–500.

124. Mobini S, Song YH, McCrary MW, Schmidt CE. Advances in ex vivo models and lab-on-a-chip devices for neural tissue engineering. *Biomaterials* 2019 Apr 1;198:146–66.

125. Hamilton L, France RM, Shakesheff KM. Development of an injectable scaffold for application in regenerative medicine to deliver stem cells and growth factors. In *J Pharm Pharmacol* 2006 Jan 1 (Vol. 58, pp. A52–A53). 1 LAMBETH HIGH ST, LONDON SE1 7JN, ENGLAND: PHARMACEUTICAL PRESS-ROYAL PHARMACEUTICAL SOC GREAT BRITIAN.

126. Heyde M, Partridge KA, Howdle SM, Oreffo RO, Garnett MC, Shakesheff KM. Development of a slow non-viral DNA release system from PDLLA scaffolds fabricated using a supercritical CO2 technique. *Biotechnol Bioeng* 2007 Oct 15;98(3):679–93.

127. Antonov EN, Bagratashvili VN, Whitaker MJ, Barry JJ, Shakesheff KM, Konovalov AN, Popov VK, Howdle SM. Three-dimensional bioactive and biodegradable scaffolds fabricated by surface-selective laser sintering. *Adv Mater* 2004 Dec 12;17(3):327.

128. Jakab K, Neagu A, Mironov V, Markwald RR, Forgacs G. Engineering biological structures of prescribed shape using self-assembling multicellular systems. *Proc Natl Acad Sci* 2004 Mar 2;101(9):2864–9.

129. Yang J, Motlagh D, Webb AR, Ameer GA. Novel biphasic elastomeric scaffold for small-diameter blood vessel tissue engineering. *Tissue Eng* 2005 Nov 1;11(11–12):1876–1886.

130. Barry JJ, Howard D, Shakesheff KM, Howdle SM, Alexander MR. Using a core-sheath distribution of chemistry through tissue engineering scaffolds to control cell ingress. *Adv Mater* 2006 Jun 6;18(11):1406–1410.

131. Sackmann EK, Fulton AL, Beebe DJ.The present and future role of microfluidics in biomedical research.*Nature* 2014 Mar 13;507(7491):181–9.

132. Squires TM, Quake SR. Microfluidics: Fluid physics at the nanoliter scale. *Rev Mod Phys* 2005;77(3):977.

133. Zhou P, He J, Huang L, Yu Z, Su Z, Shi X, Zhou J. Microfluidic high-throughput platforms for discovery of novel materials. *Nanomaterials* 2020 Dec 15;10(12):2514.

134. Zhang R, Liberski A, Sanchez-Martin R, Bradley M. Microarrays of over 2000 hydrogels–identification of substrates for cellular trapping and thermally triggered release. *Biomaterials* 2009 Oct 1;30(31):6193–201.

135. Shepherd RF, Conrad JC, Rhodes SK, Link DR, Marquez M, Weitz DA, Lewis JA. Microfluidic assembly of homogeneous and janus colloid-filled hydrogel granules. *Langmuir* 2006 Sep 15;22(21):8618–22.

136. Sebastian V, Zaborenko N, Gu L, Jensen KF. Microfluidic assisted synthesis of hybrid Au–pd dumbbell-like nanostructures: Sequential addition of reagents and ultrasonic radiation. *Cryst Growth Des* 2017 May 3;17(5):2700–10.

137. Cho SK, Moon H, Kim CJ. Creating, transporting, cutting, and merging liquid droplets by electrowetting-based actuation for digital microfluidic circuits. *J Microelectromech Syst* 2003 Feb 28;12(1):70–80.

138. Marre S, Jensen KF. Synthesis of micro and nanostructures in microfluidic systems. *Chem Soc Rev* 2010;39(3):1183–1202.

139. Hakala TA, Bialas F, Toprakcioglu Z, Bräuer B, Baumann KN, Levin A, et al. Continuous flow reactors from microfluidic compartmentalization of enzymes within inorganic microparticles. *ACS Appl Mater Interfaces* 2020;12(29):32951–32960.

140. Carneiro J, Campos JB, Miranda JM. High viscosity polymeric fluid droplet formation in a flow focusing microfluidic device–Experimental and numerical study. *Chem Eng Sci* 2019;195:442–454.

141. Juthani N, Doyle PS. A platform for multiplexed colorimetric microRNA detection using shape-encoded hydrogel particles. *Analyst* 2020;145(15):5134–5140.

142. Parthiban P, Doyle PS, Hashimoto M. Self-assembly of droplets in three-dimensional microchannels. *Soft Matter* 2019;15(21):4244–4254.

143. Hao N, Nie Y, Xu Z, Jin C, Fyda TJ, Zhang JX. Microfluidics-enabled acceleration of Fenton oxidation for degradation of organic dyes with rod-like zero-valent iron nanoassemblies. *J Colloid Interface Sci* 2020;559:254–262.

144. Cooney CG, Chen CY, Emerling MR, Nadim A, Sterling JD. Electrowetting droplet microfluidics on a single planar surface. *Microfluid Nanofluid* 2006;2:435–446.

145. Prakash S, Ashley BK, Doyle PS, Hassan U. Design of a multiplexed analyte biosensor using digital barcoded particles and impedance spectroscopy. *Sci Rep* 2020;10(1):6109.

146. Fang Z, Ding Y, Zhang Z, Wang F, Wang Z, Wang H, et al. Digital microfluidic meter-on-chip. *Lab Chip* 2020;20(4):722–733.

147. Yobas L, Martens S, Ong WL, Ranganathan N. High-performance flow-focusing geometry for spontaneous generation of monodispersed droplets. *Lab Chip* 2006;6(8):1073–1079.

148. Zhou C, Zhu P, Tian Y, Xu M, Wang L. Engineering micromotors with droplet microfluidics. *ACS Nano* 2019;13(6):6319–6329.

149. Dittrich PS, Manz A. Lab-on-a-chip: Microfluidics in drug discovery. *Nat Rev Drug Discov* 2006;5(3):210–218.

150. Agresti JJ, Antipov E, Abate AR, Ahn K, Rowat AC, Baret JC, et al. Ultrahigh-throughput screening in drop-based microfluidics for directed evolution. *Proc Natl Acad Sci* 2010;107(9):4004–4009.

151. Luni C, Serena E, Elvassore N. Human-on-chip for therapy development and fundamental science. *Curr Opin Biotechnol* 2014;25:45–50.

152. Song H, Bringer MR, Tice JD, Gerdts CJ, Ismagilov RF. Experimental test of scaling of mixing by chaotic advection in droplets moving through microfluidic channels. *Appl Phys Lett* 2003;83(22):4664–4666.

153. Straubhaar J, D'Souza A, Niziolek ZT, Budnik B. Single cell proteomics analysis of drug response shows its potential as a drug discovery platform. *Mol Omics* 2023;20:6–18.

154. Sista R, Hua Z, Thwar P, Sudarsan A, Srinivasan V, Eckhardt A, et al. Development of a digital microfluidic platform for point of care testing. *Lab Chip* 2008;8(12):2091–2104.

155. Huebner A, Bratton D, Whyte G, Yang M, Demello AJ, Abell C, et al. Static micro-droplet arrays: A microfluidic device for droplet trapping, incubation and release for enzymatic and cell-based assays. *Lab Chip* 2009;9(5):692–698.

156. Zare RN, Kim S. Microfluidic platforms for single-cell analysis. *Annu Rev Biomed Eng* 2010 Aug 15;12:187–201.

157. Gu W, Zhu X, Futai N, Cho BS, Takayama S. Computerized microfluidic cell culture using elastomeric channels and Braille displays. *Proc Natl Acad Sci* 2004 Nov 9;101(45):15861–6

158. El-Ali J, Sorger PK, Jensen KF. Cells on chips. *Nature* 2006;442(7101):403–411.

159. Oh KW, Lee K, Ahn B, Furlani EP. Design of pressure-driven microfluidic networks using electric circuit analogy. *Lab Chip* 2012;12(3):515–545.

160. Karimi M, Bahrami S, Mirshekari H, Basri SM, Nik AB, Aref AR, et al. Microfluidic systems for stem cell-based neural tissue engineering. *Lab Chip* 2016;16(14):2551–2571.

161. Chiappalone M, Vato A, Berdondini L, Koudelka-Hep M, Martinoia S. Network dynamics and synchronous activity in cultured cortical neurons. *Int J Neural Syst* 2007;17(02):87–103.

162. Pol R, Céspedes F, Gabriel D, Baeza M. Microfluidic lab-on-a-chip platforms for environmental monitoring. *Trends Anal Chem* 2017 Oct 1;95:62–8.

163. Wen H, Jung H, Li X. Drug delivery approaches in addressing clinical pharmacology-related issues: Opportunities and challenges. *AAPS J* 2015;17:1327–1340.

164. Adepu S, Ramakrishna S. Controlled drug delivery systems: Current status and future directions. *Molecules* 2021 Sep 29;26(19):5905.

165. Rawtani D, Agrawal YK. Emerging strategies and applications of layer-by-layer self-assembly. *Nanobiomedicine* 2014;1:8.
166. Preetam S, Nahak BK, Patra S, Toncu DC, Park S, Syväjärvi M, et al. Emergence of microfluidics for next generation biomedical devices. *BiosensBioelectron X* 2022;10:100106.
167. Nikoubashman A. Self-assembly of colloidal micelles in microfluidic channels. *Soft Matter* 2017;13(1):222–229.
168. Zhang L, Chen Q, Ma Y, Sun J. Microfluidic methods for fabrication and engineering of nanoparticle drug delivery systems. *ACS Appl Bio Mater* 2019 Nov 25;3(1):107–20.
169. Aresh W, Liu Y, Sine J, Thayer D, Puri A, Huang Y, et al. The morphology of self-assembled lipid-based nanoparticles affects their uptake by cancer cells. *J Biomed Nanotechnol* 2016;12(10):1852–1863.
170. Xia D, Hu C, Hou Y. Regorafenib loaded self-assembled lipid-based nanocarrier for colorectal cancer treatment via lymphatic absorption. *Eur J Pharm Biopharm* 2023;185:165–176.
171. Valencia GA, Zare EN, Makvandi P, Gutiérrez TJ. Self-assembled carbohydrate polymers for food applications: A review. *Compr Rev Food Sci Food Saf* 2019 Nov;18(6):2009–24.
172. Dali P, Shende P. Self-assembled lipid polymer hybrid nanoparticles using combinational drugs for migraine via intranasal route. *AAPS PharmSciTech* 2022;24(1):20.
173. Adams F, Merkel OM. Microfluidics for nanoencapsulation of nucleic acids using polymeric carriers. *Mat Matters* 2022;1:3.
174. Zhang H, Yang J, Sun R, Han S, Yang Z, Teng L. Microfluidics for nano-drug delivery systems: From fundamentals to industrialization. *Acta Pharm Sin B* 2023;13(8):3277–3299.
175. Wang J, Li Y, Wang X, Wang J, Tian H, Zhao P, et al. Droplet microfluidics for the production of microparticles and nanoparticles. *Micromachines* 2017;8(1):22.
176. Rezvantalab S, Moraveji MK. Microfluidic assisted synthesis of PLGA drug delivery systems. *RSC Adv* 2019;9(4):2055–2072.
177. Zhang L, Feng Q, Wang J, Sun J, Shi X, Jiang X. Microfluidic synthesis of rigid nanovesicles for hydrophilic reagents delivery. *Angew Chem* 2015 Mar 23;127(13):4024–8.
178. Zhang L, Cai LH, Lienemann PS, Rossow T, Polenz I, Vallmajo-Martin Q, et al. One-step microfluidic fabrication of polyelectrolyte microcapsules in aqueous conditions for protein release. *Angew Chem* 2016 Oct 17;128(43):13668–72
179. Song Y, Shimanovich U, Michaels TC, Ma Q, Li J, Knowles TP, et al. Fabrication of fibrillosomes from droplets stabilized by protein nanofibrils at all-aqueous interfaces. *Nat Commun* 2016 Oct 11;7(1):12934.
180. Zhao Q, Cui H, Wang Y, Du X. Microfluidic platforms toward rational material fabrication for biomedical applications. *Small* 2020 Mar;16(9):1903798.
181. Lee S, Lee TY, Amstad E, Kim SH. Microfluidic production of capsules-in-capsules for programed release of multiple ingredients. *Adv Mater Technol* 2018 May;3(5):1800006.
182. Yu Y, Chen G, Guo J, Liu Y, Ren J, Kong T, et al. Vitamin metal–organic framework-laden microfibers from microfluidics for wound healing. *Mater Horiz* 2018;5(6):1137–1142.
183. Anna SL. Droplets and bubbles in MD. *Annu Rev Fluid Mech* 2016 Jan 3;48:285–309.
184. Volpatti LR, Yetisen AK. Commercialization of MD. *Trends Biotechnol* 2014 Jul 1;32(7):347–50.
185. Lee MH, Oh SG, Moon SK, Bae SY. Preparation of silica particles encapsulating retinol using o/w/o multiple emulsions. *J Colloid Interface Sci* 2001 Aug 1;240(1):83–9.
186. Battat S, Weitz DA, Whitesides GM. An outlook on microfluidics: The promise and the challenge. *Lab Chip* 2022;22(3):530–536.
187. Whitesides GM. The origins and the future of microfluidics. *Nature* 2006 Jul 27;442(7101):368–73.

188. Eddings MA, Johnson MA, Gale BK. Determining the optimal PDMS-PDMS bonding technique for MD. *J Micromech Microeng* 2008 Apr 25;18(6):067001.

189. Lee JN, Park C, Whitesides GM. Solvent compatibility of poly(dimethylsiloxane)-based MD. *Anal Chem* Dec 1;75(23):6544–54.

190. Mohammed MI, Haswell S, Gibson I. Lab-on-a-chip or Chip-in-a-lab: Challenges of Commercialization Lost in Translation. *Procedia Technol* 2015;20:54–59.

191. Fernandes AC, Gernaey KV, Krühne U. Connecting worlds–a view on microfluidics for a wider application. *Biotechnol Adv* 2018 Jul 1;36(4):1341–66.

192. Mosadegh B, Bersano-Begey T, Park JY, Burns MA, Takayama S. Next-generation integrated microfluidic circuits. *Lab Chip* 2011;11(17):2813–2818.

193. Subramanian A. A next generation connectivity map: L1000 Platform. *Cell* 2017 Nov 30;171(6):1437–52.

194. Dekker S, Buesink W, Blom M, Alessio M, Verplanck N, Hihoud M, et al. Standardized and modular microfluidic platform for fast Lab on Chip system development. *Sensors Actuators B Chem* 2018 Nov 1;272:468–78.

195. Van Heeren H. Standards for connecting MD? *Lab Chip* 2012;12(6):1022–1025.

196. Nguyen HT, Thach H, Roy E, Huynh K, Perrault CMT. Low-cost, accessible fabrication methods for microfluidics research in low-resource settings. *Micromachines* 2018 Sep 12;9(9):461.

197. Convery N, Gadegaard N. 30 years of microfluidics. *Micro Nano Eng* 2019 Mar 1;2:76–91

198. Li H, Yang X, Cai X. Academic spin-off activities and research performance: The mediating role of research collaboration. *J Technol Transf* 2022 Aug;47(4):1037–69.

12 Application of Microfluidics in Dermal Drug Delivery System

Shiv Shankar Shukla and Bina Gidwani
Columbia Institute of Pharmacy, Raipur, India

Varsha Sahu
Utkal University, Bhubaneswar, India

Ravindra Kumar Pandey
Columbia Institute of Pharmacy, Raipur, India

Amber Vyas
Pt. Ravishankar Shukla University, Raipur, India

12.1 INTRODUCTION

The primary barrier separating the interior and exterior environments is the skin, which is the largest organ in the body, covering 20 square feet. It prevents the entry of harmful substances into the body and provides prevention from infections, and loss of water, regulates body temperature, and allows sensations like cold, heat, and touch (1). The human body's outermost layer is called skin, which works as a physical barrier against external substances, such as microorganisms, and physical, chemical, and pathogenic materials. It served as the body's initial line of defense. Additionally, it divides the blood supply and sensory nerves from the external surroundings. It is made up of the epidermis, dermis, and hypodermis as its three primary layers. (2). The keratinocytes that make up the epidermis are devoid of lymphatic and blood arteries. Blood arteries present in the underlying layers of skin provide them with nutrition and oxygen (2). They preserve the moisture content in the skin while shielding it from allergies and microbes (3). The layers that follow the stratum corneum, which is its outermost layer, are the stratum granulosum, stratum spinosum, and bottom stratum germinativum layer. A vertical column

DOI: 10.1201/9781032690926-12

of 10–30 corneocyte cells immersed in a lipid matrix makes up the structure. The main rate-limiting stage for chemical absorption from the external environment is the stratum corneum. The stratum lucidum, a thin layer of flattened keratinocytes, is the next layer of the epidermis (3). Between the stratum lucidum and stratum spinosum, there is a thin layer called the stratum granulosum. This layer is caused by the migration of granular cells that contain keratohyalin granules. Merkel cells, Langerhans cells, mature keratinocytes, and melanocytes are found in the final two layers of the epidermis, known as the stratum spinosum and basal stratum germinativum layers (2, 3). The second layer of skin is the dermis, present beneath the epidermis layer. This layer is connected through the basement membrane layer, which provides nutritional material and oxygen because it contains blood vessels, sensory nerves, and the lymphatic system. Its thickness is 0.5–5mm and contains mesenchymal stem cells, nerve endings, sweat glands, hair follicles, and sebaceous glands. The Dermis layer of the skin protects from infections and works as a water depot that provides strength and flexibility. In skin, it is the most complex structure for the development of the *invitro* skin model (2, 3). The last layer is hypodermis. It contains nerve, blood, and lymphatic vessels. It provides separation of skin from underlying organs like muscles and bones (2).

Recently, skin diseases have been the major cause of health issues because they are associated with physiological, psychological, and social factors; weak immune systems; and trapping or contact with external materials in the skin. Acne, alopecia, face pigmentation, psoriasis, eczema, and skin cancer are the most prevalent skin conditions (1, 2). The skin disease affects a large population of all ages of people. In these diseases, skin barriers are compromised, which causes water loss, susceptibility to inflammation and infections, reduced lipid production, and skin imbalance (3, 4).

As reported, psoriasis is a chronic autoimmune skin disorder that is caused by the malfunction of the immune system. Psoriasis affects 2–5% of the world population. It is a common skin disease with a damaged epidermis, associated with rough and red patches. Psoriasis is the predefined distinctive properties like thickening of the epidermis caused by increasing keratinocyte proliferation and changes in the differentiation of keratinocytes. Along with that alteration of T cells also occurs (2). Thus, their treatment is based on the reduction of inflammatory response and prohibiting keratinocyte proliferation (4, 5).

Another is acne, a long-term inflammatory condition brought on by excess sebum production in the face and upper chest sebaceous glands. Unusual keratinization, bacterial colonization, and pore obstruction were all brought on by increased sebum production. It was reported that in most cases, acne is a genetic disorder (2, 6).

Recurrent, inflammatory, and chronic dermatosis, atopic dermatitis (AD) manifests as erythema, dryness, eczema, and pruritis. In the progression of AD, the skin thickness increases, which causes persistent pruritis and scratching. AD can occur in people of all ages, and predominance in children is 12% high. It has a psychological effect on the patients. In this, on the allergens, the immune responses increased which are the pathogenic factors for the AD progression. Systemic immunosuppressive medication, topical anti-inflammatory therapy, and biotherapy are used to treat mild to severe AD (4, 7).

12.2 DERMAL DRUG DELIVERY

When treating skin diseases, transdermal or dermal medication delivery methods are the recommended approach and offer significant benefits, by managing their rate of drug release, providing self-administration, inexpensive, convenient, and avoiding gastrointestinal tract gastrointestinal tract (GIT) degradation and first-pass metabolism. Because skin has a vast number of blood arteries and lymphatic vessels that are closely connected to the entire body, it offers better techniques for drug delivery. Additionally, the skin functions as a reservoir that allows the continuous or regulated release of medications and assists in their diffusion from the skin (5, 8). It is well known that the skin acts as a barrier to protect the body from pathogens or harmful chemicals, but it also works as a hindrance to the dermal penetration of drugs. The stratum corneum of the skin is a rate-limiting step for the penetration of drugs, peptides, and DNA. Therefore, reducing or overcoming the stratum corneum resistance leads to improvement in drug permeability (1, 5).

In the last few years, various approaches have been used to overcome stratum corneum resistance. Various chemical or physical methods like iontophoresis, electroporation, thermal ablation, and chemical enhancers approaches are used to enhance the drug permeability for the treatment of skin diseases (1, 5, 9).

12.3 MICROFLUIDICS DEVICE FOR SKIN

The microfluidic system has great potential in cell culture, cell separation, chemical screening, and DNA sequencing. Microfluidic-based drug delivery system provides delivery of the molecules that are susceptible to enzymatic degradation such as proteins, peptides, and DNA. It has the potential for the fabrication of a wide range of micro/nanoscale pharmaceutical materials. Their mobile application offers chemical analysis (6, 10).

12.3.1 MICROFLUIDICS SYSTEM

Recently, microfluidics technology has gained more interest in the research field because of its wide range of applications in basic science, biomedical, and translational research. They have several applications like cloning, gene detection, drug discovery, diagnosis, and drug delivery (7). It is based on research that deals with creating tiny devices with tiny channels/chambers and managing the flow characteristics of the minute volumes of fluids included in these microchannels/chambers, which have sizes between 10 and 100 micrometers (8, 11–13).

The multidisciplinary field of microfluidics includes elements of physics, engineering, biochemistry, nanotechnology, and biotechnology. Early in the 1980s, microfluidic technologies were invented and are now being utilized in many platforms. They have multiple benefits, including the ability to transport mass and heat and reduce waste creation, response times, sample consumption, and diffusion rates. It also facilitates three-dimensional (3D) cell culture and the modeling of physiological conditions for cell-based studies. It facilitates the continuous provision of nutrients and oxygen; aids in the integration of several processes, including mixing, cell culture, cell capture, and cell lysis; and aids in detection (8).

Microfluidic has two unique properties: First, it has rapid and accurate heat transfer and diffusion properties, which are due to the surface tension, capillary effects, and laminar flow. Second, they can easily manage the small, high-density micro- or nanostructure and allow the flexible combination or integration the several operation processes (9).

The microfluidic system has the ability to fabricate reproducible, homogeneous, micro- and nano-drug carriers with particular sizes, shapes, and desired properties. This feature is particularly useful for drug screening in situ, such as cell-on-a-chip, organ-on-a-chip, and human-on-a-chip assays to determine drug responses. It is also useful for animal research. Integrating microfluidic elements, like pumps and valves, enables multiplexed drug screening and high throughput (8).

The microfluidic system uses nano- and microscale fabrication techniques for the development of the controlled and reproducible fluidic microenvironment, which provides controlled physiochemical properties, high throughput, and evaluation of the *in vitro* biomimetic activity through the microfluidic system. Because of its capacity to regulate the emulsification process and characteristics that aid in the creation of monodispersed compound droplets in the microchannel, this approach facilitates the creation of an effective tool for the synthesis of nanoparticles with desired morphologies and characteristics (10).

12.3.2 Background of Microfluidics

This field of study focuses on the processing and manipulation of tiny fluid quantities via micrometer-sized channels. Previously, it was widely used in the inkjet print head, which analyzes numerous capabilities when only a small amount of sample or reagents are used with high resolution, sensitivity, short analysis time, and low cost. Furthermore, as development with time, these are now also used in drug design, discovery, and delivery (11).

For drug delivery, the microfluidic technique offers new fundamentals such as they provide easy control of the concentration of molecules in space and time. They are also used in the production of drug carriers with different sizes, ranging from nanometers to micrometers. Along with that, this system can be used for the development and designing of the drug carrier with a preprogrammed released profile. This method helps reduce dosage and lessens pharmacological adverse effects by delivering the medication directly and locally to the intended locations (11).

The invention of microfluidic devices is attributed to four distinct research domains, including molecular analysis, molecular biology, biodefense, and microelectronics. Certain techniques, such as capillary electrophoresis, gas-phase chromatography, and high-performance liquid chromatography, are combined with optical detection in microanalysis to create a sensitive and high-resolution method for examining small amounts of samples (11).

Biodefense helps in the development of the deployable microfluidic system, which works as a detector for chemical and biological threats. If the sample volumes are very low, molecular biology requires high throughput, sensitivity, and better resolution containing analytical methods. Microelectronics is directly used in microfluidics because they use photolithography and their associated technology (11).

Over the past two decades, microfluidics has had limited application in biology. However, its application in the creation of drug delivery systems and illness treatment has increased recently. It is used in several biomedical processes, including microchip capillary electrophoresis, DNA sequencing, and cell sorting. Additionally, microfluidics is widely used in the creation of drug delivery and metabolite monitoring systems (11).

Additionally, they are employed in the creation of the lab-on-a-chip apparatus, which is utilized in drug development and carrier research. Through feedback-loop technologies, they also offer tracking of medication release and therapeutic effects concurrently (11). Because microfluidic wearable techniques rely on monitoring the skin's vital signs and key metabolites in bodily fluids like perspiration among other fluids, they are also particularly advantageous for drug delivery. As a result, these represent the most recent and novel advancements in medication delivery, discovery, and diagnosis (11, 14, 15).

12.3.3 ADVANTAGES OF MICROFLUIDICS

a) The microfluidic device provides the delivery of drugs to specific target sites.
b) This method guarantees the bioavailability of medications at particular target receptors.
c) The microfluidic system helps in reducing the production cost and, therefore, offers inexpensive formulations.
d) Recently microfluidic devices are prepared through biodegradable and biocompatible materials hence, they give low toxic formulation.
e) The microfluidic system has the ability to control the fluid flow and work with micro or nanodevices with high controllability (12).

12.3.4 FABRICATION OF THE MICROFLUIDICS DEVICE

There are various factors that affect the designing of the microfluidic device such as the type of materials used for the fabrication, the compatibility of the material with various solvents, the channel dimension, the number of inlets, mixer, and the synthesizer (8). For the development of microfluidic chips, either a single material or a combination is used. There are several materials available that are used for the microfluidic chip like polydimethylsiloxane (PDSM), poly methyl methacrylate (PMMA), polyether ether ketone, glass, quartzose, cyclic olefin copolymer (COC), polycarbonate (PC), polyimide plastic resin, and silicon. Mostly microfluidic chips are prepared using PDSM or dimethicone. It is a transparent silicon polymer, with noninflammable, nonreactive, and nontoxic properties (7).

Glass material has strong insulation, high thermal conductivity, and transparency while silicon material has unique thermal conductivity, corrosion resistance, and low transparency. The advantages of silicon and glass materials make them suitable for the extraction, biological process, and formation of systems and devices. However, their applications are limited due to their complexity, their expensiveness, their toxic by-products, their non-gas permeability, and their mixing difficulties (9, 16).

Polymers are present in various forms, with required unique properties; therefore, polymer-based microfluidic devices have been developed. The soft lithography technique provides a polymer-based microfluidic device fabrication. The PDSM overcomes the problems with glass and silicon materials and provides various advantages, such as biocompatibility, gas permeability, and low toxicity (9). Of all materials, PDSM and PMMA are the most common polymers used for the fabrication of microfluidic devices through the soft lithography technique. These materials allow the entry of oxygen. These two materials have an issue in that they are prone to swelling when exposed to powerful solvents like acetone, which interferes with fluid movement and causes uncontrollably high-carrier production. Other polymers exhibit chemical resistance to strong acids, such as COC and polytetrafluoroethylene (PTEE). These materials are employed in the hot embossing process to fabricate the microfluidic device (8). It was reported that chip-based drug delivery models have the potential for the delivery of proteins and DNA-based drug delivery (13). The materials used in the microfluidics system are discussed in Table 12.1 and Figure 12.1.

TABLE 12.1

Materials Used in the Fabrication of Microfluidics Devices

S. No.	Material Used in Microfluidic Device	Advantage	Disadvantage	References
1.	Silicon	Strong internal stability, resistance to organic solvents, and resistance to corrosion	Expensive, difficult to manage, less flexible, and opaque in color	(9, 12, 13)
2.	Glass	Transparent, insulated, and with a high heat conductivity	High price and abrasion	
3.	PDMS (polydimethylsiloxane)	Simple to assemble, extensible, transparent, appropriate for building pumps and valves, inertness, and low fabrication costs	Hydrophobic molecule absorption	
4.	Thermostat polyester	Cheap, insoluble, and incapable of absorbing biomolecules	stiff and expensive	
5.	Thermoplastics	Highly cross-linked polymer, high production at low cost	Rigidity	

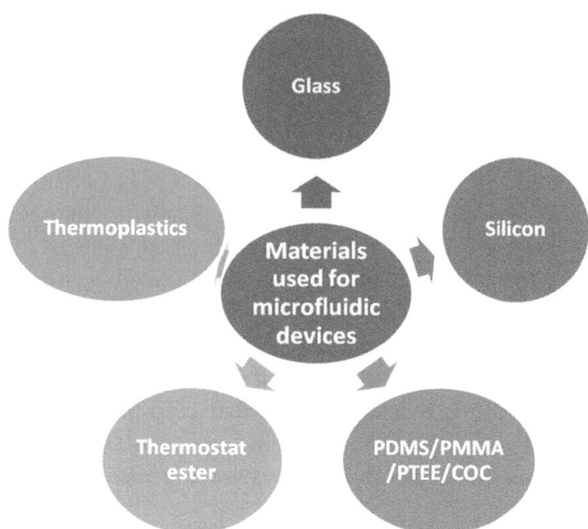

FIGURE 12.1   Materials used in the fabrication of microfluidic devices.

12.4 MICROFLUIDIC-BASED DERMAL DRUG DELIVERY SYSTEM

A fantastic tool for molecular drug efficacy monitoring is the microfluidic device. It was once employed in the detection of cancer. These instruments are employed to analyze the fluids found in channels with a micrometer-sized diameter (12). Drug delivery using microfluidic technology has a number of benefits, including accurate dosage, target-specific administration, numerous dosages, prolonged and controlled release, and minimal adverse effects. Direct drug delivery, high throughput screening, and the creation of drug carriers have all recently made use of microfluidic systems (6, 17).

As compared to the other fabricated devices it has low cost, provides better functionality, and has the ability to combine with different miniature devices. Microfluidic devices control the volume of fluid and use miniature components therefore they are capable of reducing waste, temperature control, and measuring the temperature exchange (6).

The microfluidic delivery system has the ability to improve the treatment of infectious/noninfectious diseases (7). Microfluidic provides various advantages, such as small size distribution, less polydispersity index, high encapsulation efficiency, batch-wise uniformity, and easy scale-up techniques. Particularly microfluidic chip is the very easy, simple, and most economical way to produce nanocarriers. Lipid-based, polymeric, hybrid, organic, and inorganic nanocarriers are all fabricated using microfluidic chips. Overall, the microfluidic technique has great potential for synthesizing different novel drug delivery systems (7, 10).

Renee R. Hood and a colleague created a method for preclinical research on and microfluidic production of nanoscale liposomes with adjustable sizes. They investigated liposomes' capacity to passively penetrate the skin's outer layer in order to administer drugs transdermally. Drug administration via the topical method is noninvasive and painless. In the traditional method, polydisperse liposomes are too large more than 80nm for dermal delivery, but the microfluidic technique provides monodisperse liposomes with a size of 40nm or less for size-dependent passive transdermal drug delivery system in porcine dermal tissue (14, 18).

It was observed that the microfluidic technique for nanoparticle synthesis produced nanoparticles with a smaller size, a lower diffusion coefficient, and better drug release than bulk mixing. Microfluidic-based chitosan nanoparticles have high thermal stability and reduce bactericidal concentration. This is used for the transdermal delivery of clindamycin and tretinoin (5).

It was reported that the microfluidic reactor is used for the synthesis of phospholipids-based deformable nanovesicles, which shows that changes in the input parameters like flow speed, molar concentration, and flow rate increased the entrapment efficiency of the drugs and help in tuning of size, surface charge and elasticity of the deformable nanovesicle. For determination of the deformable nanovesicle's ability to deliver the drug transdermal into the local site, they conjugated the formulation with fluorescently labeled hydrophilic bisphosphonate drug AF647 zoledronate. The formulation was lyophilized, re-suspended, and topically applied to the calvarial skin of the mice. When compared to non-deformable nanovesicles, their high-resolution fluorescence imaging and confocal microscopy demonstrate a considerable increase in the drug's encapsulated payload delivery to the target region. They also show that the synthesis of the deformable nanovesicles through a microfluidic reactor has a high yield, encapsulation efficiency, and reproducibility and acts as a good vehicle for transdermal drug delivery (15).

Sabrina Bochicchio et al. developed nanoliposomes for the delivery of D3, K2, E, and curcumin through the transdermal route. It has a high antioxidant effect and skin-curative properties. Nanoliposomes are developed through novel simil-microfluidic methods. It was the semicontinuous method that altered the problems of conventional methods, like low productivity to produce the antioxidant formulation with improved properties. This technique provides a huge production of stable antioxidant vesicles with an 84–145-nm size, negative charges, high drug loading capacity, and encapsulation efficiency. The prepared formulation was used for the cosmetic field (16). Microfluidic devices are able to manage the micro- to picoliter sample. It was reported that Loreal developed a wearable microfluidic sensor for eczema and AD that has the ability to measure the pH (17, 19, 20).

12.4.1 MICROFLUIDIC ORGAN-ON-CHIP

Recently microfluidic technology has also been used in the field of organ engineering. It is the fusion of microfluidic system advantages with tissue engineering. Additionally, this system offers a dynamic biochemical environment and a spatiotemporal chemical gradient for living organisms, enabling the creation of biomimetic tissue and organ models for use in drug discovery applications. A microfluidic device called an organ-on-a-chip is used to grow cells that mimic a specific organ or tissue. An organ-on-a-chip is a microfluidic device that mimics the complex interactions that occur between individual cells and between cells in a matrix. It is composed of different cell types grown in different layers that can interact with one another in a controlled environment. A microfluidic-based organ-on-a-chip provides an advanced architecture and network, as well as a mechanism for supporting phenotypic cell activity and the modeling of a specific organ for the development of *in vitro* disease models (2). A general microfluidic organ chip in various parts of the human body is depicted in Figure 12.2. This device contains a perfused chamber, a well, and channels with a biosensing mechanism. It can bio-mimic high-complexity human anatomical features, such as tissue and blood vessels, as well as physiological processes like blood or fluid flow and response to chemical and mechanical stimuli. They can also be constructed as spatial cell arrangements in two or three dimensions. One aim of the organ-on-a-chip is to provide personalized therapy for various ailments. Other goals include studying the architecture of the organ to reproduce the fundamental element and providing preclinical drug data, disease propagation, and toxicological data. Additionally, the apparatus simulates the vascular, lymphatic, respiratory, circulatory, digestive, and cutaneous systems (18, 21).

Recently, advancements in microelectron mechanical systems (MEMSs) have merged with microfluidic techniques. This technique combines lab-on-a-chip and cell biology to study the processes of human-derived physiology of particular organs. The microfluidic organ-on-a-chip technology shows dynamic micro and nano-scale tissue culture devices with MEMSs for the formation of multichannel microfluidic cell culture chips for bioinspired organs. To fabricate these, various materials are used like glass and silicon chips, which are conjugated with polymeric, ceramic biological matrix for the creation of specific organ microenvironment. These materials aid in controlling the device's form, surface pattern, stiffness, and small-scale architecture. Drug distribution through the skin, tissue physiology, immunology, and drug screening are all studied using the microfluidic organ-on-a-chip (19, 22). Recently, the microfluidic system has been used for testing organs like the liver, lung, heart, kidney, and skin on a microscale by investigating their properties in some physiological and pathological conditions. This system replaced the animal experiment and reduced the experimental cost. Recently, skin-on-chip devices have been used for

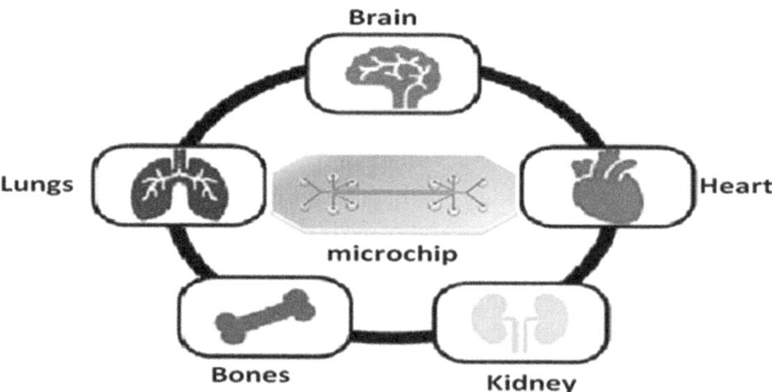

FIGURE 12.2   Microfluidic organ-on-chip in various parts of the human body.

dermal investigation (20). The vascular system is also necessary for immune cell movement from lymphoid organs to peripheral tissue and for mediating inflammatory responses. Skin-on-chips are created to emphasize the skin's vascular and perfusion systems as well as their structure and function (21).

To illustrate the trans-epithelial and trans-endothelial migration of T cells from the blood circulation to the site of skin inflammation, Ren and their colleague created a microfluidic-based skin-on-chip model. This system was built on a 3-inch-long silicon wafer that was layered with HeCaT cells, type 1 collagen gel with a porous fiber structure, and a Human umbilical vein endothelial cells human umbilical vein endothelial cells (HUVECs) layer that showed the extracellular matrix, epithelium, and endothelium components. Activated T cells in this device move toward the greater gradient of CCL20 and CXCL12 upon addition, whereby T cell transmigration is blocked by CCL20-locked dimers. Additionally, activated T cells are transmigrated via the HUVEC layer via collagen gel toward the HaCaT layer upon TNF injection into the HaCaT cell layer. This system has the ability to study the transmigration of T cells in response to drugs and inflammatory mediators (22–24).

Kwak and their team formulated a skin chip in a microfluidic chip device using fully stratified skin and mature endothelial cells. This system has a center channel that contains the epidermis, dermis as bilayered skin, and endothelial cell layers. This layer was separated through the porous membrane, which provides the fully differentiated skin in an air-liquid interface. After the endothelial and skin maturation, to reiterate the migration of leukocytes into the skin, HL-60 cells were added. Sodium dodecyl sulfate therapy resulted in an increase in the production of pro-inflammatory cytokines, specifically interleukin (IL)-6. Additionally, by incorporating dexamethasone into the device's vascular endothelium, their production was reduced. After being exposed to ultraviolet (UV) radiation, leukocytes move from the fluidic channel into the vascular layer of the skin. Therefore, this model mimics the immune response with respect to cytokine production in human skin (23, 25).

12.4.2 Microneedle Associated with Microfluidic Device for Transdermal Drug Delivery

Transdermal microfluidic-based drug delivery is simply a replacement for a hypodermic needle, associated with sensing properties, and forms multifunctional systems. It is also combined with a bioinspired reversible dry adhesive material for the formation of needles with good adhesive force and with ways to remove them (24, 26).

The microfluidic chip used for dermal administration utilizes microneedles. Recently, for the development of a microfluidic chip, different types and shapes of microneedles have been used, which provides great advances in microfluidic devices. The microneedle uses microfluidic devices for drug delivery and biomarker detection applications (7, 24).

Microneedles are solid or hollow structures with a 50–900-mm length and a less than 300-nm external diameter. They are fabricated within a patch and offer transdermal drug delivery. They are formulated to penetrate the epidermis of the skin up to a depth of 70–200mm. They are too thin and short and cannot penetrate the deeper layer of the dermis, particularly through nerves, therefore providing painless drug delivery (25).

12.4.3　Advantages of Microneedles in Transdermal Drug Delivery System

a) They are micron-sized needles placed on the patch and provide dermal drug delivery. Therefore, they offer fast healing at the injection or administered sites.

b) They easily bypass the stratum corneum and deliver the drug into the epidermis and dermis enhancing the permeability of the drugs.

c) They offer high bioavailability of drugs, especially for skin-related diseases.

d) They reduce microbial penetration compared to hypodermic needles because they are only microns in size and only rupture the epidermis.

e) The onset of action is faster with the low dose.

f) They provide painless administration of drug molecules.

g) They surpass the first-pass metabolism.

h) They can easily deliver the large molecules of the drug through a transdermal route.

i) Microneedles provide a self-administration facility therefore it has better patient compliance.

j) They provide good tolerability for long-term treatment without causing any edema and erythema (25–28).

12.4.4　Disadvantages of Microneedles

a) They have low dose accuracy.

b) They need careful attention when administered to the skin surface; if the system is not applied vertically, the dose can escape or be administered to a different degree.

c) The stratum corneum thickness varies individually; thus, their penetration depth is also different.

d) While removing the patch, the tips of microneedles break and remain within the skin.

e) Long-term or repetitive injections cause damage to veins.

f) It was also reported that the compressed dermal tissue can block the hollow microneedles (25, 29).

12.5　MATERIAL USED FOR MICRONEEDLE SYNTHESIS

For developing microneedles different materials are used. The material should provide fabrication without damaging the drug molecules, have enough mechanical strength, and provide controlled release. For their synthesis, several materials are used like silicon, metals, and glass. Microneedles fabricated from metals are expensive, brittle, and nonbiodegradable. Therefore, polymer microneedles are preferred. Various polymers are also used for the synthesis of microneedles to overcome the problem of silicon and metallic materials (25, 30). The materials used for the synthesis of microneedles are listed in Table 12.2.

TABLE 12.2

Material Used for Microneedle Synthesis (25, 31)

S. No.	Materials Used for the Microneedle Formation	Examples of Materials
1.	Metals	Silicon, Stainless steel, Titanium, and Mesoporous silicon.
2.	Biodegradable polymers	Polylactic acid (PLA), Polyglycolic acid (PGA), Polylactide-co-glycolic acid (PLGA), Polycarbonate, Polyvinylpyrrolidone (PVP).
3.	Non-biodegradable polymers	Polyvinyl acetate (PVA), Alginic acid, Gantrez AN-139, a copolymer of methylvinylether and maleic anhydride (PMVE/MA), Carbopol 971 P-NF18, Polyetherimide.
4.	Natural polymers	Thermoplastic starch, Carboxymethylcellulose, Amylopectin, Dextran, galactose, chondroitin sulfate, Maltose

Several microneedles are used like solid, porous, coated, hollow, and dissolvable. These needles are designed to painlessly penetrate the skin barrier especially the stratum corneum without affecting the nerve fibers and deliver the desired amount of liquid at the time course through the transdermal route (4, 24). They can easily puncture the skin and can be removed to form a pore, which allows the entry of the drug into the body through a rubbing lotion, cream, and gel. This provides the diffusion of drugs into the body (24, 32, 33). The materials used for the synthesis of different types of microneedles are listed in Table 12.3. Compared to other transdermal drug delivery, it improves the efficacy of the dermal delivery of the drug by minimizing the problems associated with transdermal delivery such as molecular weight, size, and lipophilicity of the biomolecules or drugs. Microneedles are a combination of transdermal delivery and injection advantages. Therefore, their use in the skin diseases or dermatology field is constantly increasing (4).

TABLE 12.3

Materials Used for the Synthesis of Different Types of Microneedles

S. No.	Type of Microneedle	Material Used for Preparation	References
1.	Solid MNs	Silicon—monocrystalline, polycrystalline silicon Metal—titanium, stainless steel, nickel Polymer—polycarbonate, Poly(lactic-co-glycolic) acid, polymethylmethacrylate, poly lactic acid	(27, 34, 35)
2.	Dissolving MNs	Natural polymer—silk, gelatin, hydroxypropyl methylcellulose Synthetic polymer—polyvinyl pyrrolidone, poly lactic acid, polyvinyl alcohol, poly(lactic-co-glycolic) acid	
3.	Hollow MNs	Ceramic, silicon, polymers, metal, and glass	
4.	Coated MNs	Polymer, stainless steel, titanium	

12.5.1 SOLID MICRONEEDLES

It was first mentioned in 1971 and used as a method for the pretreatment of the skin by the formation of pores. This involves the delivery of the medication, which is absorbed from the capillaries, through a tiny channel created by a sharp needle puncturing the skin. Because tiny pores seal up when the needle is removed, this technique makes it simple and safe to deliver the medication while lowering the risk of infection and other hazardous materials entering the body. The solid microneedle is composed of various materials, including metal, silicon, polymers, and stainless steel. These are made using lithography, micro-molding, micro-machinery, and sculpting methods. Drug delivery is made simple by conjugating a solid microneedle in a microfluidic channel (7, 36). Since the components that make up the cuticular barrier are stiff, solid microneedles have enough mechanical strength to pass through it. The drug penetration from microneedles is passive, has low delivery efficiency, and has low dose accuracy. It was also reported that the metal and silicon-based microneedles are biologically incompatible (4, 28, 37).

12.5.2 COATED MICRONEEDLES

This type of microneedle gains much interest because it can easily deliver drugs or biomolecules like proteins and DNA with minimum invasion (7). In this, the drug formulation is applied using a variety of methods, including spray-drying, molding, dip coating, inkjet printing, and inkjet deposition, to the surface of the solid microneedles. Of all these techniques, dip coating is mostly preferred. The micro-molding method provides a large production of coated microneedles and uniform and controlled drug loading. In drug delivery through coated microneedles, first, some coated microneedles are dissolved in cutaneous tissue, and the remaining microneedles are removed from the skin for recycling. The coated microneedles have low drug loading efficiency because of their thickness, needle size, nonhomogeneous coating, and premature drug loss (27, 38).

Q. Ma and their coworker developed a polyethylene glycol diacrylate (PEG-DA) microneedle and further coated it with gelation/sucrose film to increase skin permeability. The prepolymer solution was added to the mold cavity to create the microneedles, which were subsequently covered with a film made using photo-induced polymerization. The delivery and therapeutic efficacy of the produced microneedles were assessed using doxorubicin, rhodamine B, indocyanine green, and bovine serum albumin (29).

Another report shows the formation of a microfluidic system with silicon microneedles, which were further coated with Cr/Au and investigated for their chemical delivery ability (7).

12.5.3 HOLLOW MICRONEEDLES

These are micro-syringes with length and diameter at the micrometer level. They are prepared from silicon, glass, ceramic, metal, and MEMS materials. They can be formulated through deep reactive-ion etching, wet and drying etching, lithography, and 3D-printing techniques. These microneedles contain a cavity and have openings for drug delivery and extract the interstitial fluid from the skin. It provides various advantages in drug delivery (7, 39, 40).Compared to others, these microneedles give an accurate flow rate and can deliver a large dose of a drug. These microneedles are highly used for the delivery of proteins, DNA, vaccines, and drugs.

Yingjie Ren and colleagues synthesized hollow microneedles with varying diameters, heights, and shapes, as required by various drug delivery systems, using a highly precise 3D-printed master mold and dual-molding technique. In this, the hollow microneedles are prepared from biocompatible materials like light-curing resins or heat-curing polymers. Their thickness, flexibility, and rigidity were customized according to application. The drug delivery efficacy of the prepared formulation was evaluated through in-situ treatment of the psoriasis (30, 41, 42, 43).

12.5.4 DISSOLVABLE MICRONEEDLES

These microneedles are prepared from the biodegradable polymers in which drugs are encapsulated. For this microneedle, it simply penetrates the skin and releases the drugs, because this process does not require the removal of microneedles and provides one-step drug release in a controlled manner through polymer degradation (7). Dissolvable microneedles are prepared through biodegradable materials like polysaccharides, and natural or synthetic polymers by micro-molding, droplet-born air blowing, 3D printing, laser machining, and photolithography. A micro-molding method is the preferred method and is less expensive. For this, the needle or base solution is filled into a mold in centrifugal or vacuum conditions. The drug is administered into the skin by dissolving microneedles; therefore, the selection of materials used for the preparation of microneedles is important. They should have sufficient mechanical strength and good skin permeation ability. For the preparation of these microneedles, various materials are used like hyaluronic acid, polyvinyl alcohol, chitosan, dextran, and polyvinyl pyrrolidone. To increase their mechanical strength, it is coated with hyaluronidase, sucrose, and hydroxypropyl-b-cyclodextrin, which form hydrogen and electrostatic force. Dissolvable microneedles are biocompatible and suitable for long-term therapy (4, 27, 44, 45).

The primary line of treatment for psoriasis is oral methotrexate. However, it has certain adverse effects, such as hepatotoxicity and pain in the GIT. Du and his colleague developed dissolvable microneedles filled with methotrexate to treat psoriasis in order to overcome this. The preparation reduced the expression of the nucleus-related antigen (Ki67), which subsequently prevented keratinocyte proliferation and epidermal thickness. In order to reduce inflammation, it also downregulated the IL-23/IL-17 axis. When taken twice daily, the formulation effectively reduced psoriasis caused by oral methotrexate. Tekko and associates created methotrexate nanocrystals, which were then combined with dissolving microneedles, to address the poor drug loading of the product. This formulation offers continuous medication release for 72 hours and better drug loading up to a 2.48-mg microneedle patch. This conjugation shows increased drug retention in the skin and decreased systemic exposure to drugs (1, 4).

In a different study, Jing and colleagues created dissolving microneedles and combined them with pH-responsive micelles that were concealed by keratinocyte membranes to release shikonin actively. This is because the homologous targeting micelles are internalized by the HaCaT cells and show responsive release of the drug in a low acidic environment. The formulation has remarkable anti-psoriatic properties via modulating the inflammatory signals generated by IL-23/T helper 17 cells (1, 4). Triamcinolone acetonide has poor solubility and is a regularly used medication for atopic dermatitis. To overcome this, Jang and their team developed high-dose triamcinolone acetonide (TA) containing dissolving microneedles. The formulation reduced skin inflammation in mice (1, 4, 39, 46–48). A general representation of microneedles for dermal drug delivery is shown in Figure 12.3.

12.6 APPLICATIONS OF MICROFLUIDICS IN DERMAL DRUG DELIVERY

Microfluidics has gained significant advances and development in the field of dermal delivery. Tissue engineering is the key area for cell growth and regeneration in the body system. Another prime area is developing skin tissue scaffolds through microfluidics. These are discussed next.

12.6.1 MICROFLUIDIC DEVICE FOR TISSUE ENGINEERING

Tissue engineering has the potential to regenerate bioengineered tissue on the basis of cellular growth and biocompatible materials, which help in the replacement, repair, and proliferation of damaged tissue. In order to encourage tissue regeneration, bioengineered scaffolds are improving the transmission of specific cells and growth factors through tissue injury. The ready-made skin scaffolds aid in promoting cell growth proliferation, which, in turn, results in tissue vascularization. The scaffolds ought

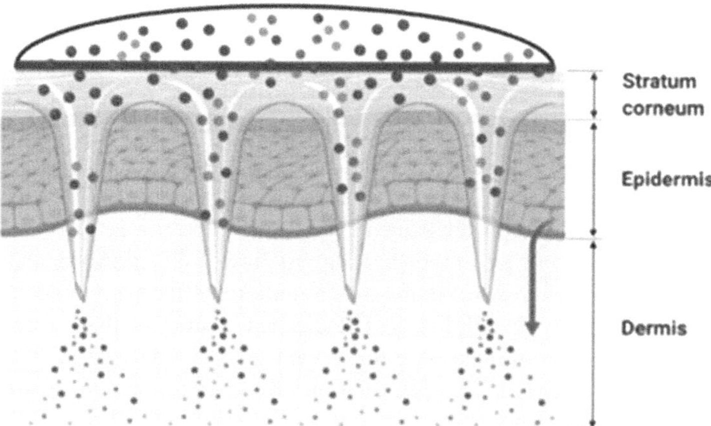

FIGURE 12.3 Microneedles for transdermal drug delivery to the skin.

to be toxic-free and biodegradable after use. According to a paper, skin scaffolds mimic the properties and functions of a certain tissue's extracellular matrix. They also imitated the mechanical, biological, and physical characteristics of the tissue (31, 49–52). Tissue-engineered skins serve the purpose of skin modeling. They can treat acute/chronic wounds, chemical permeation, clinical skin grafting, and cutaneous drug administration. Nevertheless, the tissue-engineered skin that is now available is not adequate for use in creating the skin disease model. A skin model should have many cell cultures in distinct layers that are subjected to mechanical stresses and a spatiotemporal chemical gradient. By using long-term cell culture and real-time tissue behavior monitoring in a particular controlled environment, these types of models would validate the cells' biomimetic function. (2, 53).

12.6.2 MICROFLUIDIC DEVICE FOR DEVELOPING SKIN TISSUE SCAFFOLDS

The scaffolds are a biodegradable composition that provides temporary support to the cell in new tissue growth. They can be prepared from natural and synthetic polymers. Natural polymers are widely used for scaffold preparation because of their biocompatibility and biodegradability. Scaffolds made of microparticles, microfibers, and 3D matrices have been created in recent years using the microfluidic process. Microfluidic techniques involve the manipulation, mixing, transport, separating, and control of fluids within a microchannel (32, 54, 55).

Skin tissue and cell scaffolds are the major challenges when producing biomimetic skin models, especially a dermal matrix having an *in vivo* composition and similar microenvironment that ensure their reproducibility and stability. The vessel's system of the skin is present in the dermis and performs various essential functions such as the transfer of nutrients, removing waste products from cells, helps in thermoregulation. Therefore, the vascular system also has an important role in transdermal penetration. Microfluidic advances help in the development of the perfused vascular network. In this, the pre-vascularized pattern technique is used for the development of the vascular pattern-on-chip chips (3). The skin in humans is an active organ with constant regeneration, which assures the continuous replacement of the outer layer of the cell that is exposed to the environment. The inner cell, which is produced from the skin's deeper layers, is what causes this regeneration (36). Microfluidic scaffolds have numerous advantages compared to the conventional culture and biofabrication methods. This system developed several biosensor tissues and diseased models like kidney, liver, skin, lungs, heart, cancer, and blood coagulation by using biocompatible and biodegradable materials (33, 36, 56, 57).

Although there are various advancements done on the bioengineered skin scaffolds, some hindrances occur in the preparation of bio-scaffolds limited nutrients, restriction in cell-to-cell interaction, extracellular matrix and cell interaction, and insufficient replication of physiological environment(31, 36). The identification and modulation of cellular responses based on tissue specificity are primarily influenced by extracellular matrix dynamics. Tissue growth and regeneration are significantly influenced by the extracellular matrix, as well as the healing of wounds and the advancement of disease. Because of this, systems that can replicate the dynamics of the primary tissue are frequently employed to create bio-scaffolds that aid in the study of the basic behaviors of cells (31).

Therefore, microfluidic systems are introduced into tissue engineering and scaffolds which have the potential to understand the cellular interaction with extracellular matrix in a controlled microenvironment. It was reported that the microperfusion used in the microfluidic system can easily deliver nutrients across the cells and remove the waste product from the system by providing a constant flow in the microchannels. This model also helps in mimicking the *in vivo* cellular reestablishment (31, 58, 59).

In recent years, microscopic 3D cell culture environments were generated in the microfluidic device because they provide several advantages such as provide active vasculature system, which helps in the distribution of metabolism and clearance of the waste through a scaffold system. They offer a non-disturbing mini-probe system of cells and fluids for *ex situ* analysis. They assist in tissue modulation using bioactive substances and cells, and they provide long-term microscopy validation of cells or fluids. They also provide automated spatiotemporal control in tissue development (33, 60).

12.7 CONCLUSION AND FUTURE PROSPECTS

Recently, improvements in transdermal drug delivery, numerous microfluidic drug delivery methods have been developed, microneedles, tissue engineering, skin-on-chip, and others for the treatment of various skin conditions like eczema, acne, and psoriasis. This microfluidic system provides control over drug release, time, and location, increasing drug efficiency and reducing side effects. They also offer a unique artificial skin that does not require any animal testing and is similar to human skin. Therefore, they ultimately reduce the production cost of the formulations. In this chapter, we covered the application of a microfluidic system through a transdermal route for the treatment of the skin condition. It includes the physiology of the skin, the background of a microfluidic system, materials used for their fabrication, microneedles and their details, skin-on-chip devices, and tissue scaffolds used in tissue engineering. This chapter provided knowledge of microfluidic systems with transdermal routes and their importance. Although the microfluidic system has recently gained much attention, it still needs to work on a large scale, not only a laboratory scale. They also required focusing on the treatment of various skin conditions, not only cosmetology sector but also in the treatment of the disease condition.

ACKNOWLEDGMENT

The Department of Science and Technology (DST-FIST) [SR/FST/COLLEGE/2018/418], New Delhi, is acknowledged by the authors for its financial support.

CONFLICT OF INTEREST

None.

REFERENCES

(1) Qu F, Geng R, Liu Y, Zhu J. Advanced nanocarrier- and microneedle-based transdermal drug delivery strategies for skin diseases treatment. *Theranostics* 2022;12(7):3372–3406. https://doi.org/10.7150/thno.69999

(2) Mohammadi MH, Heidary Araghi B, Beydaghi V, Geraili A, Moradi F, Jafari P, Janmaleki M, Valente KP, Akbari M, Sanati-Nezhad A. Skin diseases modeling using combined tissue engineering and microfluidic technologies. *Adv Healthc Mater* 2016;5:2459–2480.

(3) Zoio P, Oliva A. Skin-on-a-chip technology: Microengineering physiologically relevant in vitro skin models. *Pharmaceutics* 2022;14:1–30. 10.3390/pharmaceutics14030682

(4) Peng T, Chen Y, Hu W, Huang Y, Zhang M, Lu C, Pan X, Wu C. Microneedles for enhanced topical treatment of skin disorders: Applications, challenges, and prospects. *Engineering* 2023:1–20. 10.1016/j.eng.2023.05.009

(5) Sanjay ST, Zhou W, Dou M, Tavakoli H, Ma L, Xu F, Li X. Recent advances of controlled drug delivery using microfluidic platforms. *Adv Drug Deliv Rev* 2018;128:3–28. 10.1016/j.addr.2017.09.013

(6) Mancera-Andrade EI, Parsaeimehr A, Arevalo-Gallegos A, Ascencio-Favela G, Parra-Saldivar R. Microfluidics technology for drug delivery: A review. *Frontiers in Bioscience, Elite* 2018;10:74–91.

(7) Bhattacharjee G, Gohil N, Shukla M, Sharma S, Mani I, Pandya A, Chu DT, Le Bui N, Thi YV, Khambhati K, Maurya R. Exploring the potential of microfluidics for next-generation drug delivery systems. *OpenNano* 2023;12:100150.

(8) Damiati S, Kompella UB, Damiati SA, Kodzius R Microfluidic devices for drug delivery systems and drug screening. *Gene* 2018;9:103. 10.3390/genes9020103

(9) Li X, Fan X, Li Z, Shi L, Liu J, Luo H, Wang L, Du X, Chen W, Guo J, Li C. Application of microfluidics in drug development from traditional medicine. *Biosensors* 2022;12:870. 10.3390/bios12100870

(10) Ejeta F. Recent Advances of Microfluidic Platforms for Controlled Drug Delivery in Nanomedicine. In *Drug Design, Development and Therapy* 2021:15:3881–3891.

(11) Hassan S, Zhang YS. Microfluidic Technologies for Local Drug Delivery. In *Chapter 10 Microfluidics for Pharmaceutical Applications* 2019:1–25. 10.1016/B978-0-12-812659-2.00010-7

(12) Sharma IS, Thakur MO, Singh SH, Tripathi AS. Microfluidic devices as a tool for drug delivery and diagnosis: A review. *International Journal of Applied Pharmaceutics* 2021;13(1):1–8.

(13) Nielsen JB, Hanson RL, Almughamsi HM, Pang C, Fish TR, Woolley AT. Microfluidics: Innovations in materials and their fabrication and functionalization. *Anal Chem* 2020 Jan 7;92(1):150–168. 10.1021/acs.analchem.9b04986

(14) Hood RR, Kendall EL, DeVoe DL, Quezado Z, Junqueira M, Finkel JC, Vreeland WN. Microfluidic formation of nanoscale liposomes for passive transdermal drug delivery. *2013 Microsystems for Measurement and Instrumentation: Fulfilling the Promise (MAMNA)* 2013.

(15) Subbiah N, Campagna J, Spilman P, Alam MP, Sharma S, Hokugo A, Nishimura I, John V. Deformable nanovesicles synthesized through an adaptable microfluidic platform for enhanced localized transdermal drug delivery. *Hindawi Journal of Drug Delivery* 2017;2017:1–12. 10.1155/2017/4759839

(16) Bochicchio S, Dalmoro A, De Simone V, Bertoncin P, Lamberti G, Barba AA. Simil-microfluidic nanotechnology in manufacturing of liposomes as hydrophobic antioxidants skin release systems. *Cosmetics* 2020;7:22. 10.3390/cosmetics7020022

(17) Zambrano A. Market analysis and commercialization opportunities of microfluidics. *The Microfluidic Circle* 2019:1–5. 10.13140/RG.2.2.31111.04005

(18) Bendre A, Bhat MP, Lee KH, Altalhi T, Alruqi MA, Kurkuri M. Recent developments in microfluidic technology for synthesis and toxicity-efficiency studies of biomedical nanomaterials. *Materials Today Advances* 2022;13:100205.

(19) Planz V, Lehr CM, Windbergs M. In vitro models for evaluating safety and efficacy of novel technologies for skin drug delivery. *J Control Release* 2016;242:89–104. 10.1016/j.jconrel.2016.09.002

(20) Ponmozhi J, Dhinakaran S, Varga-Medveczky Z, Fónagy K, Bors LA, Iván K, Erdő F. Development of skin-on-a-chip platforms for different utilizations: Factors to be considered. *Micromachines* 2021;12:294. 10.3390/mi12030294

(21) Moon S, Kim DH, Shin JU. In vitro models mimicking immune response in the skin. *Yonsei Med J* 2021;62(11):969–980. 10.3349/ymj.2021.62.11.969

(22) Ren X, Getschman AE, Hwang S, Volkman BF, Klonisch T, Levin D, et al. Investigations on T cell transmigration in a human skinon-chip (SoC) model. *Lab Chip* 2021;21:1527–1569.

(23) Kwak BS, Jin SP, Kim SJ, Kim EJ, Chung JH, Sung JH. Microfluidic skin chip with vasculature for recapitulating the immune response of the skin tissue. *BiotechnolBioeng* 2020;117:1853–1863.

(24) Riahi R, Tamayol A, Shaegh SA, Ghaemmaghami AM, Dokmeci MR, Khademhosseini A. Microfluidics for advanced drug delivery systems, *CurrOpin Chem Eng* 2015;7:101–112. 10.1016/j.coche.2014.12.001

(25) Bariya SH, Gohel MC, Mehta TA, Sharma OP. Microneedles: An emerging transdermal drug delivery system. *J Pharm Pharmacol* 2012;64:11–29.

(26) Waghule T, Singhvi G, Dubey SK, Pandey MM, Gupta G, Singh M, Dua K. Microneedles: A smart approach and increasing potential for transdermal drug delivery system. *Biomed Pharmacother* 2019;109:1249–1258.

(27) Kulkarni D, Damiri F, Rojekar S, Zehravi M, Ramproshad S, Dhoke D, Musale S, Mulani AA, Modak P, Paradhi R, Vitore J. Recent advancements in microneedle technology for multifaceted biomedical applications. *Pharmaceutics* 2022;14:1–44. 10.3390/pharmaceutics14051097

(28) Ma Z, Li B, Peng J, Gao D. Recent development of drug delivery systems through microfluidics: From synthesis to evaluation. *Pharmaceutics* 2022;14:434. 10.3390/pharmaceutics14020434

(29) Ma Q, Cao J, Gao Y, Han S, Liang Y, Zhang T, Wang X, Sun Y. Microfluidic-mediated nano-drug delivery systems: From fundamentals to fabrication for advanced therapeutic applications, *Nanoscale* 2020;12:15512–15527.

(30) Ren Y, Li J, Chen Y, Wang J, Chen Y, Wang Z, Zhang Z, Chen Y, Shi X, Cao L, Zhang J. Customized flexible hollow microneedles for psoriasis treatment with reduced-dose drug. *BioengTransl Med* 2023;8:1–11.

(31) Gharib G, Bütün I, Muganlı Z, Kozalak G, Namlı I, Sarraf SS, Ahmadi VE, Toyran E, Van Wijnen AJ, Koşar A. Biomedical applications of microfluidic devices: A review. *Biosensors* 2022;12:1–60. 10.3390/bios12111023

(32) Rosellini E, Cascone MG. Microfluidic fabrication of natural polymer-based scaffolds for tissue engineering applications: A review. *Biomimetics (Basel)* 2023;8(1):74. 10.3390/biomimetics8010074

(33) Tong A, Voronov R. A minireview of microfluidic scaffold materials in tissue engineering. *Front Mol Biosci* 2022;8:783268. 10.3389/fmolb.2021.783268

(34) Yu F, Nivasini D, Kumar OS, Choudhury D, Foo LC, Ng SH. Microfluidic platforms for modeling biological barriers in the circulatory system. *Drug Discov Today* 2018;23:815–829.

(35) Abaci HE, Guo Z, Doucet Y, Jackow J, Christiano A. Next generation human skin constructs as advanced tools for drug development. *Exp Biol Med* 2017;242:1657–1668.

(36) Zhuge W, Liu H, Wang W, Wang J. Microfluidic bioscaffolds for regenerative engineering. *Engineered Regeneration* 2022;3:110–120.

(37) Stanton DN, Ganguli-Indra G, Indra AK, Karande P. Bioengineered efficacy models of skin disease: Advances in the last 10 years. *Pharmaceutics* 2022;14(2):319. 10.3390/pharmaceutics14020319

(38) Liu L, Zhao W, Ma Q, Gao Y, Wang W, Zhang X, Dong Y, Zhang T, Liang Y, Han S, Cao J. Functional nano-systems for transdermal drug delivery and skin therapy. *Nanoscale Adv* 2023;5:1527–1558.

(39) Giri Nandagopal MS, Antony R, Rangabhashiyam S, Sreekumar N, Selvaraju N. Overview of microneedle system: A third generation transdermal drug delivery approach. *Microsyst Technol* 2014;20:1249–1272. 10.1007/s00542-014-2233-5

(40) Nazari H, Heirani-Tabasi A, Ghorbani S, Eyni H, Razavi Bazaz S, Khayati M, Gheidari F, Moradpour K, Kehtari M, Ahmadi Tafti SM, Ahmadi Tafti SH. Microfluidic-based droplets for advanced regenerative medicine: Current challenges and future trends. *Biosensors* 2022;12:20. 10.3390/bios12010020

(41) Tomeh MA, Zhao X. Recent advances in microfluidics for the preparation of drug and gene delivery systems. *Mol Pharm* 2020;17:4421–4434. 10.1021/acs.molpharmaceut.0c00913

(42) Huang WY, Huang JP, Lin CC, Lin YS. A transdermal measurement platform based on microfluidics. *Hindawi Journal of Chemistry* 2017;2017:1–8. 10.1155/2017/9343824

(43) Desmet E, Van Gele M, Lambert J. Topically applied lipidand surfactant-based nanoparticles in the treatment of skin disorders. *Expert Opin Drug Deliv* 2016;14:109–122. 10.1080/17425247.2016.1206073

(44) Amreen K, Goel S. Review—Miniaturized and microfluidic devices for automated nanoparticle synthesis. *ECS Journal of Solid-State Science and Technology* 2021;10:017002.

(45) Zhang Y, Chen Y, Huang J, Liu Y, Peng J, Chen S, Song K, Ouyang X, Cheng H, Wang X. Skin-interfaced microfluidic devices with oneopening chambers and hydrophobic valves for sweat collection and analysis. *Lab Chip* 2020;20:2635–2645.

(46) Tabasum H, Gill N, Mishra R, Lone S. Wearable microfluidic-based e-skin sweat sensors. *RSC Adv* 2022;12:8691–8707.

(47) Sarama R, Matharu PK, Abduldaiem Y, Corrêa MP, Gil CD, Greco KV. In vitro disease models for understanding psoriasis and atopic dermatitis. *Front Bioeng Biotechnol* 2022;10:803218. doi: 10.3389/fbioe.2022.803218

(48) Kleinstreuer C, Li J, Koo J. Microfluidics of nano-drug delivery. *Int J Heat Mass Transf* 2008;51:5590–5597.

(49) Patze S, Huebner U, Liebold F, Weber K, Cialla-May D, Popp J. SERS as an analytical tool in environmental science: The detection of sulfamethoxazole in the nanomolar range by applying a microfluidic cartridge setup. *Anal Chim Acta* 2016;949:1–7.

(50) Fernandez-Carro E, Angenent M, Gracia-Cazaña T, Gilaberte Y, Alcaine C, Ciriza J. Modeling an optimal 3D skin-on-chip within microfluidic devices for pharmacological studies. *Pharmaceutics* 2022;14:1417. 10.3390/pharmaceutics14071417

(51) Maia R, Carvalho V, Lima R, Minas G, Rodrigues RO. Microneedles in advanced microfluidic systems: A systematic review throughout lab and organ-on-a-chip applications. *Pharmaceutics* 2023;15:792. 10.3390/pharmaceutics15030792

(52) Costa S, Vilas-Boas V, Lebre F, Granjeiro JM, Catarino CM, Teixeira LM, Loskill P, Alfaro-Moreno E, Ribeiro AR. Microfluidic-based skin-on-chip systems for safety assessment of nanomaterials. *Trends Biotechnol* 2023;1–17. 10.1016/j.tibtech.2023.05.009

(53) Valencia L, Canalejas-Tejero V, Clemente M, Fernaud I, Holgado M, Jorcano JL, Velasco D. A new microfuidic method enabling the generation of multi-layered tissues-on-chips using skin cells as a proof of concept. Sci Rep 2021;11:13160.

(54) Wu CH, Ma HJ, Baessler P, Balanay RK, Ray TR. Skin-interfaced microfluidic systems with spatially engineered 3D fluidics for sweat capture and analysis, *Sci Adv* 2023;9:1–14.

(55) Pérez-Salas JL, Moreno-Jiménez MR, Rocha-Guzmán NE, González-Laredo RF, Medina-Torres L, Gallegos-Infante JA. In vitro and ex vivo models for screening topical anti-inflammatory drugs. *Sci Pharm* 2023;91:20. 10.3390/scipharm91020020

(56) Hammad M, Pławiak P, ElAffendi M, El-Latif AA, Latif AA. Enhanced deep learning approach for accurate eczema and psoriasis skin detection. *Sensors* 2023;23:7295. 10.3390/s23167295

(57) Shabestani Monfared G, Ertl P, Rothbauer M. Microfluidic and lab-on-a-chip systems for cutaneous wound healing studies. *Pharmaceutics* 2021;13:793. 10.3390/pharmaceutics 13060793

(58) Xu S, Zhang Y, Jia L, Mathewson KE, Jang KI, Kim J, Fu H, Huang X, Chava P, Wang R, Bhole S. Soft microfluidic assemblies of sensors, circuits, and radios for the skin. *Science* 2014;344:70–74.

(59) Yeo JC, Lim CT. Emergence of microfluidic wearable technologies. *Lab Chip* 2016;16:4082–4090.

(60) Yu F, Nivasini D, Kumar OS, Choudhury D, Foo LC, Ng SH. Microfluidic platforms for modeling biological barriers in the circulatory system. *Drug Discov Today* 2018;23:815–829.

13 3D-Printed Microfluidic Devices with Integrated Biosensors for Dermatological Application

Astha Verma
Shri Rawatpura Sarkar Institute of Pharmacy, Durg, India

Khomendra Kumar Sarwa
Government Girls Polytechnic, Raipur, India

13.1 INTRODUCTION

Microfluids are now a well-established field of research that can be described as technology that processes small amounts of fluids (10^{-9} to 10^{-18} L) using fluidic channels of critical dimensions of 10–100 micrometers (1). Microfluidic chips are designed with several submillimeter channels that allow accurate routing of fluids providing desired features of mixing, pumping, and separating the liquid as required (2). Microfluidic technology has profound advantages, which include low sample intake and volume consumption, high sensitivity with spatial resolution, rapid processing, precise handling, and easy integration with electronic devices (3, 4). Microfluidics has a broad range of applications and includes multidisciplinary aspects involving engineering and combining domains of chemistry, physics, biotechnology, biomedicine, and bioanalysis (5). Several clinical applications of microfluidics are widely explored in the screening of cancer, single-cell analysis, biosensors, microphysiological devices, drug screening, and point-of-care (POC) diagnostics (6, 7). Microfluidics systems are intricate and the methods through which microfluidics are produced may not be suitable for mass production since they require a large working area, a distinctive clean room, and controlled sophisticated facilities to process effectively (8). Complex control systems, nonstandard user interfaces, production speed, and material modeling expenses are further drawbacks. Because of the time-consuming and expensive fabrication processes, microfluidic devices' potential expansion is thus somewhat constrained to research labs, which restricts their diffusion. As a result, increasing attempts are being made to produce microfluidic devices using simpler

DOI: 10.1201/9781032690926-13

and less expensive methods that might contribute to the development of microfluidics beyond laboratories (8, 9).

Recent technological developments have contributed to the innovation of microfluidic devices, by using three-dimensional printing (3DP) technology to create custom-based fluidic devices. Microfluidics constraints related to mass manufacturing can be overcome by 3D printing, which makes it possible to fabricate these devices more quickly and at a cheaper cost (10, 11). Three-dimensional printing, an additive manufacturing (AM) approach, is intended for the construction of a variety of structures using computer-controlled procedures based on 3D digital representations of objects intended to be printed. Digital models offer a very flexible way to create and shape objects, and the procedure involves printing subsequent layers of objects that are constructed on one another. The typical fabrication thicknesses for each printed layer range from 0.001 to 0.1 inches (11–13). With smaller space requirements, complex internal structures can be created for objects using 3DP technology, and developing parts of different sizes, from micro to macro, can be accomplished via 3DP. Thus, distinctive, patient-customized goods can be produced with extreme precision by employing computer-aided design (CAD) software to control the sequential addition of material in a 3DP process (8, 14). The first 3D-printed material was produced using a conventional planar photolithographic technique in silicon or glass, but the current availability of printable materials (such as metals, ceramics, thermoplastics, carbon-based material composites, and even living cells) has brought a broad spectrum of additional 3DP technologies, including selective laser sintering (SLS), fused deposition modeling (FDM), inkjet 3D printing (i3Dp), direct-ink writing (DIW), digital light processing (DLP) or stereolithography (SLA; 15–17). With the advancement in technologies, 3DP finds evolved and expanded use in biomedical applications, including disease modeling, bioprinting for organ transplantation, rapid prototyping of organ models, printed tissue models, in vitro substrates for cell culture, scaffolds for tissue engineering, customized fabrication of patient-specific surgical implants and prostheses, and numerous medical scenarios requiring the quick production of customized parts. Indeed, during the pandemic, 3D-printed microfluidics POC devices emerged as strong tools for determining multiple pathogen strains (18–21). The 3DP technologies characteristics features, and applications can be summarized in Table 13.1 (15–17, 19, 19–21).

Three-dimensional printing substantially facilitates the construction of multifaceted micro- and nanoscale devices that can respond to a variety of external stimuli, including optical, electrochemical, electrical, and thermal. As a result, there is now more interest in using 3DP technology for developing sensors and biosensors (22).

13.2 EMERGENCE OF 3D-PRINTED MICROFLUIDICS BIOSENSORS

The first use of biosensors was reported in cardiac pacemakers in the 1950s (23). A glucose biosensor developed by Leland Clark in 1962 marked the beginning of all the apparent interest in biosensors, which were based on an oxygen electrode (24), facilitating vital biological signal monitoring in vivo and in vitro for various applications. Since 1962, biosensors have been used in several clinical, biotechnological, biomedical, and other applications, focusing on a broad spectrum of analytes,

TABLE 13.1

Various 3D-Printed Technologies with Applications Relevant to Microfluidics

Methods	Principle/Characteristic Features	Materials	Applications	Limitations
Fused Deposition Modelling	Extrusion-based 3D printing A process that involves employing a heated nozzle to arrange thermoplastic polymeric materials in layers and extrude them onto a platform that has been cooled below its melting temperature.	Polylactic acid (PLA), Acrylonitrile, Polycarbonate (PC), Nylon, Polystyrene (PS), Polyethylene terephthalate (PET) Acrylonitrile butadiene styrene (ABS)	Tissue Scaffolds, Wearable sensors, Lab-on-chip organoids	Geometric inaccuracy, Low mechanical strength, Surface roughness
Stereolithography	Part of the Vat Photopolymerization. An ultraviolet (UV) laser beam is utilized to produce the object layer by layer after photosensitive thermoset polymers are deposited in liquid form.	ABS, polyethylene, Polypropylene nanocomposite, Photoresins, Acrylate resins, Epoxy resins	Soft robotics, Wearable sensors, Targeted drug delivery	Limited mechanical properties, Less biocompatible, Restricted to a single print material. Removal of the uncured resin remains difficult, Low resolution.
Digital Light Processing (DLP)	Also, part of the Vat Photopolymerization. UV radiation from the projector (lightbulb) cures the photopolymer resins used in the DLP process, which are processed by the printer. Each layer is formed when the light from the projector reaches the liquid polymer.	Photo resins, Ceramics	Single-cell screening and analysis	Fabrication resolution is less. Partial polymerization of the resin. Low throughput when printing large components.

(*Continued*)

TABLE 13.1
(Continued)

Methods	Principle/Characteristic Features	Materials	Applications	Limitations
Inkjet 3D Printing (i3Dp)	A stable ceramic suspension, including powdered zirconium oxide dissolved in water, is used in this approach. The suspension is pushed and dropped onto the substrate through the injection nozzle. To support further layers of printed materials, the droplets harden into a continuous pattern. Both liquid-based and wax-based inks are employed.	Hydrogels, Photoresins, Soft elastomers Liquid metals	Paper-based analytical devices (µPADs) manufacturing. Point-of-care testing (POCT) diagnostic, Scaffolds for tissue engineering.	The post-processing step requires the complete removal of solid materials.
PolyJet Process	The PolyJet method is similar to printing with an inkjet. Photopolymer droplets are directed over an integrated substrate and solidified with UV light to create objects using this 3D-printing method.	Photoresins	Measures ATP release from RBC, Fibers for cell culture	Expensive, Complex steps of manufacturing.
Selective Laser Sintering	In this process, a laser beam melts the powder and fuses it to generate multilayer shapes. Powder fusion is achieved in SLS by a variety of particle-binding techniques, including chemical processes, solid-state sintering, and absolute or partial melting.	Polystyrenes (PS), Polyamide (PA), Polycaprolactone (PCL), Polyaryletherketones (PAEK)	pH sensors Tissue scaffolds	High porosity, Do not melt all powders with a laser beam.

including minute molecules, DNA, proteins, and even whole microbes (25, 26). The recent COVID-19 pandemic has demonstrated the importance of early and precise pathogen detection, as well as the importance of their biomarkers. Furthermore, infectious diseases brought on by various viruses (such as Ebola, HIV, influenza, and hepatitis), parasites (malaria), and bacteria (tuberculosis) constitute serious global health concerns, particularly in impoverished countries (27).

A biosensor is a discrete, integrated system that generates precise quantitative or semiquantitative analytical data through a biological recognition element (biochemical receptor) in close vicinity to a physical transducer element (28). Biosensors consist of three primary components, which can be depicted in Figure 13.1: a detector: to identify the biological element or the stimulus, a transducer: to transform the input signal into detectable output, and a Signal processing system: to process the output signal in digital analog (29).

Biological sensors are broadly classified as catalytic biosensors and affinity biosensors depending on the transducer or sensing components. Catalytic sensors include various biological sensing components, such as enzymes, microorganisms, organelles, cells, and biological tissue, whereas affinity biosensors account for specific receptors, antibodies, and nucleic acids (30). The biological sensing element typically comprises one of the biocomponents indicated earlier, mounted in a transducer that can recognize the intended analyte (31). The transducing mechanism will be determined by specific types of physiological changes that result from the sensing occurrence. Transducing technologies can be divided into electrochemical (conductimetric, impedimetric,

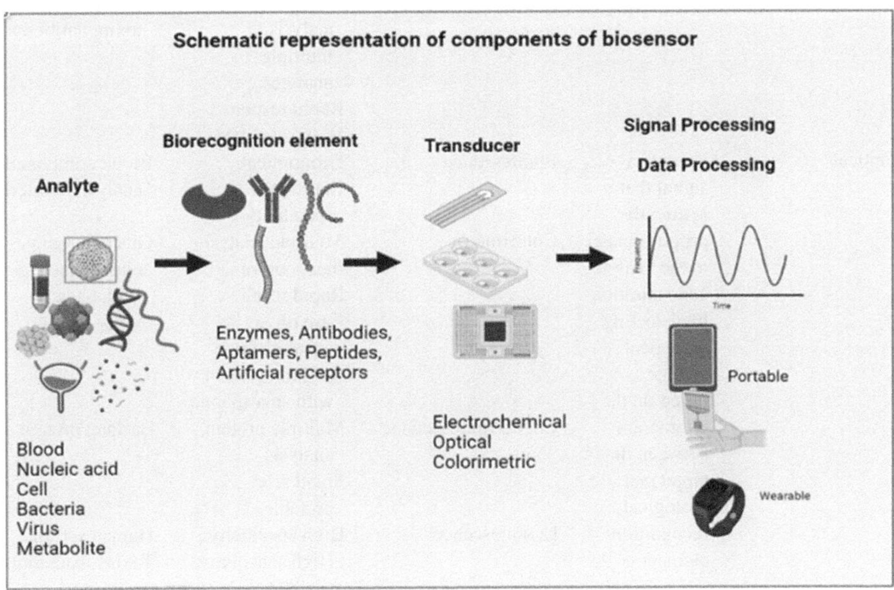

FIGURE 13.1 Schematic representation of components of a biosensor. Biosensors are typically comprised of a biorecognition element that binds with target analytes and a transducer component that converts the binding process into electrochemical or optical signals. The illustration is "created with BioRender.com."

potentiometric, and amperometric), acoustic gravimetric, optical (fluorescence, chemiluminescence, luminescence), and pyroelectric The application of various biosensors can be summarized in Table 13.2 (32–35).

Biological sensors are now multiplexed with different sensing modalities, miniaturized, and consolidated into a single device (36). The evolution of smaller devices

TABLE 13.2

3D Printed Biosensor Techniques for Diagnosis and Drug Delivery

Transducer	Principle	Techniques	Advantages	Analytes
Electrochemical	Enzyme-catalyzed reactions produce a potential or current difference	Amperometric	Simple instrumentation, Low-cost miniaturization	Glucose, nitrite, lactic acid, uric acid, dopamine, tyrosine cholesterol, and choline
		Voltammetric	Robustness Significant detection limit High specificity	Insulin, ATP, DNA, uric acid, cotinine, cancer biomarkers, catechol, dopamine, serotonin protein, and virus.
		Impedimetric	Ease of analysis, analysis of multiple analytes, Rapid response, High sensitivity	Protein, bacteria, toxin, antibody
Optical	Generate a signal that is directly proportionate to the analyte concentration by detecting an optical change based on the interaction between the target and biological recognition element.	Fluorescence	Economical, Improved specificity,	Blood component analysis, bacteria
		Colorimetric	Multiple analysis Inexpensive Rapid result Ease of customization and integration with smartphone	Glucose, lactate, nitrite, nucleic acid, bacteria, virus
		Chemiluminescence	Multiple protein analysis Small size, portable	Lactate, protein
		Luminescence	High specificity, High sensitivity, excellent enhanced substrate systems Integration with smartphone	Human serum, Toxins, bacterial pathogens

with greater functionality, the multiplexing technique, enhanced implantability in viable tissue, and reduced energy requirements is the outcome of manufacturing improvements that have led to the evolution of sophisticated biological sensors due to advancements in manufacturing processes (37). The creation of soft electronic devices with an elastic modulus similar to the tissue in the human body has also been a major development. Pacemakers, glucose-detecting electrochemical sensors, and microelectrode-based sensors are examples of devices created using conventional techniques like lithography. These strategies have been used in the field successfully for the past 50 years (38). In contrast, 3DP, one of the new AM methods, which utilizes sequential addition of materials to produce parts of the devices digitally controlled by CAD, has been used in the last decades for biomedical devices. Numerous techniques for 3DP with various polymers, ceramics, and metals were created and optimized in the 1980s and 1990s (38, 39). Later, these methods found a path in the production of biomedical devices, including the design and fabrication of customized lab-on-a-chip biosensors based on chemiluminescent and potentiometric principles led by progression in polymers-based stereolithography and micro-stereolithography techniques (40). Microfluidic biosensors that are 3D-printed offer a framework for organs-on-a-chip designs utilized in customized medicine (41). These kinds of devices provide an in vitro environment that closely resembles the physiological environment, which enables controlled, automated observation and analysis of biomedical processes with a limited analyte amount and affordable price. The quick multi-material system integration made possible by 3DP allows for elasticity to facilitate simultaneous sensor-tissue interaction (42). For human organs, soft biosensors have evolved over many centuries and have made it possible to produce drugs, model diseases, practice personalized medicine, and conduct clinical research without using animals by artificially mimicking these sensors (e.g., on a chip) (43). Organs-on-chips, a technique that intends to develop synthetic organs as an alternative to animal-based models, has undergone significant research and is successful in several biomedical sectors. Organs-on-chips are now being commercialized as the technology has advanced, and as cell self-assembly is necessary for the formation of complex tissue, organ-level organization, and functions in artificial organs, 3DP is a useful fabrication technique that can be used to control cell patterning at different extracellular matrix (ECM) layers, as well as the placement of micro-posts and other functional elements and biomaterials on a single chip medium (44).

Moreover, 3DP can be used to create ECM, live cells, tissues, and organoids layer by layer which can also include multisensory components. Several artificial sensing (or other) organs are made possible by 3DP, including liver organoids-on-a-chip, air–blood barrier, nervous system-on-a-chip, kidney organoids-on-a-chip, multiple organs-on-a-chip (liver, heart, and lung), heart, and brain organoids (45–49). These examples highlight a novel manufacturing strategy for products or devices that mimic or even build complex organs with great spatial accuracy (50). The sensors provide extremely sensitive measurements of pathogens, neurotransmitters, neurometabolites, cancer biomarkers, infectious diseases, and other biomarkers. High accuracy and specificity, a low detection limit, and a customizable database facilitate easy interface with smartphone-based readouts are further significant advantages (51–53). The brief history of the emergence of 3D-printed microfluidics biosensors can be overviewed in Table 13.3.

TABLE 13.3

Summary of Development of Microfluidic Biosensor

Time Frame	Key Target	Achievement
Early 2000s	The research focused on the development of chip on laboratory concept	The basic aim is to avoid laboratory visits. Production of real-time data. Development of a micro-sized chip for data analysis.
Mid-2000s	A prototype Wearable device	It is big and needs data analysis external unit.
Late 2000s	Microfabrication used to develop compact size device	Potential area searches in the biomedical application.
The early 2010s	The prototype is converted into an application version	The point-to-care model was developed. Continuous diagnostic chip for glucose level monitoring.
Mid-2010s	The wearable microfluidic device under investigation	Improved design. Improved miniaturization. Application enhanced in the area of fitness tracker.
The late 2010s	Startup design accepted to make better consumer-friendly products	Sweat-based analysis parameters increased. Hydration-level, lactate-level monitoring.
Early 2020s	Internet of Things (IoT) platforms and artificial intelligence involved in the detection system	Better data analysis and personalized device developed.
Ongoing	Improved advanced material used. The fluid control mechanism adopted	Compact, versatile device under investigation.

13.3 APPLICATIONS OF SKIN-INTERFACED 3D-PRINTED MICROFLUIDIC INTEGRATED BIOSENSORS

Biosensors have several potential applications in the wearables sector because of their high accuracy, rapid response, mobility, and low energy consumption. There has been a lot of interest in wearable biosensors since they can noninvasively and in situ analyze biomarkers in bodily fluids which allows real-time physiological and biochemical information suitable for health monitoring and even early medical diagnosis (54, 55).

The creation of wearable sensors is made possible by the miniaturization of microelectronics, stretchable microelectronics, and telecommunication, which opens a wide range of unique therapeutic applications. The present-day sensing technology has evolved beyond to include electrochemical, electromechanical, and transdermal (minimally invasive by evaluating fluid in between tissue) sensing in addition to electrophysiological measurements like electrocardiography (ECG), electroencephalography (EEG), and electromyography (EMG) (55, 56).

Epidermal biosensors can help with the real-time evaluation of biomarkers in biofluids and provide the capability of continuous monitoring for clinical diagnosis, therapy, and biomedical research (57). Wearable biosensors provide continuous, real-time physiological information by directly touching sampling biofluids and evaluating dynamic, noninvasive biochemical indicators without causing the wearer distress.

Wearable sensors are integrated analytical instruments that combine wireless connectivity with standard POC system characteristics in autonomously run, self-contained units (58). The substrate and electrode materials, sensing devices (for interfacing, collection, biorecognition, signal conversion, and amplification), result-concluding devices (for data gathering, interpreting, and transmission), and power devices are the fundamental elements of wearable devices (59). Different kinds of wearable technology, such as flexible wearables, textile-based wearables, and wearables based on the epidermis, have been used for this purpose. There are many bodily parts for which wearables can be used, such as the head, the eyes, and the wrist. These wearables track several psychological and physiological indicators that can be used to identify various disorders (60).

Wearable technology can be combined with various sample systems to detect various chemical parameters in physiological fluids, including saliva, blood, urine, sweat, and others. Biofluids, including saliva, tears, perspiration, and tissue fluids, are not only more convenient than analytes but also can provide continuous, real-time physiological data by exposing the body's deeper biomolecular processes. Significant biomarkers that are necessary for monitoring and diagnosis are present in body fluids like sweat, saliva, tears, interstitial fluids, and urine can be explained in Figure 13.2 (61, 62).

Human skin has multiple sensory functions and regeneration qualities and can identify different applied stimuli. These intrinsic properties have enabled researchers to develop a wide range of wearable sensors with several functions that are

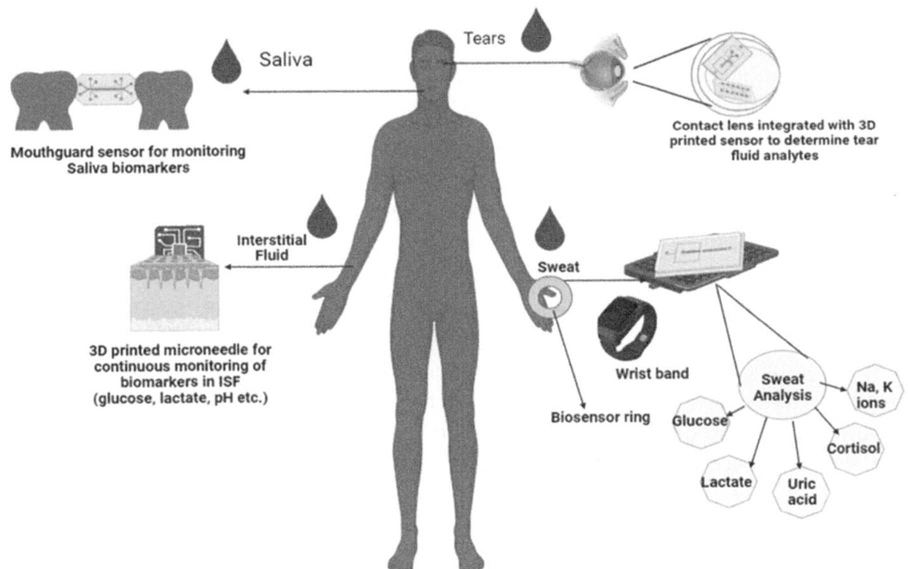

FIGURE 13.2 3D-printed microfluidic wearable sensors for monitoring analytes and biomarkers in various body fluids (sweat, saliva, tears, and interstitial body fluids). The illustration is "created with BioRender.com."

multidirectional, multimodal, self-healing, and self-powering properties. For instance, numerous glucose sensors for quantitative glucose readings have been introduced, based on optical or enzymatic electrochemical principles. They make it possible to monitor glucose levels in a variety of media, including sweat, tear fluid, physiological fluids, and even skin (63).

13.3.1 Physiological Monitoring through Sweat and Interstitial Fluids

Various 3DP techniques are used to design wearable and lightweight biosensors for measurement as well as quantification of glucose. Dias et al explain, for the first time, the designing of paper-based enzymatic reactors (PERs) that use a 3D-printed batch injection analysis (BIA) cell paired with electrochemical detection to detect glucose (Glu) in simulated serum samples. Good analytical performance, including accuracy and reproducibility below 2% and a sampling rate of 30 injections per hour at a low injection volume (10μL) was demonstrated. With the suggested method, the linear range and limit of detection (LOD) were 1–10 mmol L^{-1} and 0.11 mmol L^{-1}, respectively (64). Nesaei et al. investigated glucose biosensor microadditive fabrication. Using the direct-ink-writing (DIW) method, a specialty enzyme ink was 3D-printed on tattoo paper, and a new dual 3D-printed glucose oxidase enzyme layer and modified Prussian blue electrode for electrochemical biosensing were demonstrated. The linearity range was found in the concentration range of 100–1000 μM. The glucose biosensor's estimated sensitivity is 17.5 nA $μM^{-1}$. The printed sensors exhibited reduced material consumption, sensitivity, and specificity based on their surface characteristics and electrochemical performance (65). The 3D paper-based microfluidic electrochemical biosensor was developed by Cao et al. to measure the amount of glucose in human blood and perspiration. By immobilizing glucose oxidase on the aldehyde-based hydrophilic region and modifying the paper working electrode (PWE) with the rGO-TEPA/PB nanocomposite, an entirely new 3D paper-based microfluidic biosensor was developed. The design was predicated on the rGO-TEPA/PB nanocomposite's strong electrocatalytic reduction activity to hydrogen peroxide, which is produced by a particular enzyme–substrate reaction between glucose and glucose oxidase. This reaction releases hydrogen peroxide. The results were following the readings acquired with Roche's blood glucose meter. Strong stability, anti-interference, and repeatability were shown by the proposed 3D paper-based electrochemical device, making it extremely promising for glucose monitoring in complex biological fluids. With a detection limit of 25 μM, the suggested device can be utilized for the quantitative determination of glucose throughout a broad linear range of 0.1 mM to approximately 25 mM (66). Chiang et al developed portable and user-friendly microfluidic paper-based analytical devices (μPADs) by using 3D wax printing to create patterns of solid wax on laboratory filter paper. It emerged that the constructed μPADs offered sufficient precision and repeatability for quantitative colorimetric assessment of nitrite and glucose within ranges of concentrations applicable to the monitoring and diagnosis in human urine and saliva. Glucose detection with the μPADs produced linearity in a concentration range of 0.5–4.5 mM with the detection LOD values of 0.3 mM (67). Katseli et al. introduced a wearable device that is an electrochemical ring (e-ring), which is created utilizing a twofold extruder

3D printer in a single phase of the procedure. An electrodeposited gold layer is added to the e-ring to enable nonenzymatic glucose analysis in perspiration. The e-ring is immediately accessed by a smartphone through an Android application, and it is connected to a commercially available miniature portable potentiostat that runs in a straightforward chronoamperometric mode. The LOD was 1.2 μmol L^{-1} over the concentration range of 1.3–38.4 μmol L^{-1}(68). Advancement in continuous glucose monitoring was introduced by Liu et al by use of an assimilated microneedle (MN) biosensing device. The microneedle array (MNA) is produced using a 3DP method. With the help of microfabrication and electrochemical plating processes, the biosensing device demonstrated dependable and stable glucose detection in buffer solution, plasma, and simulated interstitial fluid (ISF). Additionally, the sensor demonstrated linear and sensitive glucose detection over a wide detection range. Additionally, the sensor was implanted into the skin's dermis layer, and it demonstrated accurate, continuous, and real-time monitoring of the subcutaneous glucose levels when food or insulin injections were consumed. The sensor exhibited a linear concentration range from 3 to 24mM with a detection limit of 48.1 μM (69). For monitoring sweat metabolites in real time, a 3D paper-based microfluidic electrochemical integrated device (3D-PMED) was presented by Cao et al. The cellulose paper was used to create the wax screen-printed patterns for the 3D-PMED. The prepatterned paper was then folded four times to create the five stacked layers that make up the electrode layer, sweat evaporator, vertical channel, transverse channel, and sweat collector. By combining the manufactured 3D-PMED with a screen-printed glucose sensor on a polyethylene terephthalate (PET) substrate, a sweat monitoring device was made possible. Red ink was used to depict the sweat flow process in 3D-PMED to show how the hydrophobicity of wax and the capillary action of filter paper can collect, analyze, and evaporate sweat. The glucose sensor was constructed with a low detection limit (5 μM) and high sensitivity (35.7 μA mM^{-1} cm^{-2}; 70). Recently Razzaghi et al. presented the fabrication of transdermal biosensors to analyze ISF, which is present in the dermis, the lowest layer of skin, to identify biomarkers by using MNAs. Microneedles (MNs) with minimal invasiveness can enter the Stratum corneum (SC) and draw out interstitial fluid via vacuum suction or capillary force. They developed 3D-printed colorimetric MNAs hydrogel composed of crosslinked poly (ethylene glycol) diacrylate (PEGDA) to extract interstitial fluid for multiplexed transdermal metabolite (specifically pH and glucose) detection. Quantitative analysis can be performed on smartphones running specifically designed apps (71). Few studies have concentrated on using noninvasive or minimally invasive devices to detect hydrogen peroxide, pH, lactate, glucose, and ethanol in interstitial fluid or other biofluids. More thorough information regarding a person's health status could be obtained through real-time dual sampling and analysis of biofluids (72). Gower et al. approached fabricating a 3D-printed microfluidic device with needle-type biosensors and FDA-approved clinical microdialysis probe integration that may be used to continuously monitor the levels of glucose and lactate in human subcutaneous tissue during cyclic exercise. The microfluidic device has integrated glucose and lactate biosensors in the form of a detachable needle that is tailored for high tissue concentrations and is housed in unique electrode holders made of 3D-printed materials (73). A multiwell plate was developed by Su et al. Using a 3D printer that used the fused deposition modeling technique. After printing, the plate was coated with platinum nanoparticles (PtNPs) that imitate peroxidase. They created an assay-based approach for measuring glucose and lactate, and the application of this method was confirmed by measuring the quantities of these two compounds in the 2.5–100µM range in urine, plasma, serum, and microdialysate from rat brain tissues. The fabrication can be used for creating multipurpose gadgets with a broader range of applications (74). Kuntawong et al. designed a wearable biosensor for continuous lactate monitoring using a conductive filament-based amperometric enzymatic flexible sensor that is 3D-printed and modified to immobilize lactate oxidase using bovine serum albumin (BSA)/glutaraldehyde (GA) crosslinking (75). Kim et al. modified 3DP technology and created and described a unique multiplex, inexpensive, and adaptable all-inclusive integrated wearable (AIIW) patch to consistently assess and evaluate these three levels of noninvasively crucial electrolytes (K+, Ca2+, and Na+) continuously in sweat. The two primary parts of the AIIW patch are the flexible wearable 3D-printed sensing unit and the flexible wearable-microfluidic sample handling unit, attached to a double-sided adhesive film that is skin compatible and forms a contour interaction with the skin to collect fresh sweat (76).

13.3.2 Physiological Monitoring through Saliva, Tear, Urine, and Blood

Biological fluids such as blood saliva, and tears are also valuable specimens for clinical diagnostic assessment, as they encompass several biomarkers that indicate human physiological conditions. Over the last decade, wearable microfluidic devices have additionally proven improved capabilities in the detection of biological fluids.

Bonacin et al. reported a nonenzymatic and metal-free ethanol sensor based on 3D PLA-graphene electrodes. They assessed the best way to activate PLA-graphene to create a sensor that can measure the amount of ethanol in saliva samples while adhering to international driving regulations. A linear detection range was seen for both the supporting electrolyte (0.990–19.3 mmol L^{-1}) and artificial saliva sample (0.990–17.4 mmol L^{-1}), with corresponding LOD of 0.135 and 0.239 mmol L^{-1}, indicating the analytical performance of the sensor that was determined by amperometric measurements (77). Sousa et al fabricated dual-µPADs as a lab-on-paper, the POC diagnosis for periodontal disease. The apparatus consists of an electrochemical and colorimetric module to achieve a dual-mode signal readout sensing approach. Hydrophobic barriers and graphite carbon-based electrodes have been developed on paper substrates using a 3D pen polymeric resin. The salivary amylase (sAA), pH, nitrite, lactate, and dual-µPAD analytical performance were assessed simultaneously. In contrast to healthy individuals (≤ 16 µmol L^{-1} and 545 U mL^{-1}), samples obtained from people previously diagnosed with periodontitis had significant levels of nitrite and sAA (>94 µmol L^{-1} and >610 U mL^{-1}) (78).

Urine contains a variety of components that can provide an abundance of information for diagnosing and tracking medical issues (79). The determination of calcium, sodium, and potassium ions in urine samples was accomplished by Dębosz et al. Using a 3D-printed multielectrode flow cell (MFC) with integrated sensors. The electrodes were ion-selective and based on cutting-edge octadecylamine-functionalized multiwalled carbon nanotube (OD-MWCNT) solid contacts. After being examined in the clinically relevant concentration range (10^{-4} to 10^{-1} mol L^{-1}), the electrodes were shown to exhibit Nernstian responses when subjected to flow injection conditions (80). Similarly, to determine uric acid in urine at the POC, a quick, easy, and sensitive 3D-printed microfluidic device coupled with smartphone-based on-chip detection was published by Dalvand et al. Using a smartphone, the 3D-printed microfluidic device was used for image-based colorimetric measurement of uric acid. It was created using a transparent photopolymer utilizing a PolyJet printer in a single pass. The uric acid was evaluated linearly over the range of 30–600 mg L^{-1} and LOD was 10.5 mg L^{-1} (81). To determine dopamine (DA), estriol (EST), and uric acid (UA) simultaneously in urine, Zhao et al. developed a simple and effective electrochemical biosensing platform based on screen-printed carbon electrode (SPCE) modified with a 3D nanocomposite built with RGO/AgNWs/AgNPs/SPCE. This composite is made of reduced graphene oxide (RGO) with the insertion of silver nanowires (AgNWs) and then the anchoring of silver nanoparticles (AgNPs). Within the ternary mixture of DA, UA, and EST, the RGO/AgNWs/AgNPs/SPCE sensor displays well-resolved oxidation peaks and enhanced oxidation peak currents. The corresponding linear response ranges for each sensor are 0.6–50 µM, 1–100 µM, and 1–90 µM, with detection limits (S/N = 3) of 0.16 µM, 0.58 µM, and 0.58 µM, respectively (82). Furthermore, Teekayupak et al. Reported the formulation of an easy-to-use 3D-printed electrochemical sensing tool for the nonenzymatic measurement of creatinine, a crucial sign of kidney health. The portable smartphone potentiostat, when used in conjunction with the modified 3D-printed electrodes, demonstrated a 0.5–35.0 mM linear detection range and a detection limit of 37.3 µM (83). A novel enzymeless electrocatalytic method for measuring cholesterol, a crucial biomarker for the early detection of atherosclerosis and cardiovascular disease, is described by Okhokhonin et al. Magnetic molecularly imprinted polymer nanoparticles were produced and placed in a 3D-printed microfluidic flow cell to enable the selective isolation and analysis of cholesterol. With a degree of extraction greater than 90% and LOD of 4 µM, cholesterol could be found in model solutions using the suggested enzymeless electrocatalytic method (84).

13.3.3 CLINICAL DIAGNOSIS OF BACTERIAL AND VIRAL PATHOGENS, ANEMIA, CANCER, PRETERM BIRTH BIOMARKERS

Wearable 3D-printed microfluidic devices have demonstrated their considerable practical uses in the monitoring of physiological signals. Additionally, given the growing desire for a healthy lifestyle, easy-to-use, point-of-noninvasive wearable technology that enables medical assessment by self and quick clinical diagnosis has a huge potential benefit (85). For example, Mosquito-borne infections affect a large portion of the world; however, many affected individuals lack access to a quick and easy diagnosis. Nielsen et al. Developed microfluidic devices with affinity monoliths that could detect viral RNA and oligonucleotides, as well as noncovalently attach a fluorescent tag. These devices were printed using a bespoke stereolithography 3D printer. They utilized an oligonucleotide sequence from the Chikungunya virus to enhance the fluorescence binding and sample load times. Approximately 10^7 loaded viral genome copies were found, a number comparable to that found in clinical samples taken during acute infection. These findings hold great potential for this 'platform's advancement into a quick and efficient approach for detecting viral pathogens carried by mosquitoes (86). For anemia diagnosis, Plevniak et al. Demonstrated the rapid fabrication of microfluidic 3D mixers, which allow reagents and blood to be mixed swiftly together by capillary force. This was achieved with 3D microfluidic simulation to guide computer design and 3D printer manufacturing. Smartphones and finger-prick blood have been effectively used to diagnose anemia at the point of treatment, with consistent results when compared to clinical assessments. This paper introduces a novel diagnostic technique with smartphone accessibility and flexibility for 3D fabrication emergence for advanced personalized medicine and mobile health care (87).

Unlike conventional enzyme-linked immunosorbent assay (ELISA), Sharafeldin et al. reported a novel flexible diagnostic device called "ELISA in a tip" that is pipet-based and has better sensitivity, quicker incubation periods, accessibility, and requires fewer volumes of analyte and reagent. Capture antibodies (Ab1) are rendered immobile by the interior walls of the pipet tip, which serves as the assay compartment into which samples and reagents are pipetted in and out. Colorimetric or chemiluminescent (CL) reagents are used to generate signals, which can then be quantified with a plate reader, CCD camera, or mobile phone. At a 25% assay cost and time savings, they employed pipet-tip ELISA to identify four cancer biomarker proteins with detection limits comparable to or lower than microplate ELISAs (88). Furthermore, Yang et al. described a technique that uses a 3D microfluidic chip to separate cancer cells in a liquid biopsy based on affinity. Three-dimensional printing and microfluidics combined; liquid biopsies can be analyzed reasonably cheaply with a chip that may be more useful than conventional microfluidic chips (89). A 3D-printed microarray designed by Sharafeldin et al. can measure the amount of proteins released after cell lysis. Desmoglein 3 (DSG3), a head and neck squamous cell carcinoma (HNSCC) metastatic biomarker, and two concurrent HNSCC biomarkers were discovered from a single-cell lysate of oral cancer cell cultures. LODs were 0.10 fg/mL for DSG3, and 0.20 fg/mL for VEGF-A, VEGF-C, and β-Tub. Quantitating these proteins secreted from single cells was made possible by the extremely low LODs. Accuracy was validated by a strong connection between the results of conventional off-line lysis, on-chip cell lysis, and ELISA (90).

One of the key contributions of 3D-printed microfluidics is the extraction of the preterm biomarker and fabrication of integrated diagnostic to detect biomarkers in maternal serum, the methodology was demonstrated by Almughamsi et al., who fabricated the multiplexed immunoaffinity extraction of preterm birth (PTB) biomarker in 3D-printed microfluidic devices. To provide biomarker-based diagnostics for PTB risk, they constructed and built 3D-printed microfluidic devices with multiplexed immunoaffinity monoliths to selectively extract different PTB biomarkers. Each monoclonal antibody's equilibrium dissociation constant concerning its intended PTB biomarker was established (91).

At the POC, rapid infectious pathogen screening is meant to be inexpensive, portable, user-friendly, and able to multiplex detect with high sensitivity. In this race, Crevillen et al. combined the advantages of electrochemical detection utilizing 3D printing technology and developed quick screening by a lab-on-a-chip system for SARS-CoV-2 sensing. This device consists of a fully 3D-printed electrochemical cell that is combined with a PDMS microfluidic channel using a 3DP pen (3DPP). An ssDNA probe that targets the N gene sequence of SARS-CoV-2 is added to the 3DPP genosensor. The mechanism of sensing is based on the electro-oxidation of adenines found in single-stranded DNA upon interaction with SARS-CoV-2 RNA. The ssDNA desorbed from the genosensor surface because the hybridization between ssDNA and target RNA reduces the sensor signal. The SARS-CoV-2/3DPP genosensor that was created exhibits quick reaction times and high sensitivity (92). Furthermore, the detection of synthetic SARS-CoV-2 at 106 copies/µL was employed using a 3D-printed microfluidic polymerase chain reaction (PCR) device by Shaka et al. With a reaction volume of about 22 nL, the microfluidic device was created using stereolithography 3DP. The microdevice demonstrated PCR amplification using primers tailored for a region specific to SARS-CoV-2 and 85 base synthetic ssDNA targets. The apparatus outperformed a qPCR instrument with a reagent capacity that was >60,000 times smaller by a factor of 2.5. A possible technique to drastically cut the cost of producing microfluidic devices for POC applications is the 3DP microdevice (93). Ding et al. developed a monolithic, 3D-printed microfluidic disc, a mini centrifuge, and a mini block heater, allowing on-site deployment for SARS-CoV-2 detection. The disc is made using a one-step 3DP technology, which eliminates the need for multiple-layer alignment and binding during the fabrication process of traditional PMMA discs. Within 50 minutes, it was possible to identify three SARS-CoV-2 genes and one inner control gene from the human genome in the disc simultaneously. The detection had great specificity (no cross-reactivity) and high sensitivity (100 copies per disc). To simplify COVID-19 diagnostics, this lab-on-a-disc device is straightforward, quick, disposable, sensitive, reliable, and multiplexed (94). The most prevalent type of infection is a respiratory infection, with a constant annual risk of disease. Mycoplasma pneumonia is a common respiratory infection that when becomes macrolide-resistant is difficult to cure. Precise medicine requires a quick and accurate determination of the mutant type of *Mycoplasma pneumonie*. To achieve this, Wang et al. proposed a novel 3D-printed device used for qPCR detection of macrolide-resistant genes of *Mycoplasma pneumonie*. The apparatus dispersed the mixture uniformly into several PCR chambers that had been preloaded with the designated primers and probes after automatically mixing the sample and reagent. After that, the apparatus was moved to the DIY qPCR setup. With remarkable speed, specificity, and ease, two types of single-base mutations of *Mycoplasma pneumonie* were found (95). Molecular diagnostics for sepsis are restricted by compounds that prevent gene amplification and bacteria present at concentrations below the detection limit. Herein, Abafogi et al. represented the development of a 3D-printed modular microfluidic device (3DpmµFD) that cleanses and preconcentrates target bacteria's genomic DNA (gDNA) in whole blood with a detection of as few as 10 *E. coli* O157:H7 CFU/mL in 2.5 mL of blood (96). Furthermore, Jóskowiak et al. described a microfluidic system that uses a 3D-printed master mold to quickly isolate and concentrate *Escherichia coli* from whole blood samples. This device can shorten the time it takes to diagnose bloodstream infections (BSIs). The device consists of a serpentine mixing channel with two inlets: one for bacterially contaminated blood samples and another for magnetic nanoparticles (MNPs) functionalized with a receptor-binding protein (RBP) unique to *Escherichia coli* (bacteriophage). A wide range of bacterial load (10^2 CFU–10^7 CFU ml^{-1}) was spiked with tenfold diluted blood, and the improved sample preparation method successfully recovered *E. coli* (on average, 66%) from the blood. By combining the proposed serpentine channel with a specific sensing element, a standalone POC device may be created, which could save a great deal of time and money on BSI diagnosis and improve the prognosis for the patients involved (97).

13.3.4 DRUG DELIVERY, WOUND HEALING, SCAFFOLDS FOR TISSUE ENGINEERING

The field of microfluidics research has experienced rapid growth because of its diverse uses, such as therapeutics delivery, cell-based analyses, and biological research. Research on the manufacture of liposomes (LPs) using 3DP to fabricate MF chips has been rare, while there are now proven microfluidic methods for preparing LPs, creating microfluidic devices is still costly and time-consuming. Additionally, the volumetric throughput of microfluidics has been severely constrained due to the conventional microchannel layout (98). To this, most notably Shan et al. provided an ultra-high volumetric throughput method for the manufacture of nano-LPs utilizing 3D-printed microfluidic chips. Microfluidic chips with crucial dimensions of 400 μm are produced using a high-resolution projection micro stereolithography (PμSL) 3D printer. The microchannels of the microfluidic chip adopt a three-layer layout, achieving a total flow rate (TFR) of up to 474 ml min^{-1}. The liposome of 80 μm was obtained. The outcomes of the experiment show that the 3D-printed integrated microfluidic chip can effectively control size and facilitate the manufacture of nano-LPs at ultra-high volumetric throughput, both of which have considerable potential in drug delivery systems (99). Furthermore, Ballacchino et al. worked to study liposome production using liquid crystal display (LCD)–printed microfluidic devices. Using semi-moon and square Y-shaped chips made by an LCD printer, curcumin-loaded LPs were produced. Curcumin LPs were evaluated for encapsulation efficiency, particle sizing, ζ-potential, and in vitro release studies at 37 °C. Three-dimensional-printed microfluidic preparation showed enhanced encapsulation efficiency in comparison to conventional and microfluidics chips (100). It is acknowledged that the formulation generated by the lab-on-a-chip device is significantly influenced by the MF channel architecture variables. To do this, Weaver et al. established a UV LCD printer to produce a progression of microfluidic chips for liposomal synthesis. The key channel characteristics for the best liposomal formulation are being studied by adjusting specific channel parameters including internal geometries and length. Liposomes measuring 120 nm in diameter and a polydispersity index of less than 0.12 can be synthesized in a repeatable manner with innovatively constructed chips. The development of smaller LPs with more regulated PDIs was correlated with channel lengthening and geometric modifications (101). Many microfluidic devices have been incorporated into drug delivery systems by scientists in recent years. It is possible to custom-design 3D-printed microfluidic devices for uses including regulating the release of medication ingredients, target-specific dosing, and minimizing side effects. Considering this, Amoyav et al. described the formulation of microspheres by a one-step 3DP-based microfluidic chip production approach for drug dissolution experiments. A modified solid-in-oil-in-water method was utilized to produce doxorubicin nonporous and porous microspheres with an average diameter of 250μm through conventional and microfluidic techniques. When compared to batch formulations, microspheres made using a microfluidics device demonstrated better drug content and encapsulation efficiency. Using two different dissolving devices with different mechanical barrier designs, the drug release characteristics of microspheres under varied pH were assessed. Finally, the chip demonstrated exceptional stability and longevity, allowing for numerous recycling operations (102). In the same lane, Noroozi et al. presented the fabrication of a microfluidic-based therapeutics delivery that produces polycaprolactone (PCL) droplets loaded with the medication dexamethasone by using stereolithography (SLA) and fused deposition modeling (FDM) 3DP. Images from a scanning electron microscope (SEM) and microscopic photos demonstrate the effectiveness with which this technique produces these droplets (103). Advances in self-propelled microdroplets, the motion of which is controlled in response to stimuli such as chemical, electrical, or magnetic fields have created new opportunities for research on smart drug delivery. Similarly, by fusing the capabilities of chemotaxis, 3DP, and microfluidic processes, a novel method to deliver the drug to specific locations at a well-controlled rate was shown. Within the drug delivery microfluidic system, a self-propelled ionic liquid ([P6,6,6,14][Cl]) microdroplet was employed as the drug carrier for the targeted delivery of the anticancer medication epirubicin. The controlled mobility, (spatial and temporal release) of the microdroplet is caused by the asymmetric release of [P6,6,6,14]$^+$ from it in the presence of an electrochemically created ion gradient inside the channel. This way, Kolsoum et al. presented an electrotactic drug delivery system that demonstrated good therapeutic payload delivery capability to the disease locations, increasing the beneficial effect and reducing the adverse consequences (104). The manufacture of different drugs and diagnostic materials that can be integrated with nanocarriers in a microfluidic environment has been made possible by recent advances in nanomedicine. By combining the synthesis of nanomaterials on a microscale platform with improved reagent manipulation, highly reproducible preparation, precisely regulated size, and low analyte volume, microfluidic devices have advanced the state-of-the-art and opened a wide range of potential applications. In this context, Kulkarni et al. developed a microfluidic system that integrates a portable, automated heat management platform with dexamethasone-loaded nano-micelles for the administration of drugs into the eyes. To create the microfluidic device, a mold was first created utilizing the SLA-based 3DP method and the polydimethylsiloxane (PDMS) soft-lithography process. Using an ex vivo cornea model, the generated dex-loaded micelles were assessed for transcorneal absorption. Ultimately, the findings showed that the suggested device can carry out a variety of controlled thermal reactions on a small platform using a downsized and integrated technique for a variety of applications (105).

Using hydrogels, therapeutic agents, living cells, and scaffolds with customizable properties, 3D microfluidic technology is widely employed in tissue regeneration and wound healing. This is because the substrate can mimic the targeted wound site with remarkable precision and resolution. Fratini et al. for the first-time combined LPs with a hydrogel to encapsulate the active pharmaceutical ingredient (API), which is then printed into a 3D scaffold for wound dressing. By using the coaxial 3D bioprinting process, two distinct bioinks have been combined into a single filament to create a scaffold with a grid pattern. The filament's inner core is a nanocomposite hydrogel made of PEGylated LPs and hydroxyethyl cellulose (HEC) encased in thyme oil (TO), which is produced via MF. A hybrid hydrogel made of cellulose and sodium alginate nanocrystals (SA/CNC) and enhanced with free TO, by comparison, represents the filament's outer shell. By doing this, the API inside the LPs is released in two separate ways: first, in bulk for the first 24 hours and, then, in a continual manner for up to 10 days (106). Despite their apparent potential for random skin tissue regeneration, biological scaffolds' limited vascularization ability and lack of responsiveness during the healing process severely limit their practical application, to overcome this Wang et al described a novel MXene-incorporated hollow fibrous (MX-HF) scaffold that uses a microfluidic-assisted 3DP technique to promote vascularization and skin flap regeneration. The scaffold has dynamically responsive channels. These MX-HF scaffolds exhibit a near-infrared (NIR)-responsive shrinkage/swelling behavior that helps cells from the surrounding environment penetrate the scaffold channels. This behavior is made possible by the photothermal conversion capacity of the MXene nanosheets and the temperature-responsive ability of the poly (NIPAM) hydrogels. Furthermore, the MX-HF scaffolds can result in enhanced endothelial cell migration, proliferation, and proangiogenic effects under NIR radiation by integrating vascular endothelial growth factor (VEGF) into the hydrogel matrix for controlled delivery. Thus MX-HF scaffolds showed diverse tissue engineering applications (107). For in vitro investigations of the interactions between blood cells and vascular endothelial cells under flow, microfluidic systems are highly beneficial. Hernández Vera et al. described a method for creating customized modular microfluidic devices that are molded in PDMS using 3D-printed molds to enable research on leukocyte adhesion to endothelial cells. TNFα stimulated one group of endothelial cells in proof-of-principle tests, while the other acted as an internal control. A microfluidic flow module was then installed in place of the barrier module, containing both endothelial populations in a single channel. The flow module was subsequently utilized to perfuse a suspension of fluorescently labeled leukocytes, and interactions between the leukocytes and TNFα-treated and endothelium cells were observed within the same field of view. The process of development resulted in modular microfluidic systems that enable regulated side-by-side analysis of adherent cell types of differing capacities to seed and activate adherent cell types and interact with cells in suspension underflow (108). In a different study, to provide a combined microperfused 3D cell culture environment for living cells, Ng et al. developed a 3D-printed microperfused culture (MPC) device integrated with a nanofibrous scaffold. In this work, the fibrous and porous characteristics of the implanted scaffold were used to replicate the structure of the ECM of a native tissue. This is the first printed gadget that has a biological component—a 3D-miniaturized porous scaffold—in its design. Research revealed that the Huh7.5 hepatocellular carcinoma model cells had thicker cell constructs on the MPC device than the static culture. A more physiologically relevant platform for the maintenance of hepatocytes has been demonstrated by the perfusion culture device described here, ensuring the possible use of 3DP (SLA) as an additive manufacturing tool for microfluidic chips with established functionalities (109). For drug delivery, the broader use of transdermal route is widely expanded by a MN, a miniature puncturing device that penetrates the epidermis and delivers a range of therapeutics, including proteins, DNA, and others, in a minimally invasive and painless manner. Economidou et al. combined 3DP of MNs and a sophisticated microelectromechanical system (MEMS) to create a 3D MN MEMS device. A device is a useful tool for treatment customization since it permits the user to have in situ control over drug administration. They proved that hollow MNs produced by SLA, an affordable 3DP technology, are consistent, repeatable, and sharp. It was discovered that the MNs could successfully pierce the skin with little loads, resulting in little discomfort and simple self-application. The MNs' exceptional fracture strength gave comfort in their application-related safety. By using cutting-edge optical imaging methods, liquid diffusion from the 3D MN MEMS into skin tissue can be viewed. It was demonstrated that the technique allowed the liquid to be widely distributed without the need for depots, speeding up the absorption of the medication. Clinical investigations conducted on diabetic rats in vivo demonstrated that the 3D MN MEMS provided painless, longer-lasting glycemic control with a somewhat faster insulin onset action than subcutaneous injection (110).

13.4 CONCLUSION

Microfluidics has been profoundly impacted by 3DP. Applications and advancements in the field indicate that 3DP will play a significant role in the production of affordable, easily accessible, compact, multipurpose, and sensitive diagnostic instruments. Using this adaptable technology, researchers with varying backgrounds have developed diagnostic assays. This technological platform allows a quicker one-step process for creating the intended chip, design flexibility, mass customization, and the capacity to produce intricate structures. A range of diagnostic tools for the detection of several clinically significant analytes, such as glucose, lactate, uric acid, glutamate, and biomarkers linked to pathogens, PTB, cancer, and more, can be made using 3DP, an emerging technology. Based on the reviewed and assembled literature, we firmly believe that the integration of 3DP technology with microfluidics could result in several advantages and opportunities for the various biomedical applications discussed in the chapter. Additionally, low LODs, excellent repeatability, and a high degree of integration of the devices are made possible by 3DP biomedical sensors, and applications for multifunctional integrated devices like wearable sensors and soft robots will flourish in the future.

ACKNOWLEDGMENT

None.

CONFLICT OF INTEREST

None.

REFERENCES

1. Gale BK, Jafek AR, Lambert CJ, Goenner BL, Moghimifam H, Nze UC, Kamarapu SK. A review of current methods in microfluidic device fabrication and future commercialization prospects. *Inventions* 2018 Aug 28;3(3):60.

2. Lee CY, Wang WT, Liu CC, Fu LM. Passive mixers in microfluidic systems: A review. *Chemical Engineering Journal* 2016 Mar 15;288:146–60.

3. Knowlton S, Yu CH, Ersoy F, Emadi S, Khademhosseini A, Tasoglu S. 3D-printed microfluidic chips with patterned, cell-laden hydrogel constructs. *Biofabrication* 2016 Jun 21;8(2):025019.

4. Lee CY, Chang CL, Wang YN, Fu LM. Microfluidic mixing: A review. *International Journal of Molecular Sciences* 2011 May 18;12(5):3263–87.

5. Sackmann EK, Fulton AL, Beebe DJ. The present and future role of microfluidics in biomedical research. *Nature* 2014 Mar 13;507(7491):181–9.

6. Maduraiveeran G, Sasidharan M, Ganesan V. Electrochemical sensor and biosensor platforms based on advanced nanomaterials for biological and biomedical applications. *Biosensors & Bioelectronics* 2018 Apr 30;103:113–29.

7. Rivet C, Lee H, Hirsch A, Hamilton S, Lu H. Microfluidics for medical diagnostics and biosensors. *Chemical Engineering Science* 2011 Apr 1;66(7):1490–507.

8. Weisgrab G, Ovsianikov A, Costa PF. Functional 3D printing for microfluidic chips. *Advanced Materials Technologies* 2019 Oct;4(10):1900275.

9. Sommonte F, Denora N, Lamprou DA. Combining 3D printing and microfluidic techniques: A powerful synergy for nanomedicine. *Pharmaceuticals* 2023 Jan 1;16(1):69..

10. Attaran M. The rise of 3-D printing: The advantages of additive manufacturing over traditional manufacturing. *Business Horizons* 2017 Sep 1;60(5):677–88.

11. Chen C, Mehl BT, Munshi AS, Townsend AD, Spence DM, Martin RS. 3D-printed microfluidic devices: Fabrication, advantages, and limitations—a mini-review. *Analytical Methods* 2016;8(31):6005–12.

12. Su CK. Review of 3D-printed functionalized devices for chemical and biochemical analysis. *Analytica Chimica Acta* 2021 May 8;1158:338348.

13. Ngo TD, Kashani A, Imbalzano G, Nguyen KT, Hui D. Additive manufacturing (3D printing): A review of materials, methods, applications, and challenges. *Composites Part B: Engineering* 2018 Jun 15;143:172–96.

14. Amin R, Knowlton S, Hart A, Yenilmez B, Ghaderinezhad F, Katebifar S, Messina M, Khademhosseini A, Tasoglu S. 3D-printed microfluidic devices. *Biofabrication* 2016 Jun 20;8(2):022001.

15. Bhattacharjee N, Urrios A, Kang S, Folch A. The upcoming 3D-printing revolution in microfluidics. *Lab on a Chip* 2016;16(10):1720–42.

16. Amin R, Knowlton S, Hart A, Yenilmez B, Ghaderinezhad F, Katebifar S, Messina M, Khademhosseini A, Tasoglu S. 3D-printed microfluidic devices. *Biofabrication* 2016 Jun 20;8(2):022001.

17. Walczak R, Adamski K. Inkjet 3D printing of microfluidic structures—on the selection of the printer towards printing your own microfluidic chips. *Journal of Micromechanics and Microengineering* 2015 Jul 22;25(8):085013.

18. Ngo TD, Kashani A, Imbalzano G, Nguyen KT, Hui D. Additive manufacturing (3D printing): A review of materials, methods, applications, and challenges. *Composites Part B: Engineering* 2018 Jun 15;143:172–96.

19. Murphy SV, Atala A. 3D bioprinting of tissues and organs. *Nature Biotechnology* 2014 Aug;32(8):773–85.

20. Salmi M, Akmal JS, Pei E, Wolff J, Jaribion A, Khajavi SH. 3D printing in COVID-19: Productivity estimation of the most promising open source solutions in emergency situations. *Applied Sciences* 2020 Jun 9;10(11):4004.

21. Deo KA, Singh KA, Peak CW, Alge DL, Gaharwar AK. Bioprinting 101: Design, fabrication, and evaluation of cell-laden 3D bioprinted scaffolds. *Tissue Engineering Parts A* 2020 Mar 1;26(5–6):318–38.

22. Xu Y, Wu X, Guo X, Kong B, Zhang M, Qian X, Mi S, Sun W. The boom in 3D-printed sensor technology. *Sensors* 2017 May 19;17(5):1166.

23. Greatbatch W. *The Making of the Pacemaker: Celebrating a Lifesaving Invention*, 2011. Prometheus Books.

24. Clark Jr LC, Lyons C. Electrode systems for continuous monitoring in cardiovascular surgery. *Annals of the New York Academy of Sciences* 1962 Oct;102(1):29–45.

25. Murugaiyan SB, Ramasamy R, Gopal N, Kuzhandaivelu V. Biosensors in clinical chemistry: An overview. *Advanced Biomedical Research* 2014;3:67.

26. Turner A. Biosensors: Then and now. *Trends in Biotechnology* 2013 Mar 1;31(3):119–20.

27. Ali MA, Hu C, Jahan S, Yuan B, Saleh MS, Ju E, Gao SJ, Panat R. Sensing of COVID-19 antibodies in seconds via aerosol jet nanoprinted reduced-graphene-oxide-coated 3D electrodes. *Advanced Materials* 2021 Feb;33(7):2006647.

28. Kawamura A, Miyata T. *Biosensors. InBiomaterials Nanoarchitectonics*, 2016 Jan 1 (pp. 157–76). William Andrew Publishing.

29. Sawant SN. Development of Biosensors from Biopolymer Composites. In *Biopolymer Composites in Electronics*, 2017 Jan 1 (pp. 353–83). Elsevier.

30. Castillo J, Gáspár S, Leth S, Niculescu M, Mortari A, Bontidean I, Soukharev V, Dorneanu SA, Ryabov AD, Csöregi E. Biosensors for life quality: Design, development and applications. *Sensors and Actuators B: Chemical* 2004 Sep 13;102(2):179–94.

31. Pearson JE, Gill A, Vadgama P. Analytical aspects of biosensors. *Annals of Clinical Biochemistry* 2000 Mar 1;37(2):119–45..

32. Borisov SM, Wolfbeis OS. Optical biosensors. *Chemical Reviews* 2008 Feb 13;108(2):423–61.

33. Marquette CA, Blum LJ. State of the art and recent advances in immunoanalytical systems. *Biosensors & Bioelectronics* 2006 Feb 15;21(8):1424–33.

34. Panjan P, Virtanen V, Sesay AM. Determination of stability characteristics for electrochemical biosensors via thermally accelerated aging. *Talanta* 2017 Aug 1;170:331–6.

35. Schreiter M, Gabl R, Lerchner J, Hohlfeld C, Delan A, Wolf G, Blüher A, Katzschner B, Mertig M, Pompe W. Functionalized pyroelectric sensors for gas detection. *Sensors and Actuators B: Chemical* 2006 Nov 24;119(1):255–61.

36. Nge PN, Rogers CI, Woolley AT. Advances in microfluidic materials, functions, integration, and applications. *Chemical Reviews* 2013 Apr 10;113(4):2550–83.

37. Ali MA, Hu C, Yttri EA, Panat R. Recent advances in 3D printing of biomedical sensing devices. *Advanced Functional Materials* 2022 Feb;32(9):2107671.

38. Ho CM, Ng SH, Li KH, Yoon YJ. 3D printed microfluidics for biological applications. *Lab on a Chip* 2015;15(18):3627–37.

39. Au AK, Huynh W, Horowitz LF, Folch A. 3D-printed microfluidics. *Angewandte Chemie, International Edition* 2016 Mar 14;55(12):3862–81.

40. Kuo AP, Bhattacharjee N, Lee YS, Castro K, Kim YT, Folch A. High-precision stereolithography of biomicrofluidic devices. *Advanced Materials Technologies* 2019 Jun;4(6):1800395.

41. Rusling JF. Developing microfluidic sensing devices using 3D printing. *ACS Sensors* 2018 Mar 1;3(3):522–6.

42. Waheed S, Cabot JM, Macdonald NP, Lewis T, Guijt RM, Paull B, Breadmore MC. 3D printed microfluidic devices: Enablers and barriers. *Lab on a Chip* 2016;16(11):1993–2013.

43. Huh D, Hamilton GA, Ingber DE. From 3D cell culture to organs-on-chips. *Trends in Cell Biology* 2011 Dec 1;21(12):745–54.

44. Ingber DE. Developmentally inspired human 'organs on chips'. *Development* 2018 Aug 15;145(16):dev156125.

45. Zhang YS, Arneri A, Bersini S, Shin SR, Zhu K, Goli-Malekabadi Z, Aleman J, Colosi C, Busignani F, Dell'Erba V, Bishop C. Bioprinting 3D microfibrous scaffolds for engineering endothelialized myocardium and heart-on-a-chip. *Biomaterials* 2016 Dec 1;110:45–59.

46. Ding C, Chen X, Kang Q, Yan X. Biomedical application of functional materials in organ-on-a-chip. *Frontiers in Bioengineering and Biotechnology* 2020 Jul 22;8:823.

47. Homan KA, Gupta N, Kroll KT, Kolesky DB, Skylar-Scott M, Miyoshi T, Mau D, Valerius MT, Ferrante T, Bonventre JV, Lewis JA. Flow-enhanced vascularization and maturation of kidney organoids in vitro. *Nature Methods* 2019 Mar;16(3):255–62.

48. Xu M, Obodo D, Yadavalli VK. The design, fabrication, and applications of flexible biosensing devices. *Biosensors & Bioelectronics* 2019 Jan 15;124:96–114.

49. Skardal A, Murphy SV, Devarasetty M, Mead I, Kang HW, Seol YJ, Shrike Zhang Y, Shin SR, Zhao L, Aleman J, Hall AR. Multi-tissue interactions in an integrated three-tissue organ-on-a-chip platform. *Scientific Reports* 2017 Aug 18;7(1):8837.

50. LináKong Y. 3D printed nervous system on a chip. *Lab on a Chip* 2016;16(8):1393–400.

51. Kadimisetty K, Mosa IM, Malla S, Satterwhite-Warden JE, Kuhns TM, Faria RC, Lee NH, Rusling JF. 3D-printed supercapacitor-powered electrochemiluminescent protein immunoarray. *Biosensors & Bioelectronics* 2016 Mar 15;77:188–93.

52. Lee W, Kwon D, Choi W, Jung GY, Au AK, Folch A, Jeon S. 3D-printed microfluidic device for the detection of pathogenic bacteria using size-based separation in helical channel with trapezoid cross-section. *Scientific Reports* 2015 Jan 12;5(1):7717.

53. Yang C, Cao Q, Puthongkham P, Lee ST, Ganesana M, Lavrik NV, Venton BJ. 3D-printed carbon electrodes for neurotransmitter detection. *Angewandte Chemie, International Edition* 2018 Oct 22;57(43):14255–9.

54. Cima MJ. Next-generation wearable electronics. *Nature Biotechnology* 2014 Jul;32(7):642–3.

55. Patel S, Park H, Bonato P, Chan L, Rodgers M. A review of wearable sensors and systems with application in rehabilitation. *Journal of Neuroengineering and Rehabilitation* 2012 Dec;9(1):1–7.

56. Wang M, Hu L, Xu C. Recent advances in the design of polymeric microneedles for transdermal drug delivery and biosensing. *Lab on a Chip* 2017;17(8):1373–87.

57. Kim J, de Araujo WR, Samek IA, Bandodkar AJ, Jia W, Brunetti B, Paixao TR, Wang J. Wearable temporary tattoo sensor for real-time trace metal monitoring in human sweat. *Electrochemistry Communications* 2015 Feb 1;51:41–5.

58. Koh A, Kang D, Xue Y, Lee S, Pielak RM, Kim J, Hwang T, Min S, Banks A, Bastien P, Manco MC. A soft, wearable microfluidic device for the capture, storage, and colorimetric sensing of sweat. *Science Translational Medicine* 2016 Nov 23;8(366):366ra165.

59. Merkoçi A, Ates HC, Brunauer A, von Stetten F, Urban GA, Güder F, Früh SM, Dincer C. Integrated devices for non-invasive diagnostics. *Advanced Functional Materials* 2021;31(15):2010388.

60. Iqbal SM, Mahgoub I, Du E, Leavitt MA, Asghar W. Advances in healthcare wearable devices. *NPJ Flexible Electronics* 2021 Apr 12;5(1):9.

61. Kim J, Campbell AS, de Ávila BE, Wang J. Wearable biosensors for healthcare monitoring. *Nature Biotechnology* 2019 Apr;37(4):389–406.

62. Su Y, Wang J, Wang B, Yang T, Yang B, Xie G, Zhou Y, Zhang S, Tai H, Cai Z, Chen G. Alveolus-inspired active membrane sensors for self-powered wearable chemical sensing and breath analysis. *ACS Nano* 2020 Apr 9;14(5):6067–75.

63. Yamamoto Y, Harada S, Yamamoto D, Honda W, Arie T, Akita S, Takei K. Printed multifunctional flexible device with an integrated motion sensor for health care monitoring. *Science Advances* 2016 Nov 23;2(11):e1601473.

64. Dias AA, Cardoso TM, Cardoso RM, Duarte LC, Muñoz RA, Richter EM, Coltro WK. based enzymatic reactors for batch injection analysis of glucose on 3D printed cell coupled with amperometric detection. *Sensors and Actuators B: Chemical* 2016 Apr 1;226:196–203.

65. Nesaei S, Song Y, Wang Y, Ruan X, Du D, Gozen A, Lin Y. Micro additive manufacturing of glucose biosensors: A feasibility study. *Analytica Chimica Acta* 2018 Dec 28;1043:142–9.

66. Cao L, Han GC, Xiao H, Chen Z, Fang C. A novel 3D paper-based microfluidic electrochemical glucose biosensor based on rGO-TEPA/PB sensitive film. *Analytica Chimica Acta* 2020 Feb 1;1096:34–43.

67. Chiang CK, Kurniawan A, Kao CY, Wang MJ. Single step and mask-free 3D wax printing of microfluidic paper-based analytical devices for glucose and nitrite assays. *Talanta* 2019 Mar 1;194:837–45.

68. Katseli V, Economou A, Kokkinos C. Smartphone-addressable 3D-printed electrochemical ring for nonenzymatic self-monitoring of glucose in human sweat. *Analytical Chemistry* 2021 Feb 9;93(7):3331–6.

69. Liu Y, Yu Q, Luo X, Yang L, Cui Y. Continuous monitoring of diabetes with an integrated microneedle biosensing device through 3D printing. *Microsystems & Nanoengineering* 2021 Sep 29;7(1):75.

70. Cao Q, Liang B, Tu T, Wei J, Fang L, Ye X. Three-dimensional paper-based microfluidic electrochemical integrated devices (3D-PMED) for wearable electrochemical glucose detection. *RSC Advances* 2019;9(10):5674–81.

71. Razzaghi M, Seyfoori A, Pagan E, Askari E, Hassani Najafabadi A, Akbari M. 3D printed hydrogel microneedle arrays for interstitial fluid biomarker extraction and colorimetric detection. *Polymers* 2023 Mar 10;15(6):1389.

72. Matzeu G, Florea L, Diamond D. Advances in wearable chemical sensor design for monitoring biological fluids. *Sensors and Actuators B: Chemical* 2015 May 1;211:403–18.

73. Gowers SA, Curto VF, Seneci CA, Wang C, Anastasova S, Vadgama P, Yang GZ, Boutelle MG. 3D printed microfluidic device with integrated biosensors for online analysis of subcutaneous human microdialysate. *Analytical Chemistry* 2015 Aug 4;87(15):7763–70..

74. Su CK, Li TW, Sun YC. Peroxidase-mimicking PtNP-coated, 3D-printed multi-well plate for rapid determination of glucose and lactate in clinical samples. *Sensors and Actuators B: Chemical* 2018 Sep 15;269:46–53.

75. Kuntawong P, Kongintr U, Promptmas C. M021 3D printed-lactate amperometric biosensor for real-time noninvasive health monitoring in human sweat. *Clinica Chimica Acta* 2022 May 1;530:S11.

76. Kim T, Yi Q, Hoang E, Esfandyarpour R. A 3D printed wearable bioelectronic patch for multi-sensing and in situ sweat electrolyte monitoring. *Advanced Materials Technologies* 2021 Apr;6(4):2001021.

77. Bonacin J, Zuben TW, Kalinke C, Janegitz B, Salles A. 3D-printed amperometric sensor for the detection of ethanol in saliva. *Electroanalysis*:e202300044, https://doi.org/10.1002/elan.202300044

78. Sousa LR, Silva-Neto HA, Castro LF, Oliveira KA, Figueredo F, Cortón E, Coltro WK. "Do it yourself" protocol to fabricate dual-detection paper-based analytical device for salivary biomarker analysis. *Analytical and Bioanalytical Chemistry* 2023 Feb 11;415:4391–400.

79. Wan QJ, Kubáň P, Tanyanyiwa J, Rainelli A, Hauser PC. Determination of major inorganic ions in blood serum and urine by capillary electrophoresis with contactless conductivity detection. *Analytica Chimica Acta* 2004 Nov 1;525(1):11–6.

80. Dębosz M, Kozma J, Porada R, Wieczorek M, Paluch J, Gyurcsányi RE, Migdalski J, Kościelniak P. 3D-printed manifold integrating solid contact ion-selective electrodes for multiplexed ion concentration measurements in urine. *Talanta* 2021 Sep 1;232:122491.

81. Dalvand K, Ghiasvand A, Keshan-Balavandy S, Li F, Breadmore M. A simple 3D printed microfluidic device for point-of-care analysis of urinary uric acid. *Australian Journal of Chemistry* 2023 Feb 10;76(2):74–80.

82. Zhao Q, Faraj Y, Liu LY, Wang W, Xie R, Liu Z, Ju XJ, Wei J, Chu LY. Simultaneous determination of dopamine, uric acid and estriol in maternal urine samples based on the synergetic effect of reduced graphene oxide, silver nanowires and silver nanoparticles in their ternary 3D nanocomposite. *Microchemical Journal* 2020 Nov 1;158:105185.

83. Teekayupak K, Aumnate C, Lomae A, Preechakasedkit P, Henry CS, Chailapakul O, Ruecha N. Portable smartphone integrated 3D-printed electrochemical sensor for non-enzymatic determination of creatinine in human urine. *Talanta* 2023 Mar 1;254:124131.

84. Okhokhonin AV, Stepanova MI, Svalova TS, Kozitsina AN. A new electrocatalytic system based on copper (II) chloride and magnetic molecularly imprinted polymer nanoparticles in 3D printed microfluidic flow cell for enzymeless and Low-Potential cholesterol detection. *Journal of Electroanalytical Chemistry* 2022 Nov 1;924:116853.

85. Matzeu G, Florea L, Diamond D. Advances in wearable chemical sensor design for monitoring biological fluids. *Sensors and Actuators B: Chemical* 2015 May 1;211:403–18.

86. Nielsen JB, Holladay JD, Burningham AJ, Rapier-Sharman N, Ramsey JS, Skaggs TB, Nordin GP, Pickett BE, Woolley AT. Monolithic affinity columns in 3D printed microfluidics for chikungunya RNA detection. *Analytical and Bioanalytical Chemistry* 2023 Oct 6;415:7057–65.

87. Plevniak K, Campbell M, Myers T, Hodges A, He M. 3D printed auto-mixing chip enables rapid smartphone diagnosis of anemia. *Biomicrofluidics* 2016 Sep 1;10(5).

88. Sharafeldin M, Kadimisetty K, Bhalerao KR, Bist I, Jones A, Chen T, Lee NH, Rusling JF. Accessible telemedicine diagnostics with ELISA in a 3D printed pipette tip. *Analytical Chemistry* 2019 May 3;91(11):7394–402.

89. Yang Y, Griffin K, Villareal S, Pappas D. Isolation of Cancer Cells from Liquid Biopsies Using 3D-Printed Affinity Devices. In *Microfluidic Systems for Cancer Diagnosis*, 2023 Jun 11 (pp. 233–240). Springer US.

90. Sharafeldin M, Chen T, Ozkaya GU, Choudhary D, Molinolo AA, Gutkind JS, Rusling JF. Detecting cancer metastasis and accompanying protein biomarkers at single cell levels using a 3D-printed microfluidic immunoarray. *Biosensors and Bioelectronics* 2021 Jan 1;171:112681.

91. Almughamsi HM, Howell MK, Parry SR, Esene JE, Nielsen JB, Nordin GP, Woolley AT. Immunoaffinity monoliths for multiplexed extraction of preterm birth biomarkers from human blood serum in 3D printed microfluidic devices. *Analyst* 2022;147(4):734–43.

92. Crevillen AG, Mayorga-Martinez CC, Vaghasiya JV, Pumera M. 3D-Printed SARS-CoV-2 RNA genosensing microfluidic system. *Advanced Materials Technologies* 2022 Jun;7(6):2101121.

93. Shaka K, Jones K, Putzke A, Measor P. A 3D Printed Microfluidic PCR Device towards Detecting SARS-CoV-2. In *Optical Diagnostics and Sensing XXIII: Toward Point-of-Care Diagnostics*, 2023 Mar 16 (Vol. 12387, pp. 60–62). SPIE.

94. Ding X, Li Z, Liu C. Monolithic, 3D-printed lab-on-disc platform for multiplexed molecular detection of SARS-CoV-2. *Sensors and Actuators B: Chemical* 2022 Jan 15;351:130998.

95. Wang A, Wu Z, Huang Y, Zhou H, Wu L, Jia C, Chen Q, Zhao J. A 3D-printed microfluidic device for QPCR detection of macrolide-resistant mutations of mycoplasma pneumoniae. *Biosensors* 2021 Oct 29;11(11):427.

96. Abafogi AT, Kim J, Lee J, Mohammed MO, van Noort D, Park S. 3D-printed modular microfluidic device enabling preconcentrating bacteria and purifying bacterial DNA in blood for improving the sensitivity of molecular diagnostics. *Sensors* 2020 Feb 21;20(4):1202.

97. Jóskowiak A, Nogueira CL, Costa SP, Cunha AP, Freitas PP, Carvalho CM. A magnetic nanoparticle-based microfluidic device fabricated using a 3D-printed mould for separation of Escherichia coli from blood. *Microchimica Acta* 2023 Sep;190(9):356.

98. Jahn A, Vreeland WN, Gaitan M, Locascio LE. Controlled vesicle self-assembly in microfluidic channels with hydrodynamic focusing. *Journal of the American Chemical Society* 2004 Mar 10;126(9):2674–5.

99. Shan H, Lin Q, Wang D, Sun X, Quan B, Chen X, Chen Z. 3D printed integrated multilayer microfluidic chips for ultra-high volumetric throughput nanoliposome preparation. *Frontiers in Bioengineering and Biotechnology* 2021 Oct 11;9:773705.

100. Ballacchino G, Weaver E, Mathew E, Dorati R, Genta I, Conti B, Lamprou DA. Manufacturing of 3D-printed microfluidic devices for the synthesis of drug-loaded liposomal formulations. *International Journal of Molecular Sciences* 2021 Jul 28;22(15):8064.

101. Weaver E, Mathew E, Caldwell J, Hooker A, Uddin S, Lamprou DA. The manufacturing of 3D-printed microfluidic chips to analyse the effect upon particle size during the synthesis of lipid nanoparticles. *The Journal of Pharmacy and Pharmacology* 2023 Feb 1;75(2):245–52.

102. Amoyav B, Goldstein Y, Steinberg E, Benny O. 3D printed microfluidic devices for drug release assays. *Pharmaceutics* 2020 Dec 23;13(1):13.

103. Noroozi R, Kashtiban MM, Taghvaei H, Zolfagharian A, Bodaghi M. 3D-printed microfluidic droplet generation systems for drug delivery applications. *Materials Today Proceedings* 2022 Jan 1;70:443–6.

104. Dalvand K, Ghiasvand A, Gupta V, Paull B. Chemotaxis-based smart drug delivery of epirubicin using a 3D printed microfluidic chip. *Journal of Chromatography B* 2021 Jan 1;1162:122456.

105. Kulkarni MB, Velmurugan K, Nirmal J, Goel S. Development of dexamethasone loaded nanomicelles using a 3D printed microfluidic device for ocular drug delivery applications. *Sensors and Actuators A: Physical* 2023 Aug 1;357:114385.

106. Fratini C, Weaver E, Moroni S, Irwin R, Bashi YH, Uddin S, Casettari L, Wylie MP, Lamprou DA. Combining microfluidics and coaxial 3D-bioprinting for the manufacturing of diabetic wound healing dressings. *Biomaterials Advances* 2023 Oct 1;153:213557.

107. Wang X, Yu Y, Yang C, Shang L, Zhao Y, Shen X. Dynamically responsive scaffolds from microfluidic 3D printing for skin flap regeneration. *Advanced Science* 2022 Aug;9(22):2201155.

108. Hernández Vera R, O'Callaghan P, Fatsis-Kavalopoulos N, Kreuger J. Modular microfluidic systems cast from 3D-printed molds for imaging leukocyte adherence to differentially treated endothelial cultures. *Scientific Reports* 2019 Aug 5;9(1):11321.

109. Ng FL, Cen Z, Toh YC, Tan LP. A 3D-printed micro-perfused culture device with embedded 3D fibrous scaffold for enhanced biomimicry. *International Journal of Bioprinting* 2023 Jul 11;10;0226.

110. Economidou SN, Uddin MJ, Marques MJ, Douroumis D, Sow WT, Li H, Reid A, Windmill JF, Podoleanu A. A novel 3D printed hollow microneedle microelectromechanical system for controlled, personalized transdermal drug delivery. *Additive Manufacturing* 2021 Feb 1;38:101815.

14 Regulatory Perspective on Microfluidics in Dermaceuticals

Krishna Yadav
Rungta College of Pharmaceutical Sciences and Research,
Bhilai, India

J John Kirubakaran and S Princely Ebenezer Gnanakani
Parul University, Waghodia, India

Manju Rawat Singh, Deependra Singh, and Rakesh Tirkey
Pt. Ravishankar Shukla University, Raipur, India

Sunita Minz
Indira Gandhi National Tribal University, Amarkantak, India

Wasim Raza
Chhattisgarh Council of Science and Technology, Raipur, India

Nagendra Singh Chauhan
Government Ayurvedic College, Raipur, India

Pravin Kumar Sahu
Chouksey Engineering College, Bilaspur, India

Madhulika Pradhan
Gracious College of Pharmacy, Abhanpur, India

DOI: 10.1201/9781032690926-14

14.1 INTRODUCTION

The fast development of microfluidic technology over the last several decades has resulted in a multitude of applications in the area of life sciences, notably in the field of dermatology. Benefits such as high analytical throughput, enhanced analytical performance, increased sensitivity, easy parallelization through multiplexing, and the ability to manage reduced reagent volumes while significantly reducing instrumental footprints are some of the advantages that microfluidics offers. These advantages are driven by the advantages of system miniaturization (1).

The field of microfluidics has emerged as a transformational force in the intricate terrain of drug development, which encompasses drug discovery, preclinical studies, and clinical trials. The pharmaceutical analysis process, which is an essential part of the drug development process, is plagued by difficulties such as the consumption of time, poor throughput, and the inefficiency of cost. The field of microfluidics offers a solution to these difficulties by delivering analytical efficiency and high-throughput capabilities without sacrificing accuracy or automation. By using tiny devices, microfluidics plays a significant role in the development of drug applications by facilitating the acceleration of drug screening and analysis. This, in turn, results in decreased expenses and reagent usage (2).

Microfluidic chip devices have dimensions that range from micrometers to millimeters. These devices have minimum volumes and integrated functionality inside microscopic chips. As a result, the consumption of samples and reagents may be accomplished at nanoliter and picolitre levels. Designs that use multichannel and array architectures make it possible to achieve high-throughput capacities, which, in turn, speeds up screening and lowers total expenses. Not only does microfluidic technology transform the process of drug discovery, but it also solves difficulties that have been present in pharmaceutical analysis for a very long time (3).

Since it was first developed in the early 1990s, microfluidic technology has been utilized in a wide range of research fields. Some of these fields include chemical synthesis, single-cell analysis, proteomics, tissue engineering, environmental analysis, high-throughput screening, and medical diagnostics. These platforms not only assist the efficient development of pharmacological analyses but also give insights into the processes that occur in biological systems. It is becoming more common to make use of microfluidic technology in order to generate in vitro models for lead compounds that are capable of providing more accurate predictions of effectiveness, cost-effective toxicity, and pharmacokinetics in human subjects. The development of novel screening assays, the conservation of space and resources, and the provision of extra benefits via miniaturization are all things that may be accomplished with its assistance. This chapter focuses on the regulatory and authorization aspects of microfluidic technology in the field of dermaceuticals (4, 5).

14.2 UNDERSTANDING THE REGULATORY LANDSCAPE

Products for the skin may be divided into two primary categories: cosmetics and chemicals that have been authorized by the Food and Drug Administration (FDA), which includes medications and "cosmeceuticals." A product or ingredient is classified according to the FDA rules based on the purpose for which it is intended to be used. In accordance with the Federal Food, Drug, and Cosmetics Act of 1938, cosmetics are defined as materials that are intended to be applied to the human body in order to cleanse, beautify, increase attractiveness, or adjust appearance without having an effect on the structure or functions of the body (6).

A substance that is intended for the diagnosis, cure, mitigation, treatment, or prevention of illness and that changes the structure or function of the body is what the FDA considers to be a drug according to its definition. With the purpose of cleansing, beautifying, enhancing beauty, or altering one's appearance, cosmetics are designed to be applied in a variety of different ways. Products that go beyond the concept of cosmetics, such as acne treatments that need a prescription, are regarded to be medications when they are sold. It is possible for some medications to have cosmetic effects, such as antiperspirant deodorants and shampoos that treat dandruff. In addition to medical equipment that is used for services like microdermabrasion and hair removal, skin-protectant drug products are an important category of substances that may be purchased without a prescription.

A cosmetic product can claim to do things like "moisturizes, soothes, smoothing, rubbing, friction, and lubrication," as stated in a 2003 monograph, which verified that these kinds of claims are allowed. The categorization of skin care products is largely impacted by the purpose for which they are meant to be used. The Wheeler–Lea Act gives the Federal Trade Commission (FTC) the authority to oversee advertising claims made by nonprescription personal care goods that are regulated by the FDA. The FDA may issue a warning notice if a skin care product is marketed with a drug claim or vice versa (7, 8).

This means that an over-the-counter (OTC) product that has been authorized by the FDA has an "active" component that has the ability to change the structure or function of the skin. The word *cosmeceutical*, which was first put forth by Dr. Albert Kligman, is used to describe cosmetic substances that include components that are physiologically active. A skin care routine that includes both OTC medications and cosmetics has the potential to provide considerable advantages. There is a blurring of the boundary between cosmetics and medications since the categorization of a product is determined by the ingredients that it contains as well as the purpose for which it is intended.

There are a number of characteristics of the epidermis and dermis that contribute to the perception of healthy skin. These characteristics include the density of the extracellular matrix, the distribution of cells within connective tissue, the appearance of cornified cells, and natural fluorescence variations. A number of visible diseases, including xerosis, acne, and aberrant pigmentation, may be brought on by alterations in the physiology of the skin. When it comes to assisting customers in regaining the health and attractiveness of their skin, a skincare routine that includes both OTC and cosmetic items is of critical importance (9, 10).

The evolution of regulations in the skincare and pharmaceutical industries has been influenced by scientific advancements, consumer concerns, and the changing healthcare landscape. Regulatory bodies like the FDA have played a crucial role in establishing and refining guidelines to ensure the safety, efficacy, and quality of skincare and pharmaceutical products. The regulatory framework has adapted to encompass a more comprehensive understanding of product ingredients, manufacturing processes, and their potential impact on consumer health. Balancing innovation and consumer protection, regulations have addressed challenges such as the intersection of cosmetics and drugs, the advent of novel technologies, and the globalization of the industry.

The emergence of microfluidics has introduced transformative approaches to drug development and skin care applications. Microfluidic technology, characterized by its miniature scale and precise control of fluids, has enabled advancements in the formulation and delivery of dermaceutical products. The integration of microfluidics in dermaceutical research presents regulatory implications as authorities navigate the challenges and opportunities posed by this novel technology. Regulatory frameworks must adapt to address issues related to process miniaturization, increased analytical efficiency, and the need for precise control over formulations. As microfluidics becomes more integral to dermaceutical innovation, regulatory standards are likely to evolve to ensure the safety, efficacy, and quality of these products. This reflects a commitment to fostering advancements while safeguarding consumer health and well-being. The dynamic interplay between the emergence of microfluidics and regulatory considerations underscores the importance of an agile and responsive approach to governing the evolving landscape of dermaceuticals (11, 12).

14.3   THE ROLE AND BENEFITS OF STANDARDS AND GUIDELINES

Standardization in microfluidics, particularly in the pharmaceutical domain, can effectively address the challenges outlined in the preceding section. While the topic of microfluidics standardization is not widely discussed, it holds significant potential for advancing the field and promoting the development of microfluidic-based technologies in health care. Although the focus here is on medical devices, the principles discussed may have applicability to other areas utilizing microfluidic technologies. It is crucial to clarify that this chapter primarily addresses testing strategies to assist product developers in propelling the microfluidics field forward rather than specific technical requirements for design fulfillment, which fall under product standards (13).

Adhering to standards and guidelines in microfluidics for pharmaceuticals offers several key advantages:

Harmonization

- The implementation of standardized norms lowers the amount of duplication and disputes that occur in the testing techniques that are established by various research and development laboratories.
- The provision of a dependable instrument for product assessment, as well as the facilitation of development and approval, is of critical importance to both the industry and regulatory bodies.
- Participates in the development of preclinical knowledge by means of bench testing or simulations that are both cost-effective and efficient, with the ability to reduce dependence on clinical data and animal investigations (14).

Safety and Performance

- Reducing duplication and conflicts in testing procedures established by various research and development laboratories is one of the key benefits of establishing standardized criteria.
- An essential component for both the business sector and regulatory authorities, offering a trustworthy instrument for product assessment and making the process of creation and approval easier.
- Bench testing or simulations that are both cost-effective and efficient contribute to preclinical learning, which may result in a reduction in the dependence on clinical data and animal investigations (15).

Early-Stage Product Development

- One way to avoid instances of duplication and conflicts in testing procedures produced by various research and development laboratories is to set standardized norms that are consistent.
- Because it offers a trustworthy instrument for product assessment and makes the process of development and approval easier, it is essential for both the industry and regulatory bodies.
- This stage allows for more cost-effective lab testing or simulations, which contributes to preclinical learning and has the potential to reduce dependence on clinical data and animal research (15–17).

Development of a Supply Chain

- Standards covering materials, manufacturing, and testing contribute to the establishment of industrial supply chains.
- Costs are reduced for everyone involved, from basic researchers to manufacturers of the end product.

Acceleration of Newcomers into the Field

- Standards make it possible for users who are not experts to make use of microfluidic components as tools without necessitating an in-depth comprehension of the mechanics that are embedded within the system.
- It makes it easier for new people and organizations to enter the industry, which, in turn, encourages innovation and cooperation via the process.

Overall, adherence to standards ensures a streamlined development process, enhances safety and performance assessments, encourages broader participation in the field, and contributes to the establishment of efficient supply chains.

14.4 NEED FOR STANDARDS AND GUIDELINES

The absence of standardized practices in microfluidics for pharmaceuticals can pose challenges to product development, particularly for small businesses. The lack of universally accepted test methods may hinder the ability of these businesses to develop and validate their own methods, making it challenging to comply with regulatory requirements. Regulatory bodies, such as the U.S. FDA, may resort to engaging with individual companies to formulate device-specific test plans as an alternative. However, this approach is inefficient in terms of cost and resources. Additionally, it introduces complexities in the interpretation of test results for both manufacturers and regulatory reviewers. Standardization is crucial to streamline the development process, ensure regulatory compliance, and facilitate a more efficient and transparent evaluation of microfluidic devices for pharmaceutical applications (18).

Due to the increasing commercialization of microfluidics-based devices, as depicted in Figure 14.1, as well as the growing number of submissions to regulatory agencies such as the FDA, there is an urgent requirement for evaluation methods that are consistent, well defined, and streamlined for similar device types. This is especially true in the field of pharmaceutical microfluidics. At the moment, diagnostics make up a significant fraction of the microfluidic device applications that are under consideration. Despite the consistent expansion of the market and the development of innovative applications for point-of-care diagnostics and initial drug efficacy assessment, there has been limited progress in the standardization of fundamental aspects of microfluidic-based technologies. These aspects include flow and interconnections. The lack of standardized practices poses challenges for regulatory evaluation and hinders the broader adoption and integration of microfluidics into pharmaceutical applications. Addressing these issues through the establishment of standardized approaches is essential for ensuring the reliability, safety, and efficacy of microfluidic devices in pharmaceutical development and regulatory processes (19).

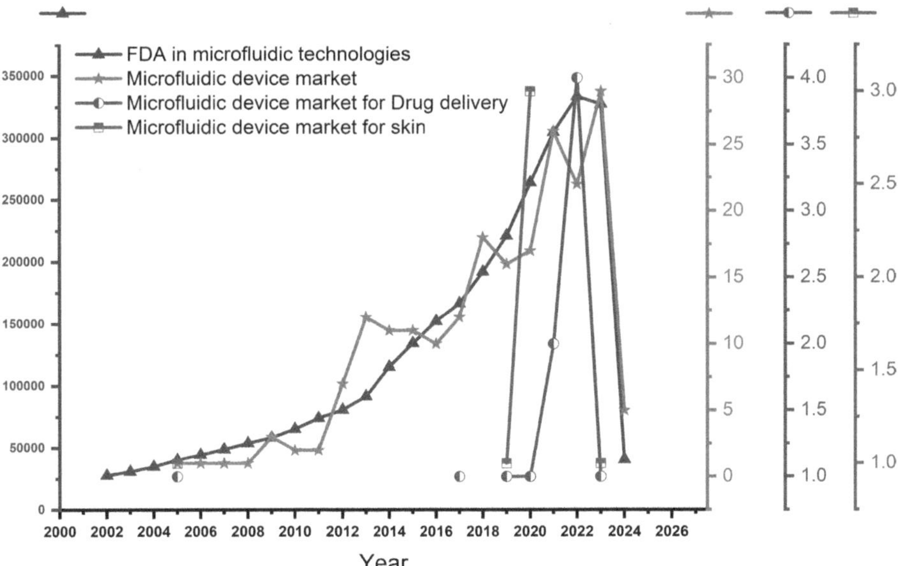

FIGURE 14.1   Illustrative diagram depicting the continuous expansion of the microfluidic devices market across various application domains. (Data from PubMed and NIH NLM, 1 Feb 2024.)

Recognizing the opportune moment for the microfluidics community to embrace standardization, we propose the establishment of test methods for common aspects of microfluidic devices. These standardized practices not only contribute to propelling the commercialization of this emerging field but also ensure a more consistent submission process to regulatory agencies, including the FDA and the European Medicines Agency (EMA). The adoption of standardized test methods is crucial to maintaining momentum and fostering regulatory alignment within the dynamic landscape of microfluidics for pharmaceutical applications.

14.5 CURRENT REGULATORY STANDARDS

Creating skin care products through microfluidics, especially in the context of "skin-on-a-chip" approaches, involves adhering to specific rules and checks to ensure safety and efficacy. In the skin-on-a-chip method, microfluidic systems are combined with models that replicate human skin, requiring careful examination to verify functionality, the use of safe materials, and scalability. Evaluating these small systems is essential to understand their impact on product quality, shelf life, and effectiveness.

Rigorous testing is crucial to validate the advantages of microfluidics, such as improved analysis and faster processing. As regulations evolve to accommodate these technologies, it is vital to promote innovation while ensuring that skin care products meet high-quality standards and are safe for use, particularly in the context of the skin-on-a-chip approach (20).

14.5.1 STANDARDIZATION OF MICROFLUIDICS-BASED DEVICES

The realization of the urgent need for standardization in the area of microfluidics-based devices for cutaneous applications has been going on for a considerable amount of time within the community. Interfaces, interconnections, materials necessary for fluidic sealing, bonding methods, materials within the flow path, and considerations regarding achievable pressure are some of the areas that have been identified as having the potential to undergo significant improvement through the implementation of standardization. Due to the fact that these knowledge gaps were identified, the group known as SEMI (Semiconductor Equipment and Materials International) decided to launch a microfluidic standardization initiative.

In spite of the fact that four standards were published that addressed high-pitch microfluidic linkages, the influence of these standards remained restricted since almost little participation from the microfluidics community occurred throughout the process of developing these standards. In addition, more fundamental recommendations that do not include comprehensive specifications have been made available (21). Publicly available specifications and international working agreements are two examples of the alternate distribution paths that Tantra et al. presented for consensus-based methods. Although it is possible that they are not formally recognized as standard papers, they do provide benefits in terms of the speed with which they may be published and the possibility of catering to a more extensive audience.

A nonprofit organization has been established in order to further the cause of fostering and advocating for microfluidics standards. Additionally, an International

Organization for Standardization (ISO) task force, ISO/CD 22916 Laboratory Equipment—Interoperability of microfluidic devices, has been formed in order to further this cause. This effort has also been vigorously explored in order to expand into allied technological domains, such as organ-on-chip technologies, which include the extension of this program. In the past, attempts to standardize have mostly focused on improving dependability in relation to different types of failure modes.

In addition, in order to accomplish the objective, several interested parties, such as regulatory stakeholders, academic researchers, and representatives from the industry, take part in the activities of standardization. Interconnections in microfluidic systems have been the subject of various standards that have been issued by SEMI and the ISO. These standards are presented in Table 14.1. A few of them are still in the process of being developed. Microfluidics that have been standardized are of tremendous assistance in the process of constructing a device that is controlled and harmonized for derma medicines (19). In the following, a comprehensive discussion on the standardization of a variety of microfluidic devices has been provided.

14.5.1.1 Standardization of Materials

The lack of uniformity in the areas of material selection, process development, and tool design, as stated by Klapperich, is a key obstacle that must be overcome in the field of biomedical diagnostics. The materials and methods that are popular in product development, which are known for their design flexibility and prototyping advantages, are not the same as those that are preferred by the industry (e.g., COC, which stands for cyclic olefin copolymer; PMMA, which stands for poly(methyl methacrylate), polystyrene; and glass), which are better suited for mass production

TABLE 14.1

Various Standards for Employing Microfluidic Technology in Dermaceuticals

Association	Standards of Interest	Status
ISO/DIS	22916 Microfluidic Devices—Interoperability Requirements for Dimensions, Connections, and Initial Device Classification	Under Development
ISO	IWA 23:2016 Interoperability of Microfluidic Devices—Guidelines for Pitch Spacing Dimensions and Initial Device Classification	Published
ISO/AWI TS 6417	Microfluidic Pumps—Symbols and Performance Communication	Under Development
SEMI	SEMI MS11 Specification for Microfluidic Port and Pitch Dimensions	Published
SEMI	SEMI MS6-0308 Guide for Design and Materials for Interfacing Microfluidic Systems	Published
SEMI	SEMI MS7-0708 Specification for Microfluidic Interfaces to Electronic Device Packages	Published
SEMI	SEMI MS9-0611 Specification for High-Density Permanent Connections Between Microfluidic Devices	Published

Note: SEMI: Semiconductor Equipment and Materials International; ISO: International Organization for Standardization.

techniques such as injection molding or wafer-level manufacturing. Due to the fact that the performance of the device may be considerably impacted by the materials that are used, this mismatch becomes especially troublesome throughout the process of scaling up. Regrettably, there has been very little progress made in this field, with the exception of the fact that university academics now have access to contemporary additive manufacturing methods, such as three-dimensional (3D) printing. With the use of these technologies, it may be possible to close the gap that exists between prototype and mass manufacturing.

Point-of-care, environmental, and food safety applications have all found uses for paper-based microfluidic devices that have shown to be useful. Capillary forces are used for analyte transport in their principal biosensor detection system, which employs a detection strategy that is based on a catalytic cycle and colorimetric detection. As a result of the fact that the operating processes of paper-based microfluidics are unique from those described in this study, paper-based microfluidic devices are classified as a separate category of microfluidic devices (22).

Cracking and delamination are two different types of material-related failure mechanisms that are common. Nevertheless, it is of the utmost importance to recognize that the conditions surrounding the storage, transportation, and the use of microfluidic devices might be drastically different from those of typical electrical equipment. The failure mode of fluid leakage is often caused by fractures and delamination; hence, performing leakage tests may be able to capture some characteristics of this failure mode.

14.5.1.2 Standardization of Chemical Resistance and Biocompatibility

In the context of microfluidic devices, it is important to take into account the chemical resistance and biocompatibility of the materials. In spite of the fact that the majority of these devices use noncorrosive solutions at or close to room temperature, the significance of chemical resistance is predominantly associated with a certain group of biomedical applications. In the context of microreaction technology applications, an exception occurs when certain polymer devices come into contact with high quantities of organic solvents.

The testing of chemical resistance is one of Wilhelm's recommended methods. This approach comprises the continuous flow of several solvents at a consistent rate for a period of five hundred minutes. By comparison, this protocol has not been well accepted within the community. This mostly owes to the fact that the majority of microfluidic devices are built for shorter use durations, and as a result, the practicality of such an approach has not been widely adopted.

The ISO standard that outlines the consequences of product immersion in liquid chemicals does not seem to be directly relevant to a significant number of microfluidic devices. In contrast, the ISO 10993 standard, which focuses on the biocompatibility testing of medical devices, is considered to be applicable for the majority of blood-contacting medical devices, regardless of the size of the device. Using the concepts defined in ISO 10993, it is possible to carry out the biological evaluation of all components that are in touch with the fluid inside a biomedical microfluidic system. This can be done without the need to change these well-known test procedures (1, 19).

14.5.1.3 Standardization of Electrodes

Electrodes are distinguished by the fact that, in principle, they are capable of doing their own self-testing. One of the test options designed to monitor and correct drifts in the electronic measurements, included impedance that uses low frequencies to determine the structural deterioration of electrodes. This process was backed by physical measurements taken from electrode arrays that were used in drug testing experiments on cells. The second method included conducting a mid-frequency oscillation test that was based on changes in capacitance between a bio-fluid and the electrodes. The purpose of this test was to determine whether the electrodes had acquired contamination, deterioration, or fouling (23, 24).

No official attempts have been made toward the establishment of standard procedures for electrical and electrochemical measurements in microfluidic applications, despite the fact that these efforts have been undertaken. In order to design such standard procedures, it is necessary to take into consideration the frequent flaws that occur with electrodes. These faults include cracking or delamination from the substrate, deteriorated gate voltages, particle obstructions in the channel, and leakage. Various other failure modes that could have a negative impact on electrode performance include trapped bubbles, foreign particles or particle precipitation during dilution or mixing steps, bubbles that result from leakage or electrolysis, manufacturing and design tolerances, and operation that exceeds the normal limits. These failure modes represent a mismatch between the requirements of the user and the technical limitations of the design (1).

14.5.1.4 Standardization of Long-Term Reagent Storage in Modularity and Interconnections

When it comes to the storage of devices, one of the most persistent problems with dependability is the progressive loss of medium over the course of the product's shelf life. The microfluidics community has the ability to promote standards in this field by using the information that is already available about blister packets. This knowledge can be derived from the fact that blisters are used for the storage of reagents in other areas of the life sciences. It is possible to readily test liquid storage reservoirs for reagent loss after they have been held for lengthy periods of time at extreme temperatures. This capability is comparable to that of blisters.

Research on delamination, which involves the examination of the detachment of material from fluid-contacting surfaces of reservoirs where a reagent was held, was carried out by the business Schott in accordance with the recommendations provided by USP 166043. The usage of two distinct formulations, namely a solution of potassium chloride at a concentration of 15 percent and a solution of sodium thiosulfate at a concentration of 10 percent, led to the recall of merchandise owing to problems with delamination. In addition, established buffers or formulations that are employed in the process of drug development were put through testing. These include ultra-pure water, citrate buffer, phosphate buffer, sodium bicarbonate buffer, and EDTA (ethylenediaminetetraacetic acid). Despite this, the extent to which this study may be used in microfluidics applications is still largely unknown and is highly dependent on the application that is currently being considered (25).

14.5.1.5 Validation of New Microfluidic Models for Clinical Use

The primary aim of functional microfluidic models is to improve patient outcomes, particularly in dermatology. Future studies dedicated to identifying and validating clinically relevant models and readouts in dermatological applications are expected to contribute significantly to this objective. Drug response analysis will involve exploring various configurations of functional models and aligning the results with patient responses to identify the most predictive setup and readouts.

It is imperative to assess the specificity and sensitivity of microscale functional models, especially when compared to traditional dermatological methods like the transwell assay. Ongoing studies are already venturing into this direction, exploring the capabilities of microscale models in dermatology (26).

Upon successful validation, these dermatology-specific studies will provide crucial data to initiate biomarker clinical trials. These trials will involve integrating functional models into patient treatment decisions alongside other molecular approaches, promoting a comprehensive approach to dermatological care. The development of personalized models in dermatology should prioritize incorporating the minimum biological complexity necessary for predicting patient responses while eliminating unnecessary features that may complicate the system. Customizing these personalized dermatological models requires an individualized approach for each condition, involving the identification of indispensable organs, tissues, components, and biological functions necessary to predict patient responses and anticipate common complications of treatment. The process of determining optimal configurations and readouts calls for collaborative efforts from multidisciplinary teams, bringing together dermatologists, scientists, engineers, and data analysts (27).

The foundation for such collaborative teams is already evident in emerging molecular tumor boards within major dermatological centers. These boards, currently composed of dermatologists, surgeons, pathologists, and other specialists, convene to discuss the most effective treatment strategies for dermatological cases. Expanding the composition of these boards to include experts in functional models holds the potential for significant synergies, advancing precision dermatology and improving patient outcomes in the field of dermatological care.

14.5.2 REGULATION OF NANO-BIOMATERIALS USED IN MICROFLUIDIC TECHNOLOGY-BASED DERMACEUTICALS

14.5.2.1 European Commission

14.5.2.1.1 Definition and Harmonization Efforts

In the context of cosmetic goods, the definition of nanoparticles may be found in Regulation 1223/2009 of the European Commission (EC). This rule defines nanoparticles as "insoluble or bio-persistent 3d purposely created material, having one or more exterior dimensions, or an internal structure, on the scale from 1 to 100 nm." Nanomaterials are characterized by their ability to be insoluble or bio-persistent. In order to guarantee uniformity across a wide range of applications, this definition underwent further refinement via the implementation of EC Recommendation 2011/696.

A nanomaterial is defined as a "natural, incidental, or manufactured material containing particles, where, for fifty percent or more of the particles in the number size distribution, one or more external dimensions are in the size range of one to one hundred nanometers," according to the most recent recommendation. According to this definition, some nanoparticles, such as fullerenes, graphene flakes, and single-wall carbon nanotubes, are specifically recognized to be nanomaterials. It is crucial to highlight that these nanomaterials have exterior dimensions that are less than 1 nanometer. This regulatory framework intends to provide precise guidelines for the characterization of nanomaterials in cosmetic goods as well as their application in manufacturing cosmetics (28).

14.5.2.1.2 *Regulatory Governance and Labeling*

Legislation 1223/2009 of the EC, which was enacted in 2009, is the regulation that governs cosmetic items inside the European Union (EU). A significant contribution is made by the Scientific Committee on Consumer Safety (SCCS), which does so by offering direction, in particular concerning the evaluation of the safety of components that are used in cosmetic items. In situations where there are questions about the safety of a nanomaterial, the EC has the ability to seek an opinion from the SCCS, which is required to provide a response within a period of six months. The EC has the authority to order the responsible party to deliver the required information within a predetermined and non-extendable deadline in the event that critical data are unavailable. When it comes to the use of nanomaterials in cosmetic goods, the views of the SCCS help to creating an environment that is transparent and allows for informed decision-making (29).

Additionally, the legislation provides certain criteria for the labeling of cosmetic items that include nanomaterials. An explicit listing of each nanomaterial must be included in the product's components list, followed by the word "nano" surrounded in brackets. This is necessary to ensure that the product is transparent. In addition, within the EU, every single cosmetic product is required to have a designated responsible person who is in charge of monitoring compliance. Each and every cosmetic product is required to submit an electronic report to the EC via the Cosmetic Products Notification Portal (CPNP) prior to its introduction onto the market. Because of the importance of market monitoring, this reporting obligation is very necessary. A regulatory framework has been established in the EU with the purpose of ensuring the safety and transparency of cosmetic goods that incorporate nanomaterials.

Compliance with European Commission standards is of the utmost importance when it comes to the usage of microfluidic nanoparticles in cosmetic products. If a cosmetic product includes novel nanomaterials that have not been subjected to a complete risk assessment by the SCCS, the responsible person for the product is obligated to furnish the European Commission with an electronic notice. In this notification, which should be submitted six months before the product is released to the market, specific information should be included. This information should include the identification of nanomaterials, physicochemical characterization, estimated annual market quantity, toxicological profile, safety data, and exposure conditions. This stringent reporting method is in line with larger regulatory frameworks, which place an emphasis on transparency and safety in the inclusion of microfluidic nanoparticles into cosmetic items that are sold in the European market (30).

14.5.2.1.3 SCCS Guidance and Safety Evaluation

The eleventh version of the "Scientific Committee on Consumer Safety (SCCS) notes of guidance for the testing of cosmetic components and their safety assessment" was published by the SCCS in 2021. This amendment emphasizes that the safety evaluation is dependent on the safety of the components of the ingredient, which is based on risk assessment and exposure limits that are derived by toxicological data. Considering that the EU does not permit the testing of cosmetic components on animals, it is permissible to make use of data from related fields, given that there is enough support and reason offered (29).

According to SCCS/1628/21, the safety evaluation is in accordance with the principles and techniques of chemical risk assessment that are used in the EU. Four primary components make up this all-encompassing evaluation: (1) the identification of risks, (2) the examination of dose-response relationships, (3) the evaluation of exposure, and (4) the characterization of risks. Within the context of the risk assessment process, the recommendations pay particular attention to nanoparticles and place an emphasis on the peculiar issues that pertain to them.

The SCCS has published a paper with the title "Guidance on the Safety Assessment of Nanomaterials in Cosmetics." This document was officially issued in 2019. This guide is a version of the paper that was used for the Nanomaterial Safety Assessment in 2012, and it demonstrates a commitment to embracing improvements in nanomaterial safety issues. By taking into account recent advancements, it is intended to provide applicants and risk assessors with assistance in the process of compiling safety assessment dossiers for nanomaterials. The primary emphasis of this guidance is on the identification of risks, the use of physicochemical characterizations, and the evaluation of exposure as fundamental components for the safety evaluation of nanomaterials.

In addition, the paper that was labeled "Scientific advice on the safety of nanomaterials in cosmetics" was amended by SCCS/1611/19. The purpose of this recent publication is to identify specific physicochemical and exposure aspects that raise concerns for consumer safety. This will help bridge gaps in previous safety assessments and contribute to the ongoing discourse on the safety of microfluidic nanomaterials in cosmetic applications.

Certainly, adherence to the SCCS guidelines is crucial in the context of microfluidic nanomaterials. The safety evaluation of cosmetic products incorporating these innovative materials requires meticulous consideration of risk factors, exposure levels, and toxicity data. Aligning microfluidic nanomaterials with established risk assessment practices ensures compliance with EU regulations, emphasizing the commitment to safety and responsible innovation in cosmetic formulations. This approach not only facilitates regulatory compliance but also underscores the dedication to consumer safety in the development and use of novel cosmetic technologies (30, 31).

14.5.2.2 United States

14.5.2.2.1 Definition of Nanomaterial and Regulating Authorities

Nanomaterials do not have a specific regulatory definition in the United States, unlike in the EU, where they are regulated by the FDA. The current safety evaluation methodology, according to the FDA, may be modified to accommodate a wide range of materials, including nanomaterials (32). On the other hand, according to major groups like the International American Society for Testing and Materials (ASTM), a world leader in establishing international standards, nanomaterials are implicitly characterized as being in the 1–100-nm range within the American scientific community. Specifically, the National Nanotechnology Initiative (NNI) and the ASTM both place an emphasis on the study, creation, and manipulation of materials on the nanoscale in their respective 2006 definitions of nanotechnology.

Nanotechnology in cosmetics is regulated by the FDA in the United States under the Federal Food, Drug, and Cosmetic Act (FFDCA), which covers a wide range of items including food and medications (33). In order to evaluate potential methods of nanotechnology product regulation, the FDA formed the National Nanotechnology Initiative (NNI) and the Nanotechnology Task Force (NTF). It is the legal obligation of cosmetics companies selling their wares in the United States to guarantee the safety and accurate labeling of all components, including those operating at the nanoscale. Except for colors, cosmetic ingredients in the United States do not need regulatory clearance, unlike in the EU. Cosmetics companies have the option to voluntarily comply with the FDA's regulations on the labelling of nanomaterials, even though the agency does not require such labels owing to concerns that they do not conform to toxicity profiles. In addition, the Voluntary Cosmetic Registration Program (VCRP) and the FDA's Personal Care Products Council (PCPC) have established rules for the voluntary registration of cosmetic components and the reporting of adverse reactions. This initiative allows manufacturers to stay informed about materials with known risks, enabling them to make informed decisions and enhance the safety of their finished products. This regulatory approach in the United States, although differing from the EU's, underscores the commitment to ensuring the safety and transparency of cosmetic products, including those incorporating microfluidic nanomaterials (34, 35).

14.5.2.2.2 FDA-Released Documents

The FDA published three comprehensive guideline documents in June 2014, with a particular emphasis on two publications that were important to cosmetics. These documents addressed safety issues linked to nanotechnology. The advice included in these publications is extremely helpful, despite the fact that they do not constitute legally obligatory duties.

The article, which is titled "Considering Whether an FDA-Regulated Product Involves the Application of Nanotechnology," provides an overview of two primary considerations that should be taken into account when determining whether or not FDA-regulated items, such as cosmetics, use nanotechnology (36). These topics surround the size of particles and the qualities and phenomena that are reliant on the size of the particles. To be more specific, the evaluation takes into account materials that are designed to have dimensions in the nanoscale range (about 1–100 nm), as well as materials that are designed to display size-related features or phenomena, even if they are not in the nanoscale range, all the way down to one micrometer (1000 nm). Due to the fact that features that are critical for safety, effectiveness, and regulatory status might extend beyond the normal nanoscale range, this understanding is extremely important.

When it comes to ensuring the safety of nanoparticles in cosmetic products, the second paper, which is headed "Guidance for Industry—Safety of Nanomaterials in Cosmetic Products," places an emphasis on the significance of classifying nanomaterials and assessing their different chemical and physical characteristics (37). The FDA emphasizes the necessity of extensive particle characterization, which includes surface qualities, morphological traits, and other physical properties such as solubility, dimensional distribution, agglomeration, and possible contaminants. Toxicology considerations and evaluations of absorption, distribution, metabolism, and excretion (ADME) of nanomaterials in cosmetics entail examining routes of exposure, uptake/absorption, and conducting toxicity testing. These are all aspects of the ADME process. An approach that is comparable to the one used for evaluating exposure to non-nano components is utilized for the evaluation of nanoparticles. When it is required, the FDA suggests making adjustments to established tests and developing new alternative procedures. This is especially true for nanomaterials that are insoluble or partially soluble, which is a regular occurrence due to the fact that nanoparticles have a tendency to form bigger agglomerates that are intractable. This regulatory framework is in line with efforts to assure the safety of microfluidic nanoparticles in cosmetic goods and to conduct an accurate assessment of their chemical composition (29).

14.5.2.3 Other Countries

According to the definition provided by Health Canada, nanomaterials are substances or products that show nanoform traits or phenomena, independent of their size, or that have nanometric dimensions in at least one exterior dimension, an interior dimension, or surface structure within the nanoscale (38). The rule places an emphasis on the necessity of avoiding the marketing of cosmetic goods that include substances that are dangerous to health. It is supported by a list of cosmetic compounds that were restricted or forbidden in 2007.

Without making a clear distinction between nanoparticles and bulk compounds, the National Industry Chemicals Notification and Assessment Scheme (NICNAS) in Australia is responsible for ensuring the safety of cosmetic ingredients. NICNAS, which is located in Australia, describes nanomaterials as industrial materials that are purposefully manufactured and generally have diameters ranging from 1 to 100 nanometers. Although New Zealand agrees with the EU's definition of nanomaterials, the country suggests postponing the labeling of nanomaterials explicitly in order to bring it in line with international norms.

In Brazil, there are no particular rules that control nanoparticles; nonetheless, debates regarding nanomaterials were begun by ANVISA in 2012, and the Internal Committee of Nanotechnology (CIN) was officially established in 2013.

While the Drugs and Cosmetics Act 1940 and Rules 1945 govern cosmetics generally, no specific legislation governs cosmetics including nanomaterials in India. The Bureau of Indian Standards (BIS) has formed a Nanotechnology Sectional Committee to strive for the harmonization of nanotechnology rules.

The Health Administration Department of the State Council (SFDA) requires all cosmetics to undergo safety and health quality testing for microbiological, toxicological, chronic toxicity, and carcinogenicity before they may be issued a hygiene license or record-keeping certificate to sell in China. Adherence to these many regulatory frameworks is necessary in the context of microfluidic nanoparticles because it guarantees compliance, safety, and uniform methods across all worldwide markets (39).

14.6 CONCLUSION

The regulatory viewpoint on microfluidics in dermaceuticals exposes a dynamic environment that is molded by increasing norms and rules. A dynamic landscape is revealed. The need for new dermatological solutions is expected to continue to increase, and regulatory agencies are playing an increasingly important role in guaranteeing the safety, effectiveness, and compliance of formulations that are based on microfluidic molecules. When it comes to establishing standardized procedures that are capable of addressing the specific issues that are offered by microfluidic technologies, collaboration between academic institutions, industry, and regulatory bodies becomes very necessary. The pursuit of internationally harmonized laws encourages responsible innovation in the dermaceutical industry, as well as promotes transparency, enables market access, and facilitates market access among consumers. Moving forward, it will be vital to maintain a discourse and collaborate across disciplines in order to adapt regulatory frameworks to the dynamic nature of microfluidics. This will ensure that there is a balance between fostering innovation and protecting public health. A unified strategy that is beneficial to all stakeholders in the dermaceutical environment is advocated for in this publication, which makes a contribution to the ongoing discussion on regulatory issues in the field of microfluidics.

ACKNOWLEDGMENT

All the authors want to credit their affiliated institutes.

CONFLICT OF INTEREST

None.

REFERENCES

1. Deliorman M, Ali DS, Qasaimeh MA. Next-generation microfluidics for biomedical research and healthcare applications. *Biomed Eng Comput Biol* 2023;14: 11795972231214388.
2. Kang L, Chung BG, Langer R, Khademhosseini A. Microfluidics for drug discovery and development: From target selection to product lifecycle management. *Drug Discov Today* 2008 Jan;13(1–2):1–13.
3. Cui P, Wang S. Application of microfluidic chip technology in pharmaceutical analysis: A review. *J Pharm Anal* 2019 Aug;9(4):238–47.
4. Jia X, Yang X, Luo G, Liang Q. Recent progress of microfluidic technology for pharmaceutical analysis. *J Pharm Biomed Anal* 2022 Feb;209:114534.
5. Kashaninejad N, Moradi E, Moghadas H. Micro/nanofluidic devices for drug delivery. *Prog Mol Biol Transl Sci* 2022;187(1):9–39.

6. Geoffrey K, Mwangi AN, Maru SM. Sunscreen products: Rationale for use, formulation development and regulatory considerations. *Saudi Pharm J* 2019 Nov;27(7):1009–18.

7. Toklu HZ, Antigua A, Lewis V, Reynolds M, Jones J. Cosmetovigilance: A review of the current literature. *J Family Med Prim Care* 2019 May;8(5):1540–5.

8. Ribet V, Albinet Claudin L, Brinio E, Berthier A, Millet V, Halbeher C, et al. Surveillance of dermo-cosmetic products: A global cosmetovigilance system to optimise product development and consumer safety. *Eur J Dermatol* 2021 Aug;31:463–69.

9. Bowler PJ. Impact on facial rejuvenation with dermatological preparations. *Clin Interv Aging* 2009;4:81–9.

10. Katz LM, Lewis KM, Spence S, Sadrieh N. Regulation of cosmetics in the United States. *Dermatol Clin* 2022 Jul;40(3):307–18.

11. Cornell EM, Janetos TM, Xu S. Time for a makeover-cosmetics regulation in the United States. *J Cosmet Dermatol* 2019 Dec;18(6):2041–7.

12. Halachmi S, Marquart L. Regulation of medical devices for dermatology. *Dermatol Clin* 2022 Jul;40(3):297–305.

13. Chan HF, Ma S, Leong KW. Can microfluidics address biomanufacturing challenges in drug/gene/cell therapies? *Regen Biomater* 2016 Jun;3(2):87–98. https://doi.org/10.1093/rb/rbw009

14. Zima T. Accreditation of medical laboratories - System, process, benefits for labs. *J Med Biochem* 2017 Sep;36(3):231–7.

15. Silverio V, Guha S, Keiser A, Natu R, Reyes DR, van Heeren H, et al. Overcoming technological barriers in microfluidics: Leakage testing. *Front Bioeng Biotechnol* 2022;10:958582.

16. Gharib G, Bütün I, Muganlı Z, Kozalak G, Namlı I, Sarraf SS, et al. Biomedical applications of microfluidic devices: A review. *Biosensors (Basel)* 2022 Nov;12(11):1023.

17. Petrie K, Cox CT, Becker BC, MacKay BJ. Clinical applications of acellular dermal matrices: A review. *Scars Burn Heal* 2022;8:20595131211038310.

18. Natu R, Herbertson L, Sena G, Strachan K, Guha S. A systematic analysis of recent technology trends of microfluidic medical devices in the United States. *Micromachines (Basel)* 2023 Jun;14(7):1293.

19. Reyes DR, van Heeren H. Proceedings of the first workshop on standards for microfluidics. *J Res Natl Inst Stand Technol* 2019;124:1–22.

20. Damiati S, Kompella UB, Damiati SA, Kodzius R. Microfluidic devices for drug delivery systems and drug screening. *Genes (Basel)* 2018;9(2). https://www.mdpi.com/2073-4425/9/2/103

21. Chang YJ, You H. Progress of microfluidics based on printed circuit board and its applications. *Chin J Anal Chem* 2019;47(7):965–75. https://www.sciencedirect.com/science/article/pii/S1872204019611692

22. Musile G, Grazioli C, Fornasaro S, Dossi N, De Palo EF, Tagliaro F, et al. Application of paper-based microfluidic analytical devices (PAD) in forensic and clinical toxicology: A review. *Biosensors* 2023;13:743.

23. Slaninova N, Fiedorova K, Selamat A, Danisova K, Kubicek J, Tkacz E, et al. Analysis and testing of a suitable compatible electrode's material for continuous measurement of glucose concentration. *Sensors (Basel)* 2020 Jun;20(13):3666.

24. Cong H, Zhang N. Perspectives in translating microfluidic devices from laboratory prototyping into scale-up production. *Biomicrofluidics* 2022 Mar;16(2):21301.

25. Pfreundt A, Andersen KB, Dimaki M, Svendsen WE. An easy-to-use microfluidic interconnection system to create quick and reversibly interfaced simple microfluidic devices. *J Micromech Microeng* 2015 Sep;25(11):115010. https://doi.org/10.1088/0960-1317/25/11/115010

26. Costa S, Vilas-Boas V, Lebre F, Granjeiro JM, Catarino CM, Moreira Teixeira L, et al. Microfluidic-based skin-on-chip systems for safety assessment of nanomaterials. *Trends Biotechnol* 2023;41(10):1282–98. https://www.sciencedirect.com/science/article/pii/S0167779923001567

27. Ayuso JM, Virumbrales-Muñoz M, Lang JM, Beebe DJ. A role for microfluidic systems in precision medicine. *Nat Commun.* 2022;13(1):3086. https://doi.org/10.1038/s41467-022-30384-7

28. Ferreira L, Pires PC, Fonseca M, Costa G, Giram PS, Mazzola PG, et al. Nanomaterials in cosmetics: An outlook for European regulatory requirements and a step forward in sustainability. Cosmetics 2023;10:53.

29. Halla N, Fernandes IP, Heleno SA, Costa P, Boucherit-Otmani Z, Boucherit K, et al. Cosmetics preservation: A review on present strategies. *Molecules* 2018 Jun;23(7):1571.

30. Gautam P, Ganghas D, Mittal P, Gupta V, Dhiman K. Regulatory framework of cosmetic in the European Union. *Toxicol Commun* 2022;4(3):13.

31. Gupta V, Mohapatra S, Mishra H, Farooq U, Kumar K, Ansari MJ, et al. Nanotechnology in cosmetics and cosmeceuticals-A review of latest advancements. *Gels* 2022 Mar;8(3):173.

32. Sahu KK, Kaurav M, Bhatt P, Minz S, Pradhan M, Khan J, et al. 5 - Utility of Nanomaterials in Wound Management. In: Solanki PR, Kumar A, Pratap Singh R, Singh J, Singh RB, editors. *Nanotechnological Aspects for Next-Generation Wound Management*. Academic Press; 2024. p. 101–30. https://www.sciencedirect.com/science/article/pii/B978032399165000006X

33. Singh D, Pradhan M, Shrivastava S, Murthy SN, Singh MR. Chapter 11 - Skin Autoimmune Disorders: Lipid Biopolymers and Colloidal Delivery Systems for Topical Delivery. In: Grumezescu AMBTN in GF and C, editor. William Andrew Publishing; 2016. p. 257–96. https://www.sciencedirect.com/science/article/pii/B9780323428682000115

34. Ferraris C, Rimicci C, Garelli S, Ugazio E, Battaglia L. Nanosystems in cosmetic products: A brief overview of functional, market, regulatory and safety concerns. *Pharmaceutics* 2021;13:1408.

35. Dhapte-Pawar V, Kadam S, Saptarsi S, Kenjale PP. Nanocosmeceuticals: Facets and aspects. *Future Sci OA* 2020 Aug;6(10):FSO613.

36. Yadav K, Singh D, Singh MR, Minz S, Sahu KK, Kaurav M, et al. Dermal nanomedicine: Uncovering the ability of nucleic acid to alleviate autoimmune and other related skin disorders. *J Drug Deliv Sci Technol* 2022;73:103437. https://www.sciencedirect.com/science/article/pii/S1773224722003471

37. Yadav K, Singh D, Singh MR, Minz S, Sahu KK, Kaurav M, et al. Dermal nanomedicine: Uncovering the ability of nucleic acid to alleviate autoimmune and other related skin disorders. *J Drug Deliv Sci Technol* 2022;73:103437. https://www.sciencedirect.com/science/article/pii/S1773224722003471

38. Pradhan M, Alexander A. Development and validation of a robust RP-HPLC method for analysis of calcipotriol in pharmaceutical dosage form. *Res J Pharm Technol* 2019;12(2):579–83.

39. Włodarczyk R, Kwarciak-Kozłowska A. Nanoparticles from the cosmetics and medical industries in legal and environmental aspects. *Sustainability* 2021;13:5805.

Index

Pages in *italics* refer to figures and pages in **bold** refer to tables.

A

acrylonitrile, 237, **305**

additive manufacturing, 1, 31, 56, 67, 84, 101, 125, 157, **167**, 178, 197, 235, 321, 336

aerospace, 2–3, 25, **59**, 87, 90, 159, **168**

agarose, 32–3, **34**, **57**, 212

alginate, 33, **34**, 36–8, 42, **57–8**, 73, 90, 92, 94, 106, 114, 128, 136, 142–3, 174, 177, 259–60, 265, 320

Alzheimer's Association International, 67

American Society for Testing and Materials, 341

anatomical models, 4, 16, 74, 103–4

antimicrobial, 13, **35**, 37, 90–4, 129, **145**, **199**, 220

artificial skins, 169

B

binder jetting, 2, **58**, 89

bioactive bandages, 13

biocompatible materials, 4, 6–7, 22, 140, 265, 295–6

bioengineering, 1, 70, 134, 136, 170

bioink, 4, 30–47, 56, **58**, 66, 87, 106, 112, 115, 125, 129–30, 132, 134–40, 143, 148, 150, 163, 172, 175, 177, 259, 320

biomaterial, 4, 7, 11, 31–3, **34**, 36, 38, 40–3, 56, 60, 63–4, 67, 70–1, 73, 81, 100, 103, 106, 111, 126–9, **131**, 132, 134–8, *141*, 144, 146, 149–50, 158, 163, **167**, 206, 220, 231–3, 247, 270, 309, 338

bio-printed skin, 135

bioreactors, 132, 179, 257, 259

biosensors, 100, 206, 248, 303–4, 307–13

blood-vessel-on-chip, 259

bone marrow-derived mesenchymal stem cells, 258

bone regeneration, 20, **59**, 64, 130, 146, 148

bovine serum albumin, 294, 314

brain-on-a-chip, 256

burn injuries, 5, 44, **45**, 142

C

cancer, 10, 15, 19, 21, 44, 61, 67, 71, 109, 114, 126, 142, 149, 170, 173, 201, 220, 226, 248–52, 259, 283, 288, 297, 303, **308**, 309, 315–16, 319

carbon nanowires, 166

cardiomyocytes, 71, 254, 256

cardiovascular diseases, 248

cell aggregates, 39, 67, 135

cell culture, 61, 106–10, 134, 149, 171, 173–4, 179, 209–10, 214, 229–30, 232, 250, 254, 259, 270, 284, 290, 297–8, 304, **306**, 320

Cell Incorporation Functional Integration, 7

cell-on-a-chip, 285

chitosan, **35**, 36–7, 43, **57**, 68, 90, 94, 129, **131**, 150, 165, 170, 174, 289

collagen, 6–7, 31–4, **35**, 36–7, 39, 42–3, **45**, 73, 91, 93, 106, 113, 115, 127–9, **131**, 134, 138, 143, 146–8, 170, 174, 214, **215–18**, 220, 239, 255, 291

complex procedure visualization, 16

composite nanoparticles, 60

computed tomography, 157, 176, 250

computer-aided design, 2, 32, 44, 56, 82, 87, 110, 112, 125, 157, 194–5, *195*, 304

continuous inkjet, 85, *86*, 132

continuous liquid interface production, 87

copolymer, 62, 93, 112, 127, 130, 171, 174, 286, **293**, 335

cord derived mesenchymal stem cells, 258

cosmetic, 132, 143, 330, 338–42

COVID, 250

customized medical devices, 24

customized wound care, 8

cytochrome P450, 114

D

dermaceuticals, 329, 331, **335**, 338, 343

dermal drug delivery, 66, 82, 88, 92, 95, **118**, 149, 174, 208, 284, 288–9, 291–3, 296, 298

digital light processing, 3, **59**, 87, 139–40, 158, 235, 304

digital microfluidic, 237, 250, *262*

direct ink writing, 32, 89, 158

direct metal laser sintering, 2

direct powder extrusion, **59**, 89

droplet-by-droplet, 132

drop on demand, 32, 85, *86*, 132

drug delivery devices, 19, 67, 105, 108, 158, 200

drug-eluting implants, 158

drug-eluting patches, 158

drug-eluting scaffolds, 62

drug release profile, 82, 95, **117–19**, 193

drug screening, 12, 46, 59, 100, 143, 149, 240, 254, **264**, 270, 285, 290, 303, 329